Atlas of Emergency Radiology

Rita Agarwala

Atlas of Emergency Radiology

Vascular System, Chest,
Abdomen and Pelvis,
and Reproductive System

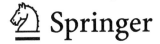 Springer

Rita Agarwala
Department of Radiology
John H Stroger Jr Hospital of Cook County
Chicago, IL
USA

ISBN 978-3-319-13041-5   ISBN 978-3-319-13042-2   (eBook)
DOI 10.1007/978-3-319-13042-2
Springer Cham Heidelberg New York Dordrecht London

Library of Congress Control Number: 2015932668

Printed on acid-free paper

Springer is part of Springer Science+Business Media (www.springer.com)

Acknowledgments

I greatly appreciate the time spent by

Dr. Amrita Sikka, MD
Dr. Dheeraj Reddy Gopireddy, MD, MPH, MBA
Dr. Anita Kelekar, MD

for reviewing the material in this book. They have made important corrections and have given me useful suggestions.

Contents

Part II   Chest

Part III   Abdomen and Pelvis

Part IV Reproductive System

Abbreviations

AA	Abdominal aorta
AAA	Abdominal aortic aneurysm
AIDS	Acquired immunodeficiency syndrome
APS	Anterior pararenal space
ARDS	Acute respiratory distress syndrome
CBD	Common bile duct
CECT	Contrast enhanced computed tomography
COP	Cryptogenic organizing pneumonia
CT	Computed tomography
DVT	Deep venous thrombosis
EEC	Endometrial echo complex
GB	Gallbladder
GGO	Ground glass opacity
GIST	Gastrointestinal stromal tumor
GSW	Gunshot wound
HIV	Human immunodeficiency virus
HP	Hypersensitivity pneumonitis
IEP	Interstitial edematous pancreatitis
IJ	Internal jugular
ILD	Interstitial lung disease
IMA	Inferior mesenteric artery
IMH	Intramural hematoma
IPF	Idiopathic interstitial fibrosis
IUD	Intrauterine device
IVC	Inferior vena cava
IVDA	Intravenous drug abuse
IVDU	Intravenous drug use
JRA	Juvenile rheumatoid arthritis
LAD	Lymphadenopathy
LAM	Lymphangioleiomyomatosis
LP	Lymphoid interstitial pneumonia
LUL	Left upper lobe
MIP	Maximum intensity projection
MRI	Magnetic resonance imaging
NET	Neuroendocrine tumor
NSCLC	Non small cell lung cancer
NSIP	Nonspecific interstitial pneumonia

PD	Pancreatic duct
PE	Pulmonary embolus
PID	Pelvic inflammatory disease
PJP	*Pneumocystis jiroveci* pneumonia
PPS	Posterior pararenal space
PRF	Posterior renal fascia
PTC	Percutaneous transhepatic cholangiography
RA	Right atrium
RB-ILD	Respiratory bronchiolitis-associated ILD
RCC	Renal cell carcinoma
RLL	Right lower lobe
RLQ	Right lower quadrant
RML	Right middle lobe
RUL	Right upper lobe
SB	Small bowel
SBO	Small bowel obstruction
SMA	Superior mesenteric artery
SMV	Superior mesenteric vein
TB	Tuberculosis
TCC	Transitional cell carcinoma
TI	Terminal ileum
TSC	Tuberous sclerosis complex
UIP	Usual interstitial pneumonia
UPJ	Ureteropelvic junction
US	Ultrasound
UV	Uretero-vesical
UVJ	Uretero-vesical junction
VP	Ventriculo-peritoneal
WON	Walled-off necrosis
XGC	Xanthogranulomatous cholecystitis

Part I

Vascular System

Contents

R. Agarwala, *Atlas of Emergency Radiology:*
Vascular System, Chest, Abdomen and Pelvis, and Reproductive System,
DOI 10.1007/978-3-319-13042-2_1, © Springer International Publishing Switzerland 2015

Thrombotic Embolism

Diagnosis
Acute Pulmonary Embolus

Imaging Features
1. Intraluminal filling defect
2. Occluded artery larger than the adjacent patent arteries
3. Doughnut sign in short axis, tram track sign in long axis of artery, thrombus surrounded by contrast-filled blood
4. Eccentric filling defect forming acute angle with wall

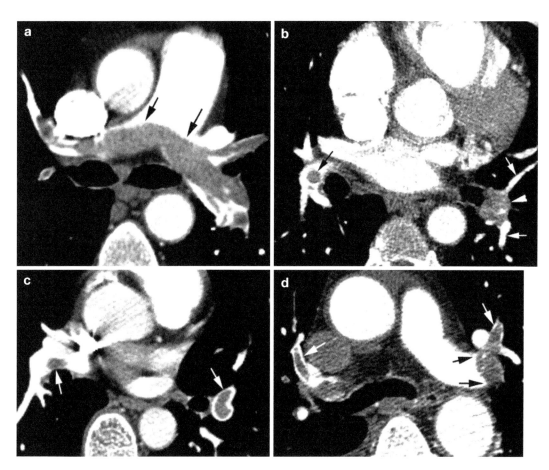

Fig. 1.1 Acute pulmonary embolus. CECT axial images show (**a**) saddle thrombus (*thin black arrows*) involving the right and left main pulmonary arteries across the bifurcation. (**b**) Enlarged left lower lobe pulmonary artery (*arrowhead*) filled with thrombus and larger than adjacent patent arteries (*white arrows*). Doughnut sign in the right lower lobe pulmonary artery (*black arrow*). (**c**) Doughnut sign in the right and left lower lobe pulmonary arteries (*arrows*). (**d**) Eccentric thrombus causing filling defect with acute angle with wall in the left lower lobe pulmonary artery (*black arrows*). Tram track sign in both upper lobe pulmonary arteries (*white arrows*)

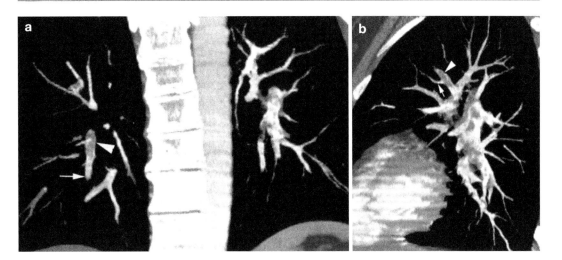

Fig. 1.2 Acute pulmonary embolus. (**a**) Coronal and (**b**) sagittal reformatted CT shows portion of artery with thrombus larger (*arrowhead*) than the distal portion and the adjacent arteries (*thin white arrow*)

Ancillary findings of acute pulmonary embolus

1. Hampton's hump—pleural-based, wedge-shaped areas of consolidation may represent infarction

2. Linear atelectasis, regional oligemia, pleural effusion

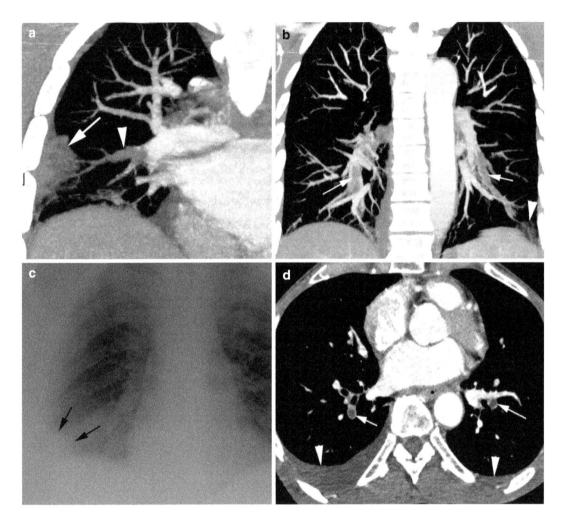

Fig. 1.3 Hampton's Hump. (**a**) Axial CT shows thrombus in the right lower lobe pulmonary artery (*arrowhead*) with peripheral wedge-shaped pleural-based increased density due to infarction (*arrow*) forming Hampton's hump. (**b**) Coronal reformatted image shows thrombus in multiple lower lobe arteries bilaterally (*arrows*) with wedge-shaped infarction in left costophrenic angle (*arrowhead*), the Hampton's hump. (**c**) Chest X-ray of Hampton hump in a different patient with history of PE shows a convex blunting of right costophrenic angle (*black arrows*). (**d**) Axial CT in different patient shows embolus in the lower lobe pulmonary artery bilaterally (*arrow*) with pleural effusion (*arrowheads*) bilaterally more on the right side

Assessment of severity and prognosis of PE—right heart strain

1. Short axis ratio of RV/LV in diastole at the level of valves >1 and >1.5 indicates severe episode.
2. Leftward bowing of interventricular septum.
3. Reflux of contrast into IVC.
4. Diameter of MPA more than 29 mm.

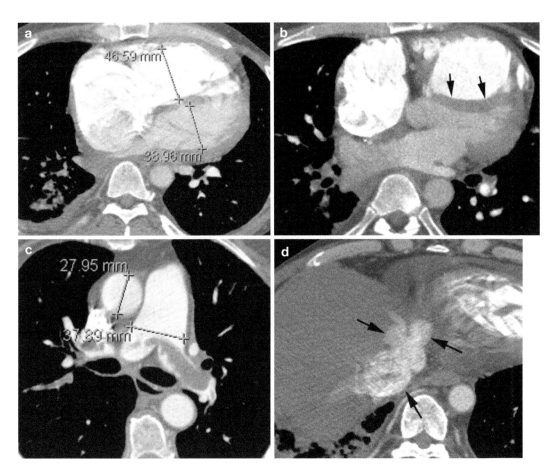

Fig. 1.4 Right heart strain. Axial CT (**a**) short axis ratio of the right ventricle and left ventricle at the level of the valves is more than one. (**b**) Leftward deviation of the interventricular septum (*arrows*). (**c**) Pulmonary artery-to-aorta ratio greater than one and with saddle thrombus. (**d**) Reflux of contrast into IVC and hepatic veins (*arrows*)

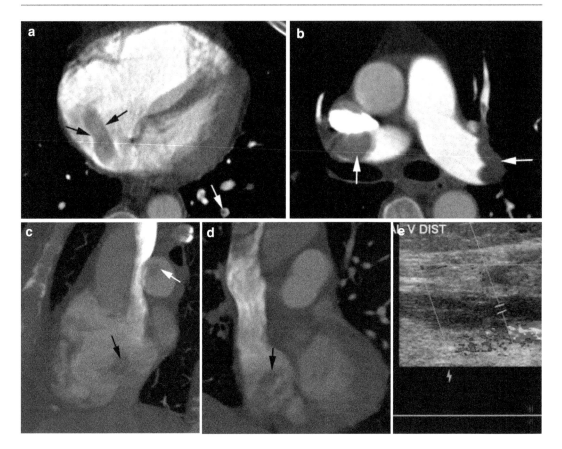

Fig. 1.5 Acute PE with thrombus in RA and popliteal vein. (**a**) Axial CT shows thrombus in RA as well marginated filling defect (*black arrows*). Thrombus is also seen in the lower lobe pulmonary artery (*white arrow*). (**b**) Axial CT shows thrombus in both main pulmonary arteries (*arrows*). (**c**, **d**) Sagittal and coronal reformatted images show thrombus in the RA (*black arrow*) and right main pulmonary artery (*white arrow*). (**e**) Doppler US shows echogenic thrombus distending the left popliteal vein (*cursor*) with lack of color and spectral flow

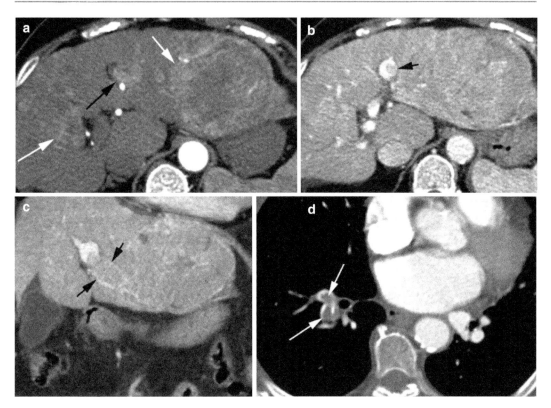

Fig. 1.6 Hepatocellular carcinoma (HCC) invading the left portal vein with PE in the right lower lobe. Axial CT: (**a**) Arterial phase shows enhancing tumor thrombus in the left portal vein (*black arrow*). Multicentric HCC is seen in the rest of the liver (*white arrows*). (**b**) Portal venous phase shows high-density thrombus in the portal vein (*arrow*). (**c**) Coronal reformatted image shows tumor vessels in the tumor extending into the portal vein (*arrows*). (**d**) Axial CT shows pulmonary emboli in the right lower lobe pulmonary arteries (*arrows*)

Diagnosis
Chronic PE
A. Vascular CTPA signs
1. Pulmonary artery findings:
   (i) Complete obstruction
   (ii) Partial filling defects:
      (a) Organized thrombus runs parallel to arterial lumen, causing thickened wall and irregularity of intima
      (b) Obtuse angle with vessel wall in transverse plane
      (c) Poststenotic dilatation or aneurysm can occur
      (d) Abrupt vessel narrowing by recanalization or stenosis by organized thrombus
      (e) Bands and webs
      (f) Calcification within chronic thrombus
2. Pulmonary hypertension signs:
   (a) Enlarged pulmonary artery diameter more than 29 mm.
   (b) Ratio of MPA to aorta is more than 1:1.
   (c) Wall of pulmonary arteries may show atherosclerotic calcification.
   (d) Hypertrophy and enlargement of the right atrium and right ventricle. Right ventricle: left ventricle short axis ratio more than 1:1 and right ventricular myocardial thickness more than 4 mm.
   (e) Small pericardial effusion or thickness.
   (f) May have lymphadenopathy.
3. Systemic collateral signs:
   (a) Bronchial arteries dilated (more than 2 mm proximally) and tortuous due to increased flow
   (b) Nonbronchial systemic arteries, commonly the inferior phrenic, intercostal, and internal mammary arteries, dilate
B. Parenchymal signs
   (a) Scars often multiple from pulmonary infarcts showing as wedge-shaped or linear subpleural opacities, more in the lower lobes in areas of decreased lung attenuation
   (b) Mosaic pattern with decreased perfusion in areas of stenotic arteries and increased attenuation in redistributed vascular flow with larger vessels
   (c) Cylindrical bronchiectasis of segmental and subsegmental bronchi adjacent to severely stenotic or obstructed pulmonary arteries

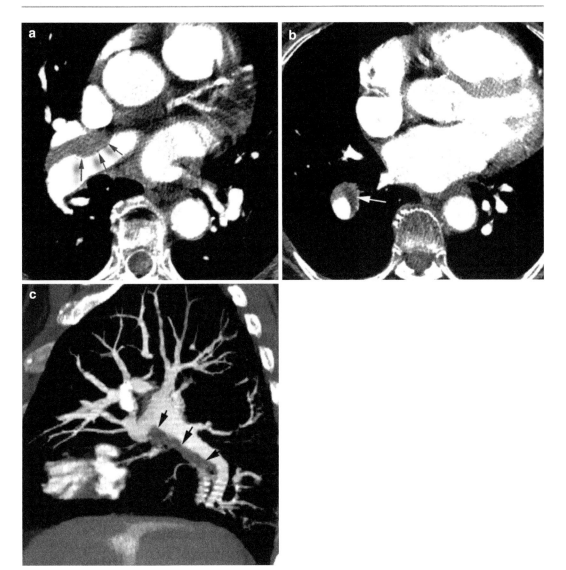

Fig. 1.7 Chronic thrombus in the right main and lower lobe pulmonary artery with narrowing of lumen. (**a**) Axial CT shows eccentric thrombus having obtuse angle (*arrows*) with contrast-filled lumen. (**b**) Large eccentric thrombus (*arrow*) in the right lower lobe branch in axial plane. (**c**) Eccentric organized thrombus parallel to lumen and irregularity of intimal surface in sagittal reformatted image (*arrows*)

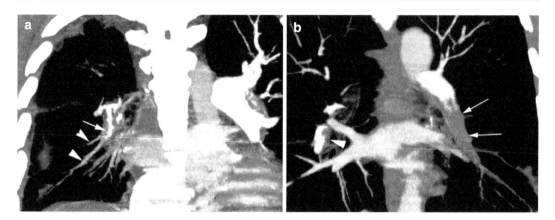

Fig. 1.8 Acute and Chronic PE. Coronal reformatted images show (**a**) recanalization of thrombus at the proximal right lower branch pulmonary artery (*arrow*) with complete obstruction of the distal branches (*arrowheads*). (**b**) Acute PE at the left lower lobe pulmonary artery with thrombosed vessel larger in size (*arrows*). Chronic thrombus in the right lower lobe pulmonary artery with peripheral thrombus (*arrowhead*) parallel to the lumen

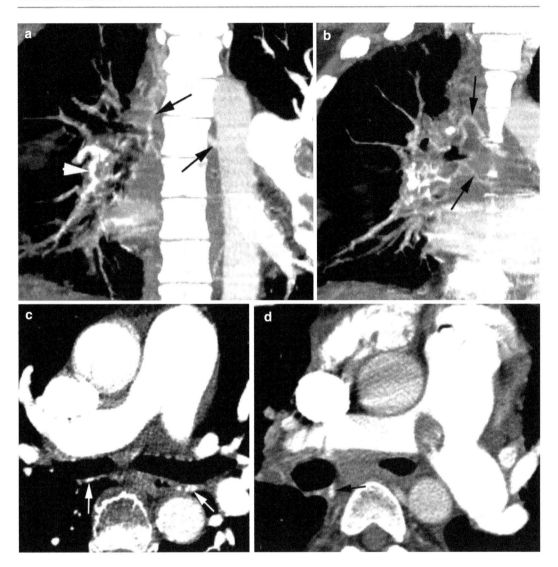

Fig. 1.9 Chronic PE with collateral circulation: (**a–e**) Coronal reformatted and axial images show dilated and tortuous bronchial arteries (*arrows*). Partial recanalization of the right lower lobe pulmonary artery thrombus with contrast flowing through the center of the thick artery (*arrowhead*). (**f, g**) Axial and coronal reformatted CT shows dilated intercostal arteries (*arrows*). (**h**) Dilated inferior phrenic arteries (*arrows*)

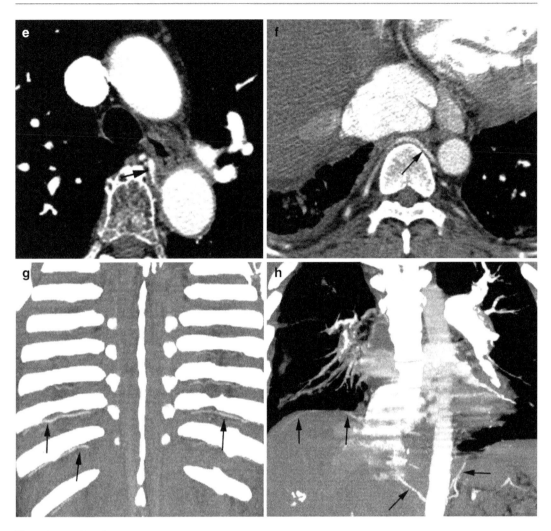

Fig. 1.9 (continued)

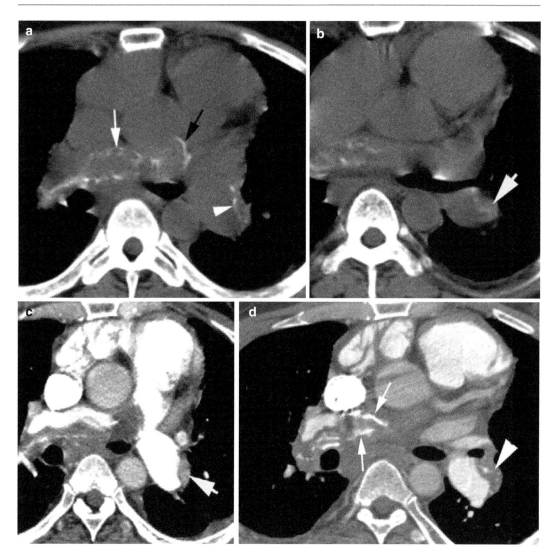

Fig. 1.10 Chronic PE with atherosclerotic calcification of pulmonary artery and calcification of thrombus. (**a**) Non-contrast axial CT shows calcification in the wall of the right main pulmonary artery (*white arrow*), bifurcation of the main pulmonary artery (*black arrow*) and proximal left main pulmonary artery (*arrowhead*). (**b, c**) Axial non-contrast and post-contrast axial CT shows high-density wall thickening of the left PA (*arrow*) due to calcification of chronic thrombus. (**d**) Post-contrast axial CT shows atherosclerotic calcification of the right main pulmonary artery wall (*arrows*). Calcification of left pulmonary artery wall is seen surrounding the chronic thrombus (*arrowhead*)

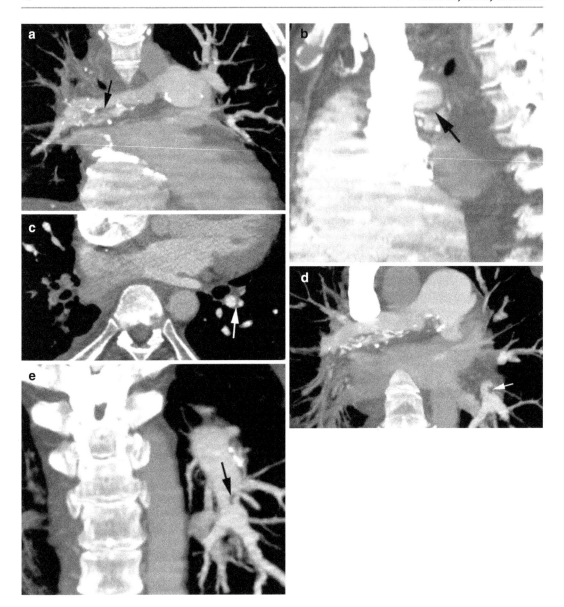

Fig. 1.11 Chronic PE with band. Same patient as in Fig. 1.9. (**a**, **b**) Coronal and sagittal reformatted images show linear band in the right main pulmonary artery (*black arrow*).(**c–e**) Axial, oblique coronal MIP, and coronal reformatted images show band in the left lower lobe pulmonary artery (*arrow*)

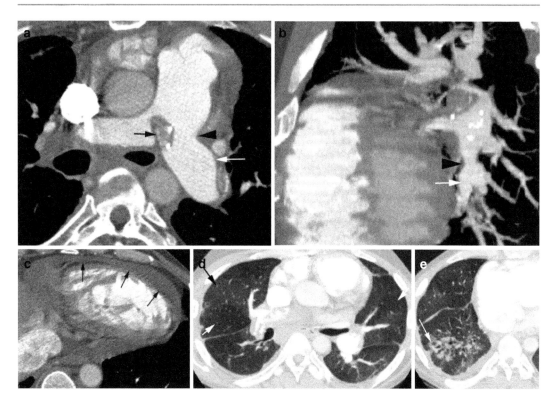

Fig. 1.12 Chronic PE with pulmonary artery stenosis, poststenotic dilatation, mosaic perfusion, and bronchiectasis. (**a**) Axial CT shows stenosis origin of the left main pulmonary artery (*arrowhead*) by chronic thrombus with calcification (*black arrow*) and with poststenotic dilatation (*white arrow*). (**b**) Sagittal reformatted image shows stenosis of the left lower lobe pulmonary artery (*arrowhead*) and poststenotic dilatation (*arrow*). (**c**) Axial CT lower thorax shows small pericardial effusion (*arrows*). (**d**) Axial CT with lung windowing shows mosaic perfusion. Vessels within the ground glass densities are larger in size (*black arrow*) than in the areas of decreased attenuation (*white arrows*). (**e**) Axial CT shows fibrotic changes with bronchiectasis in the right lower lobe (*arrow*)

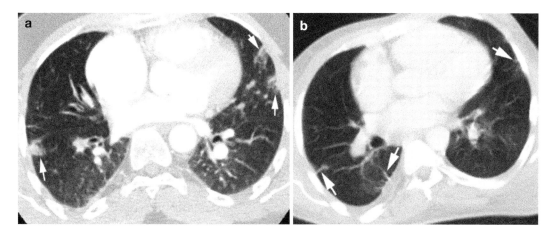

Fig. 1.13 Chronic PE with pulmonary scar of patient in Fig. 1.7. Axial CT (**a**) show chronic infarctions with subpleural wedge-shaped scar bands (*white arrows*). (**b**) Irregular peripheral linear fibrosis (*arrows*)

Diagnosis
Pulmonary Hypertension

Imaging Features
Chest radiography
1. Prominent main pulmonary artery in frontal chest radiograph
2. Reduced retrosternal air space in lateral chest radiograph from right ventricular dilatation
CT pulmonary angiogram
1. Dilated main pulmonary artery at bifurcation 29 mm or more

2. Main pulmonary artery diameter more than the ascending aorta in patients younger than 50 years
3. Dilated segmental pulmonary arteries with artery-to-bronchus ratio of 1:1 or more in three to four lobes
4. Straightening or leftward bowing of the interventricular septum
5. Right ventricular dilatation with right ventricle-to-left ventricle diameter ratio more than 1:1 at mid-ventricular level on axial images
6. Dilatation of IVC and hepatic veins
7. Pericardial effusion

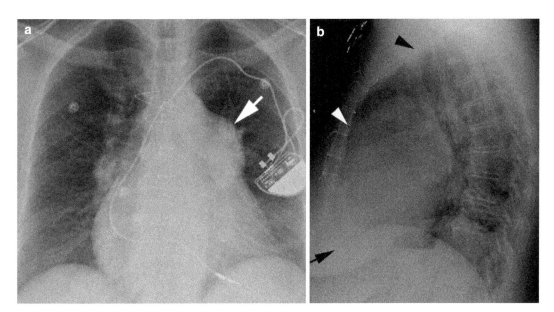

Fig. 1.14 Radiographic and CT findings of pulmonary hypertension. (**a**) Frontal chest radiograph shows prominent main pulmonary artery (*arrow*). (**b**) Lateral chest radiograph shows filling of retrosternal space (*white arrow*) by the dilated right ventricle which is in contact with more than one third of the distance from the sterno-diaphragmatic angle (between *black arrow* and *white arrowhead*) to the junction of trachea and sternum (*black arrowhead*). Axial CT (**c**) shows dilated main pulmonary artery, and the pulmonary artery-to-aorta ratio is more than 1. (**d**) Mild leftward bowing of the interventricular septum (*arrow*). The right ventricular lumen diameter is larger than that of the left ventricle. (**e**) Reflux of contrast into IVC and intrahepatic veins (*arrows*). (**f**) The ratio of segmental bronchus to adjacent pulmonary artery is greater than one (*arrow*)

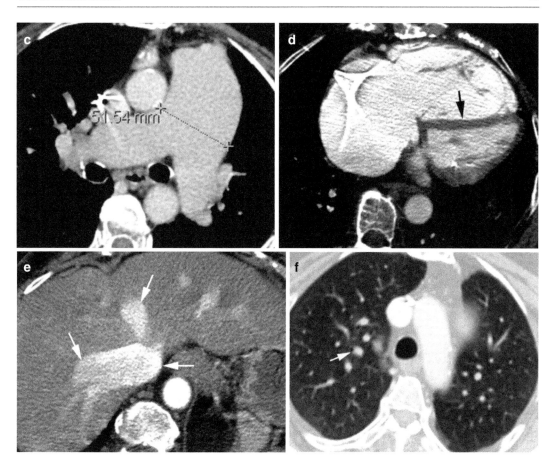

Fig. 1.14 (continued)

Septic Embolism

Diagnosis
Septic Embolism

Imaging Findings
1. Multiple lung nodules, poorly marginated, usually bilateral, peripheral, and subpleural location.

2. Vary in size indicating repeated episodes of embolic showers.
3. Varying degrees of cavitation and can have air fluid levels.
4. Multiple wedge-shaped peripheral areas of increased attenuation.
5. In most cases, feeding vessel can be seen.

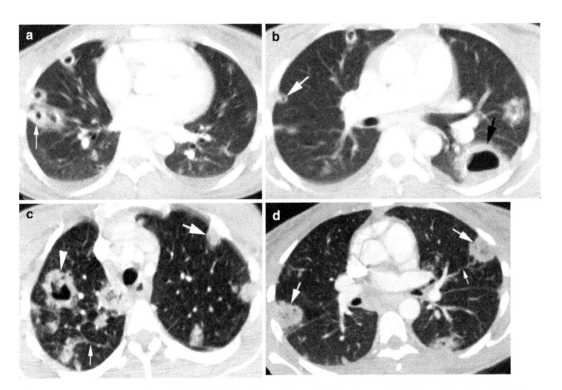

Fig. 1.15 Septic emboli. (**a, b**) Axial CECT of the chest in a patient with bacterial endocarditis shows multiple peripheral cavitating nodules of varying size (*white arrow*), air/fluid level in one nodule (*black arrow*). (**c, d**) Axial CECT in a patient with history of IV drug abuse shows bilateral peripheral ill-marginated necrotic nodules (*thick white arrows*) with abscess formation (*arrowhead* in **c**). (**e**) Frontal chest radiograph of the same patient shows multiple peripheral nodules indicating vascular dissemination (*arrows*). (**f**) Non-enhanced axial CT in a patient with gunshot injury shows bilateral septic emboli (*black arrowheads*) with small cavitation, focal consolidation around some cavitating nodules (*thick white arrow*), left pneumothorax (*white arrowhead*), and small right empyema (*thin black arrow*). Pleura fluid and blood cultures showed MRSA infection. Feeding vessels are seen in multiple nodules (*thin white arrows* in **c, d, f**)

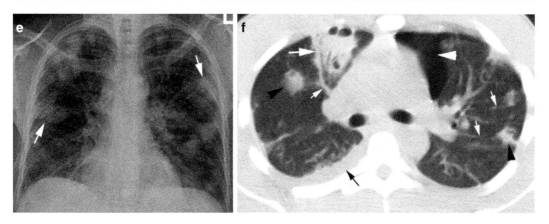

Fig. 1.15 (continued)

Tumor Embolism

Diagnosis
Tumor Embolus

Imaging Findings
1. Lobulated heterogeneous filling defect in enhanced pulmonary artery
2. Tree-in-bud appearance from either tumor embolus in centrilobular pulmonary arteries or tumor thrombotic microangiopathy

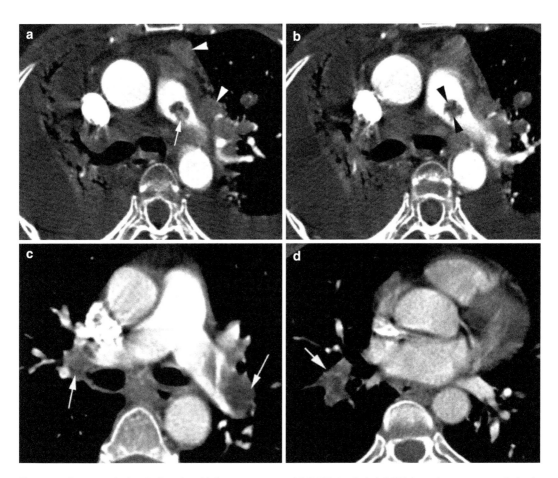

Fig. 1.16 Tumor embolus. Patient 1: with lung cancer. (**a**, **b**) Axial CT chest shows the tumor embolus in the left main pulmonary artery to have soft tissue attenuation (*black arrowhead* in **b**) similar to the mediastinal lymph nodes. Central vessel is seen (*arrow* in **a**) within the embolus. Metastasis is seen to pericardium, hilar, and mediastinal lymph nodes (*white arrowheads*). Patient 2: with RCC. (**c**, **d**) Axial CT chest shows tumor embolus in bilateral main and right lower lobe pulmonary arteries (*arrows*) with multiple faint linear densities within the emboli. (**e**, **f**) Axial and coronal reformatted CT of the upper abdomen show large necrotic left renal mass (*white arrow*) with tumor extending through the renal vein (*arrowhead*) into the IVC (*black arrow*)

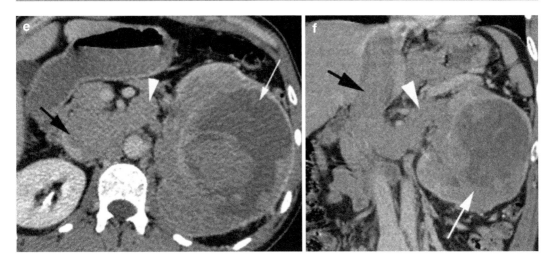

Fig. 1.16 (continued)

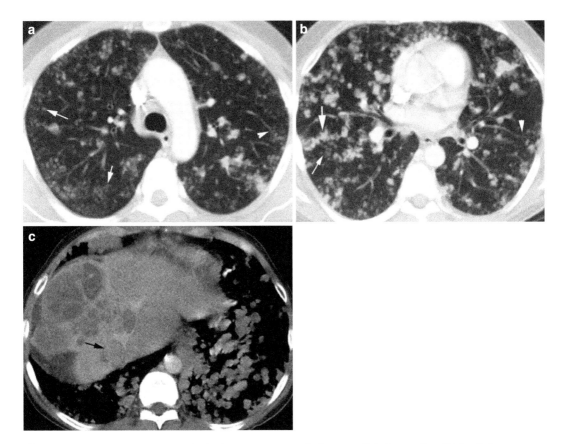

Fig. 1.17 Tumor embolus with tree-in-bud appearance from HCC. Axial CT (**a**, **b**) shows diffuse pulmonary centrilobular nodules (*thin white arrows*) some in diffuse tree-in-bud distribution (*arrowhead*) due to emboli to centrilobular arteries. (**b**) Beaded appearance of pulmonary artery (*thick white arrow*) can be from microangiopathy. (**c**) HCC invading IVC (*black arrows*) with soft tissue density distending IVC

Non-pulmonary Artery Thrombus

2

Contents

R. Agarwala, *Atlas of Emergency Radiology:*
Vascular System, Chest, Abdomen and Pelvis, and Reproductive System,
DOI 10.1007/978-3-319-13042-2_2, © Springer International Publishing Switzerland 2015

Venous Thrombosis

Diagnosis
Acute Deep Vein Thrombosis

Imaging Findings
Ultrasound:

1. Acute DVT can be sonolucent, spongy, loosely attached to the vessel wall, have an expanded vessel lumen and with no collaterals.
2. Chronic DVT is more echogenic, attached to a vein wall; veins are irregular and smaller, and with collaterals.
3. No color flow in complete occlusion and minimal peripheral flow around thrombus in incomplete occlusion.
4. Spectral Doppler ultrasound shows absence of flow in complete occlusion and spontaneous and continuous flow with absent or dampened respiratory phasicity in incomplete occlusion.

CT:
Filling defect in the vein in CETC

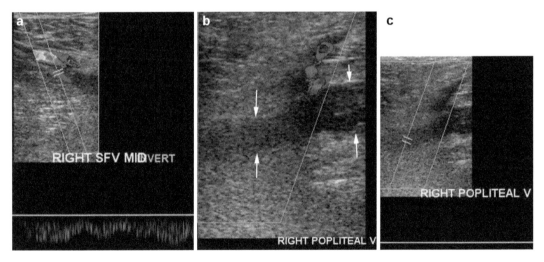

Fig. 2.1 Ultrasound of thrombus in the popliteal vein. Ultrasound of (**a**) the mid-superficial vein shows color flow and spontaneous phasic flow. (**b**) The popliteal vein shows echogenic thrombus distending the vein with no color flow (*arrows*). Flow is seen in the popliteal artery. (**c**) Absence of spectral flow in the popliteal vein

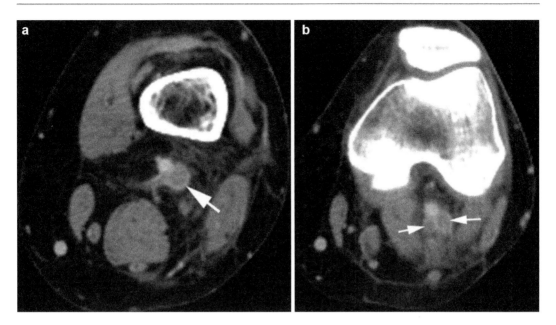

Fig. 2.2 Acute thrombus in the popliteal vein. Axial CECT (**a**, **b**) shows thrombus completely filling and distending the popliteal vein and its bifurcation (*arrows*) with edema in surrounding adipose tissue in the popliteal fossa

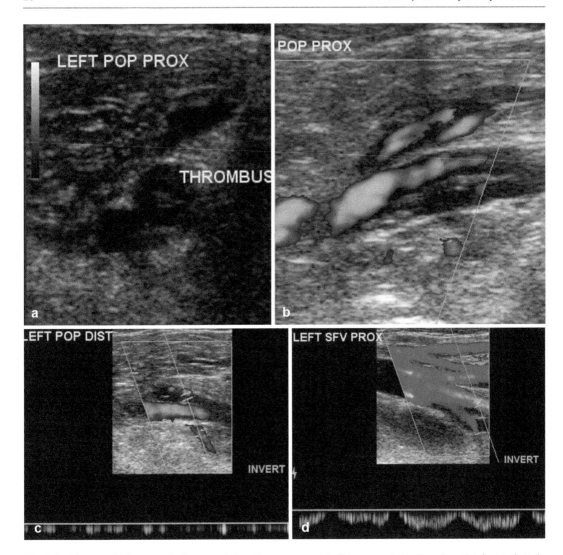

Fig. 2.3 Ultrasound of a nonocclusive central thrombus. (**a**) Transverse grayscale US shows echogenic central thrombus in the popliteal vein. (**b**) Longitudinal color Doppler sonogram of the popliteal vein shows reduced antegrade flow around the thrombus. (**c**) Spectral study shows continuous flow with no respiratory phasicity. (**d**) Normal antegrade flow in the superficial vein with spectral waves showing normal respiratory phasicity

Diagnosis

Thrombus in the Inferior Vena Cava

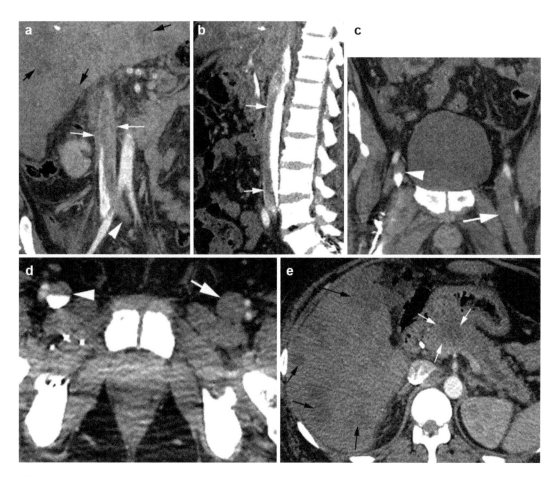

Fig. 2.4 Thrombus IVC with pancreatic carcinoma. CECT (**a**) coronal reformatted image shows thrombus in the IVC (*thin white arrow*) extending to the left common iliac vein (*arrowhead*). (**b**) Sagittal reformatted image shows thrombus contrast level with thrombus floating above the contrast. (**c**, **d**) Coronal and axial CT of the pel-vis shows thrombus completely distending the left femoral vein (*arrow*) and partially filling the right femoral vein (*arrowhead*). (**e**) Axial CT shows low-density mass at head of the pancreas (*white arrows*) obstructing the pancreatic duct and diffuse nodular liver metastasis (*black arrows* also in **a**)

Diagnosis
Thrombus in the Superior Mesenteric Vein

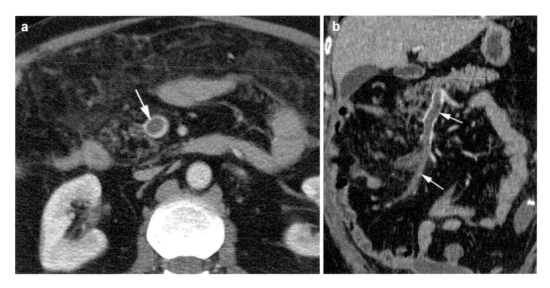

Fig. 2.5 Thrombus in the superior mesenteric vein—acute. (**a**, **b**) Axial and coronal reformatted CECT shows acute thrombus in SMV in a patient with recent bowel surgery. The vein is distended by the thrombus with peripheral rim of contrast flow (*arrows*) proximally. The distal vein is completely thrombosed

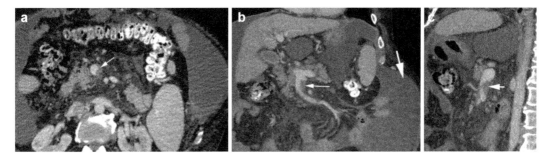

Fig. 2.6 Thrombus in the SMV—chronic. History of cirrhosis and hemoperitoneum. (**a–c**) CECT axial, coronal, and sagittal reformatted images show eccentric chronic thrombus in distal SMV (*thin arrow*). High-density hemorrhagic ascites is distending the abdomen (*thick arrow*)

Diagnosis
Bilateral Gonadal Vein Thrombus

Imaging Findings
1. Dilated gonadal veins bilaterally distended with thrombus.
2. Thin rim of contrast flow at the periphery.
3. Veins are at the anterior and medial aspect of the psoas muscles.

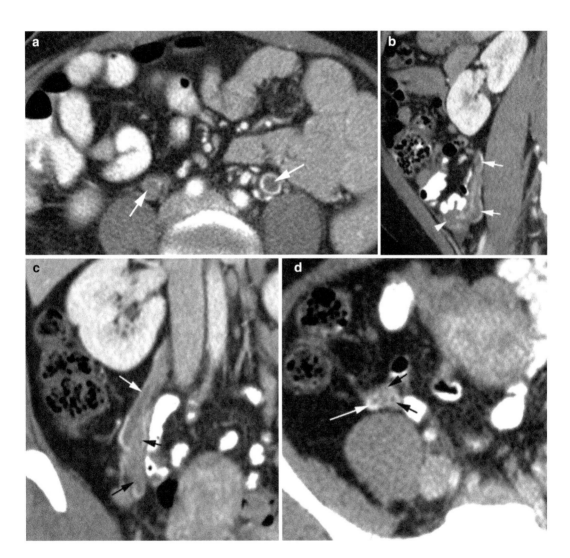

Fig. 2.7 Thrombus in gonadal veins. Patient 1: CECT (**a**) axial image shows bilateral gonadal vein thrombus (*arrows*) with rim of contrast around the thrombus. Patient 2: (**b**) Sagittal reformatted image shows thrombus in the right ovarian vein (*arrows*) extending from the ovary (*arrowhead*). (**c, d**) Coronal and axial CT shows thrombus in multiple ovarian venous plexus (*black arrows*) which unite higher with the main ovarian vein (*white arrow*)

Diagnosis
Renal Vein Thrombus

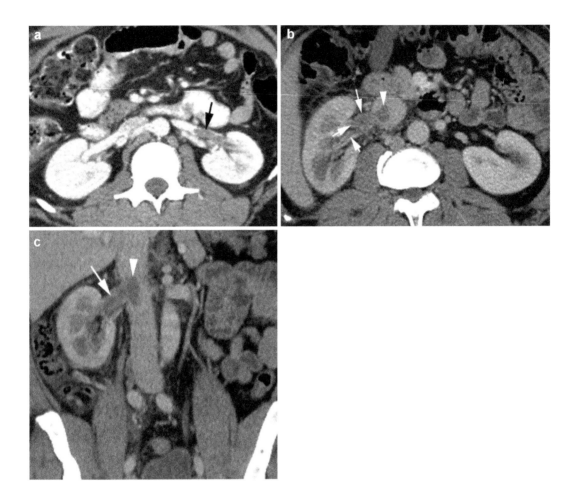

Fig. 2.8 Renal vein thrombus. Patient 1: HIV positive with parvovirus infection, severe anemia, and left flank pain. (**a**) Axial CT shows thrombus in distal left renal vein (*arrow*). Patient 2: right flank pain. (**b**, **c**) Axial and coronal reformatted CT shows thrombus in the right renal vein and its branches (*arrows*) extending to the IVC (*arrowhead*). Ureteral and bladder washes were negative for cancer

Diagnosis
Chronic DVT

Imaging Findings

1. Grayscale ultrasound shows echogenic thrombus adherent to the wall of the vein.
2. Color Doppler shows irregular thickening and filling defect of the wall with no luminal filling defect.

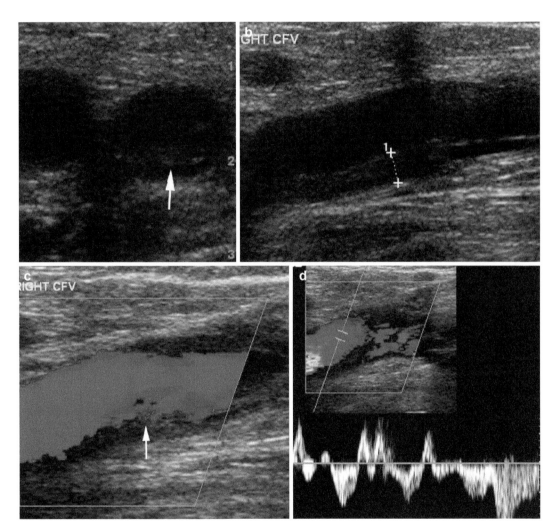

Fig. 2.9 Chronic DVT. (**a**, **b**) Transverse and longitudinal views of grayscale ultrasound of the CFV shows echogenic thrombus adherent to the inferior wall of the CFV (*arrow* in **a**, *caliper* in **b**). (**c**) Color Doppler shows no central filling defect of the vein. Irregular wall thickening of the inferior wall of the CFV is again seen (*arrow*). (**d**) The spectral wave shows arterial pulsation from tricuspid regurgitation. (**e**) Axial CT shows dilated IVC (*arrow*). (**f**) Axial CT shows reflux of contrast into the hepatic veins (*arrow*)

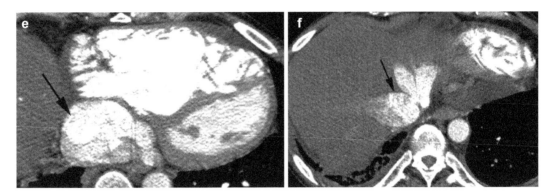

Fig. 2.9 (continued)

Diagnosis

Acute Thrombus in the Internal Jugular Vein

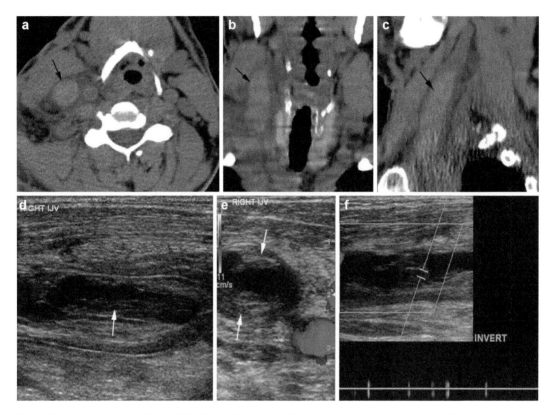

Fig. 2.10 Acute thrombus in the right internal jugular vein—sonolucent and echogenic thrombus. (**a–c**) Noncontrast axial, coronal, and sagittal reformatted CT shows the right IJ to be distended with acute high-density thrombus (*arrow*). (**d**) Longitudinal grayscale ultrasound shows echogenic thrombus at the periphery (*arrow* also in **e**) and sonolucent thrombus at the center distending the internal jugular vein. (**e**) No color flow in transverse color Doppler study. (**f**) Spectral study shows absent spectral waves

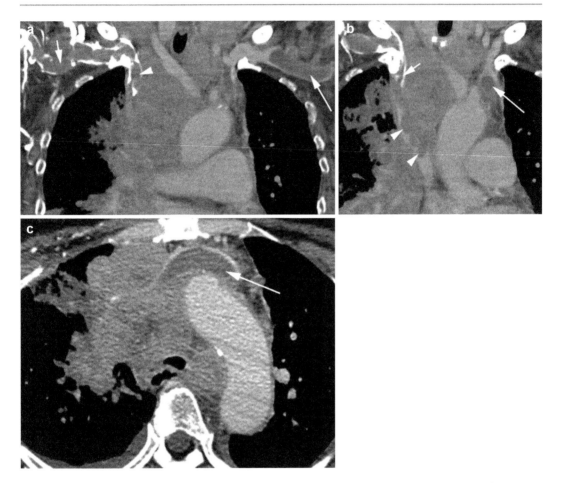

Fig. 2.11 Thrombus brachiocephalic veins. Patient with small-cell lung cancer. CECT (**a**) coronal reformatted image shows thrombus in the right (*short arrow*) and left (*long arrow*) subclavian veins and in the right innominate vein (*arrowhead*). (**b**) Coronal reformatted image shows lobulated low-density tumor (*arrowheads*) invading the SVC causing filling defect of the contrast-filled lumen. Bland thrombus is seen in the right (*short arrow*) and left (*long arrow*) innominate veins having lower density than tumor thrombus. (**c**) Axial CT shows the left innominate vein obstructed by the mediastinal mass and distended by low-density bland thrombus (*arrow*)

Diagnosis

Thrombus in the Right Pulmonary Vein

Imaging Features

1. Elongated filling defect in the right pulmonary vein

2. Infarctions in the spleen and both kidneys

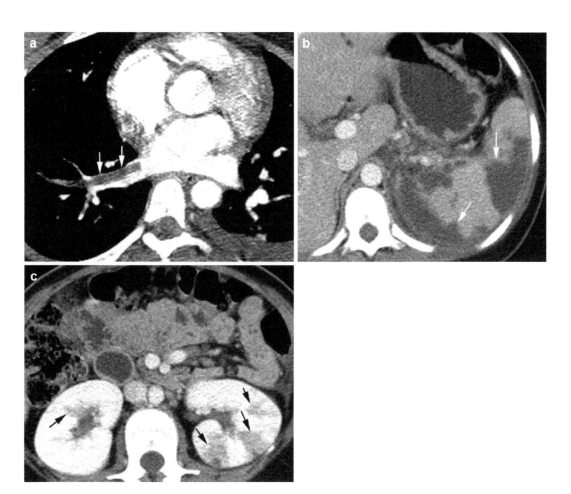

Fig. 2.12 Thrombus in the right pulmonary vein. A patient being treated for severe iron deficiency anemia. Axial CT (**a**) shows thrombus in the inferior right pulmonary vein (*arrows*), (**b**) splenic infarctions (*arrows*), and (**c**) multiple infarctions in both kidneys (*arrows*)

Acute Cardiac Thrombus

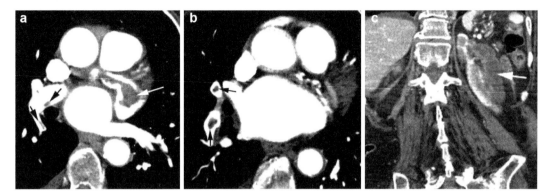

Fig. 2.13 Thrombus in the left atrium. CECT (**a**, **b**) axial images show thrombus in the left atrium (*white arrow*) and pulmonary emboli in the right main and its segmental branches (*black arrows*). (**c**) Coronal reformatted image shows partial infarction of the left kidney (*arrow*)

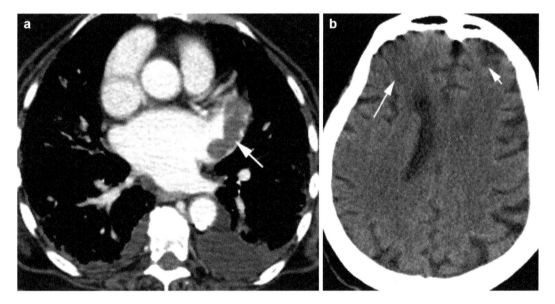

Fig. 2.14 Thrombus in the left atrium with cerebral infarction. (**a**) CECT axial image of the chest shows large thrombus in the left atrial appendage (*arrow*). (**b**) Axial CT of the head shows faint low-density acute infarction of frontal lobes (*arrows*) larger on the right side

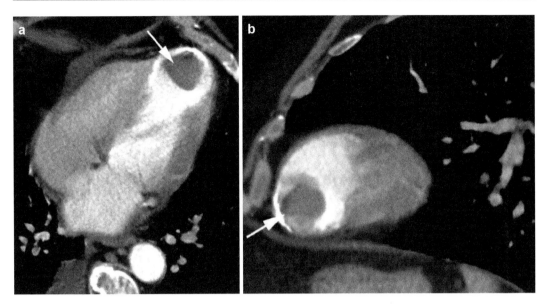

Fig. 2.15 Thrombus in left ventricular aneurysm. CECT (**a**) axial and (**b**) sagittal reformatted images show large thrombus (*arrow*) as filling defect in the true aneurysm of the left ventricle with a widemouthed connection with the ventricular lumen

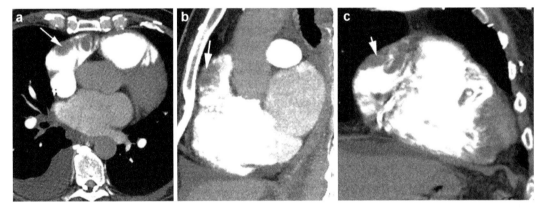

Fig. 2.16 Thrombus in the right atrium. History of ischemic cardiomyopathy and low ejection fraction. CECT (**a**) axial, (**b**) sagittal, and (**c**) coronal reformatted images show large lobulated thrombus in the right atrium (*arrow*)

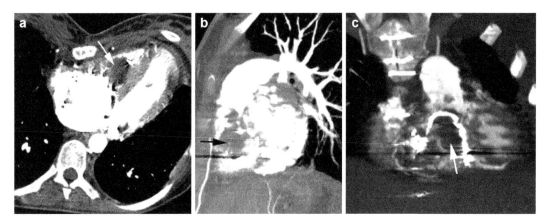

Fig. 2.17 Thrombus in the right ventricle. Patient with history of IVDA, fungal endocarditis with tricuspid valve replacement, and mitral valve vegetation. CECT (**a**) axial, (**b**) sagittal, and (**c**) coronal reformatted images show large thrombus (*arrow*) as filling defect in the right ventricle. Beam-hardening artifacts are seen from the tricuspid valve replacement

Chronic Venous Thrombus

Diagnosis
Chronic IVC Thrombus

Imaging Findings
1. Eccentric high density with a speck of calcification in focal chronic IVC thrombus

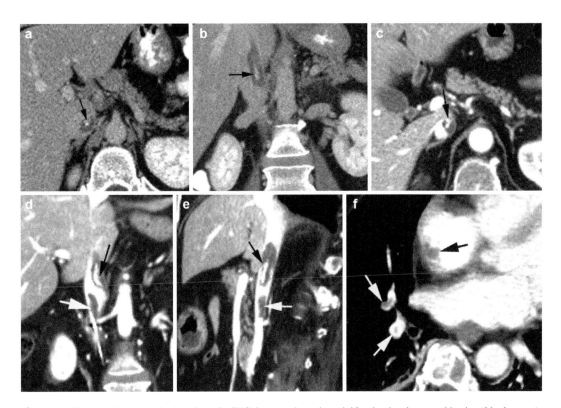

Fig. 2.18 Chronic thrombus in intrahepatic IVC in a patient with unresectable anaplastic astrocytoma. (**a, b**) Axial and coronal reformatted views in delayed venous phase show high-density chronic thrombus (*arrow*) with calcification surrounded by low-density thrombus adherent to the IVC wall. (**c–e**) Axial, coronal, and sagittal reformatted images in venous phase done 2 years later show the calcification has increased in size (*black arrow*). Low-density eccentric chronic thrombus has also increased in size with a second new acute IVC thrombus (*white arrow*). (**f**) Axial CT of the lower chest shows thrombus in the right atrium (*black arrow*) and in some pulmonary arteries (*white arrows*)

Diagnosis
Diffuse IVC Calcification

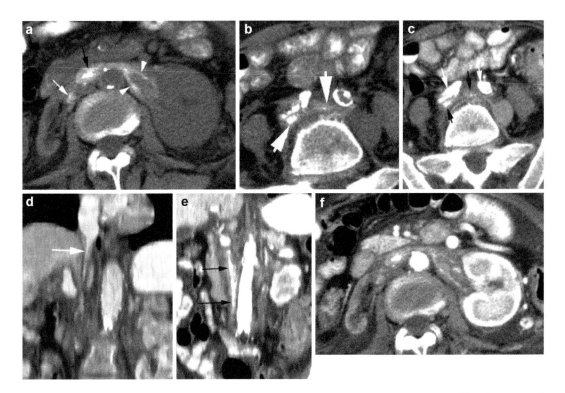

Fig. 2.19 Diffuse IVC calcification from unknown cause. (**a**, **b**) Noncontrast axial CT shows large IVC calcification (*black arrow*). The calcification involves the right (*thin white arrow*) and left renal veins (*arrowheads*) and bilateral common iliac veins (*thick white arrow*). Atherosclerotic calcification is also seen in the aorta and iliac arteries. (**c–f**) Postcontrast axial, coronal reformatted, and axial images show contrast filling the aorta and iliac arteries (*white arrows*) with negligible contrast in the IVC (*black arrows*). The left kidney shows good enhancement with poor enhancement of the right kidney. The intrahepatic IVC shows slit-like narrowing (*arrow* in **d**) with no calcification

Fig. 2.20 Chronic thrombus in the SVC due to mediastinal mass. (**a**) Chronic thrombus in the SVC (*long arrow*) due to compression by mediastinal mass (*ellipse*). Dilated vasa vasorum (*short arrows*) around the thrombosed SVC are draining into the azygos vein. Esophageal veins (*black arrow*) are also dilated. (**b**) Coronal reformatted view shows collateral flow through dilated pericardiophrenic vein (*long white arrow*), dilated SVC vasa vasorum (*short white arrows*) around SVC thrombus (*thick arrow*), and dilated intercostal veins (*arrowhead*) and tracheal veins (*black arrow*). (**c**) Sagittal reformatted view shows esophageal varices (*black arrow*), dilated collateral veins between the posterior wall of the thrombosed SVC (*arrowhead*) and trachea (*white arrow*), and dilated superior epigastric vein (*thin white arrow*) and azygos vein (*thin black arrow*)

Diagnosis

Chronic Thrombus in SVC Causing Right-to-Left Shunt

Imaging Findings

1. Absent contrast in lumen of SVC
2. Collateral connection between the innominate veins and superior pulmonary veins via the bronchial venous plexus around the airways, hilar vessels, and pleura

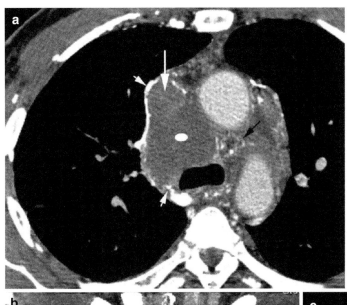

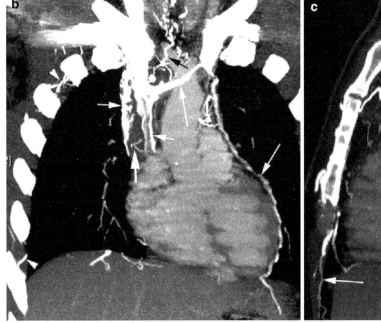

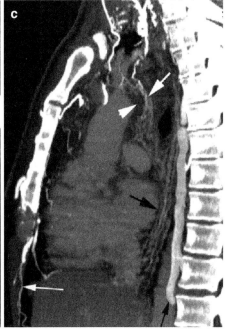

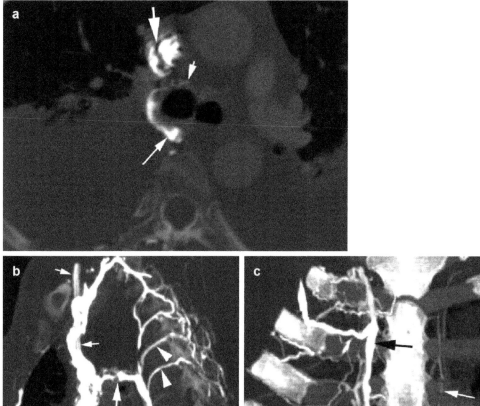

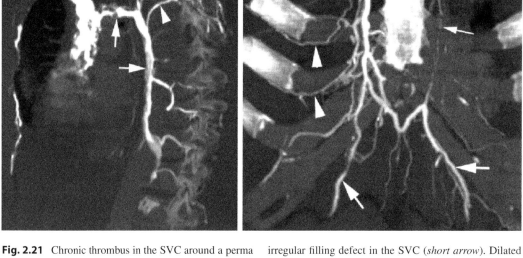

Fig. 2.21 Chronic thrombus in the SVC around a perma catheter. (**a**) Axial CT shows irregular filling defect in the SVC caused by perma catheter coated with thrombus (*thick white arrow*) within contrast-filled SVC. Dilated bronchial veins (*short thin white arrow*) connecting to the azygos vein (*long thin white arrow*). (**b**) Sagittal reformatted image shows perma catheter with thrombus causing irregular filling defect in the SVC (*short arrow*). Dilated azygos vein with arch (*white arrows*) and dilated posterior intercostal veins (*arrowheads*). (**c**) Dilated right internal thoracic vein (*black arrow*), anterior intercostals veins (*arrowheads*), and bilateral musculophrenic veins (*thick white arrows*). The left internal thoracic vein is not dilated (*thin white arrow*)

Diagnosis

Cavernous Transformation of the Portal Vein

Imaging Features

1. Dilated vasa vasorum enhancing the wall of the portal vein with thrombus in the lumen
2. Dilated paracholedochal veins around the thrombosed portal vein
3. Portosystemic collateral varices

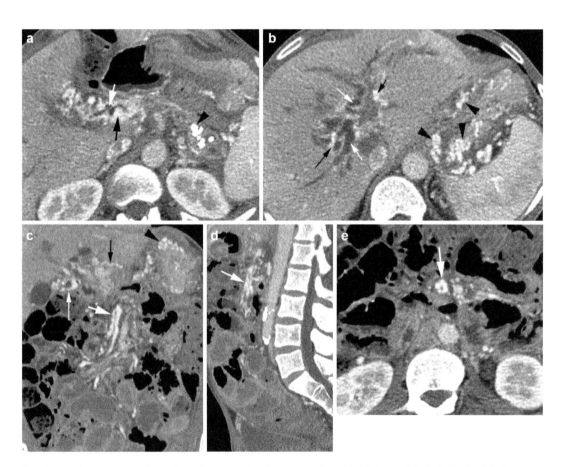

Fig. 2.22 Cavernous transformation of the portal vein and superior mesenteric vein. A patient with chronic pancreatitis and portal vein thrombosis. (**a**) Axial CT shows thrombus in the main portal vein (*white arrow*) with dilated vasa vasorum enhancing the thick wall of the portal vein (*thin black arrow*). Calcification in the pancreas from chronic pancreatitis (*black arrowhead*). (**b**) Axial CT shows thrombus in intrahepatic portal veins (*white arrows*) with dilated paracholedochal veins (*black arrows*) around the portal vein and varicose veins in the stomach (*arrowheads*). (**c**–**e**) Coronal, sagittal reformatted images and axial CT show vasa vasorum in the wall of the thrombosed SMV (*thick white arrow*) and in the wall of the thrombosed portal vein (*thin white arrow*). Gastric varices (*arrowhead*) and varicose vein in ligamentum venosum draining into the left gastric vein (*thin black arrow*)

Diagnosis

Obliterative Portal Venopathy (Idiopathic Portal Hypertension)

Imaging Features

1. Noncirrhotic portal hypertension
2. Nodular regenerative hyperplasia
3. Varying degree of thrombosis, fibrosis, and sclerosis of portal vein branches

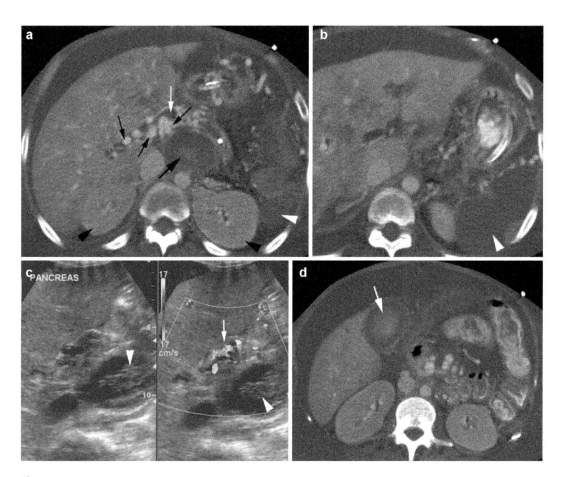

Fig. 2.23 Obliterative portal venopathy in a 34-year-old male patient with chronic pancreatitis and coagulopathy. (**a**, **b**) Axial CT shows cavernous transformation of the portal vein with dilated paracholedochal veins (*thin black arrows*) around chronic portal thrombus (*white arrow*), diffuse ischemia of the liver showing poor enhancement, diffuse infarction of both kidneys (*black arrowheads*) and the spleen (*white arrowhead*), and with high-density hemorrhage in a pseudocyst (*thick black arrow*). (**c**) Color

Doppler ultrasound shows color flow in the dilated para-choledochal veins around the thrombus of the portal vein (*white arrow*). Echogenic hemorrhage is seen in the pseudocyst (*arrowhead*). (**d**) Axial CT shows hemorrhage in the gall bladder (*arrow*). (**e**) Ultrasound done a few weeks later shows gangrenous cholecystitis with sloughing of the mucosa (*arrows*). (**f**) Ultrasound of the infarcted spleen shows coarse echogenicity (*arrows*) of the splenic parenchyma

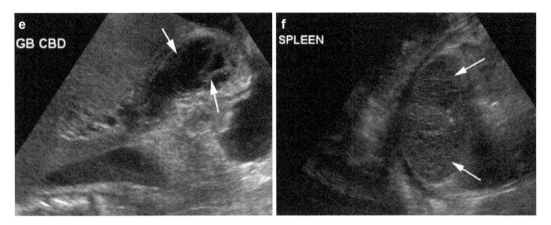

Fig. 2.23 (continued)

Tumor Thrombus

Diagnosis
Tumor Thrombus in the IVC

Imaging Findings
1. Density of tumor thrombus higher than thrombotic thrombus
2. Neovascularity within the thrombus

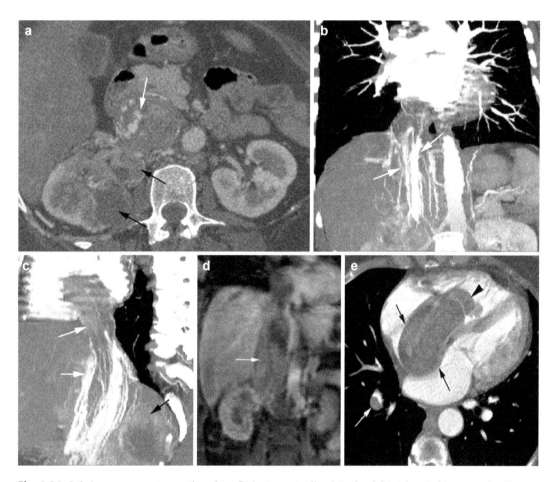

Fig. 2.24 Inferior vena cava tumor thrombus. Patient with RCC. (**a**) Axial CT shows RCC of the right kidney (*black arrows*) invading into the IVC. The IVC is distended with tumor thrombus showing dilated vessels within the tumor extension (*white arrow*). (**b–d**) Coronal, sagittal reformatted CT and coronal post-gad MRI show linear vascularity within the tumor within the IVC and extending into the right atrium (*white arrows*) with neovascularity extending from necrotic RCC (*black arrow* in **c**). (**e**) Axial CT shows tumor thrombus with central neovascularity extending through the right atrium (*black arrows*) into the right ventricle (*arrowhead*). A tumor embolus is seen at the lower lobe pulmonary artery (*white arrow*)

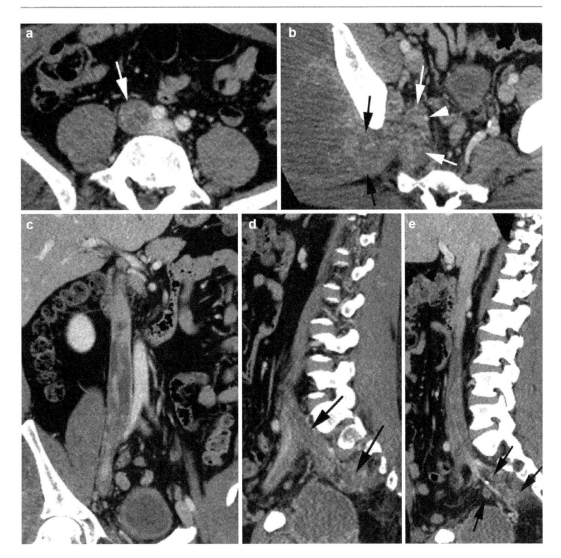

Fig. 2.25 Tumor thrombus in the IVC from sarcoma of the right gluteal muscle extending through the gluteal veins. (**a**) Axial CT shows tumor thrombus in the IVC showing heterogeneous density with tumor neovascularity (*arrow*). (**b**) Tumor extending via the gluteal veins through the sciatic foramen (*black arrows*) involving the piriformis muscle. Internal iliac artery (*arrowhead*) medial to the tumor-invaded veins (*thick white arrows*). (**c**) Coronal reformatted CT shows the IVC distended with tumor thrombus having neovascularity. (**d**) Sagittal reformatted images show the internal iliac vein distended with irregular soft tissues from tumor invasion (*arrows*). (**e**) Sagittal reformatted image shows superior and inferior gluteal veins with irregular tumor thrombus (*arrows*)

Diagnosis
Tumor Thrombus Portal Vein

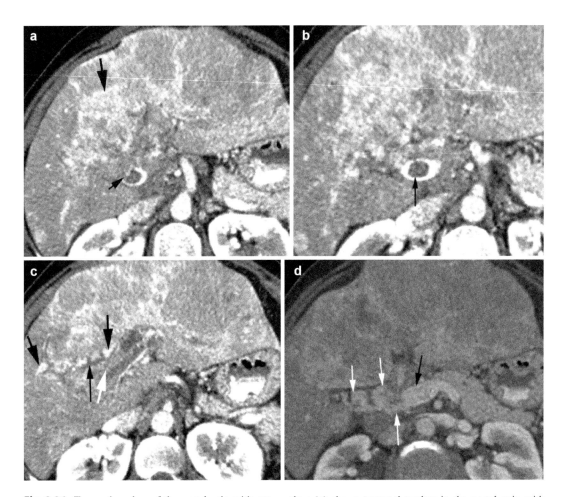

Fig. 2.26 Tumor thrombus of the portal vein with cavernous transformation. Hepatocellular carcinoma invading the portal vein with chronic thrombus in portal branches in the right lobe of the liver resulting in cavernous transformation. The dilated paracholedochal veins around the thrombosed right main portal vein and its branches drain into the main portal vein. (**a**) Axial CT shows HCC (*thick black arrow*) in the right lobe of the liver invading into the portal vein with destruction of portal wall (*thin black arrow*). (**b**) Axial CT at lower plane than (**a**) shows tumor thrombus in the portal vein with small vessels within the thrombus (*black arrow*). (**c**) Cavernous transformation of a right lobe portal vein with dilated paracholedochal veins (*thick black arrows*) in the anterior wall of the portal vein which contains central-enhancing tumor thrombus (*white arrow*) surrounded by low-density bland thrombus (*thin black arrow*). (**d**, **e**) Axial CT and (**f**) coronal reformatted image show paracholedochal veins (*white arrows*) draining into the portal vein (*black arrow*)

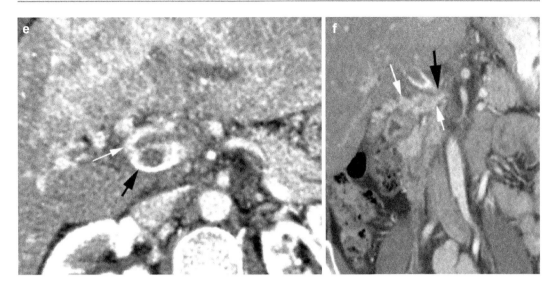

Fig. 2.26 (continued)

Gas Embolism

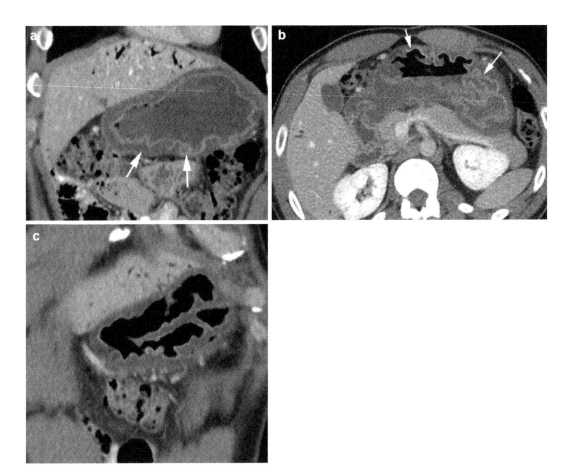

Fig. 2.27 Gas embolus in portal veins. History of ingestion of hydrogen peroxide and abdominal pain. (**a**) Coronal reformatted CT, (**b**) axial, and (**c**) coronal reformatted CTs show thick edematous gastric wall, undulating gastric mucosa with gas entrapped between the gastric folds (*arrows*). Diffuse portal venous gas is seen more in the left liver lobe

Aortic Thrombus

Diagnosis

Thrombus Lumen of the Aorta Without Significant Atherosclerosis

Imaging Features

1. Thrombus occluding the aorta below the origin of the SMA with partial obstruction of renal arteries and extending to common iliac arteries
2. Collateral flow through dilated celiac artery, SMA, and IMA
3. Patchy areas of infarction of the right kidney and poor enhancement of the left kidney

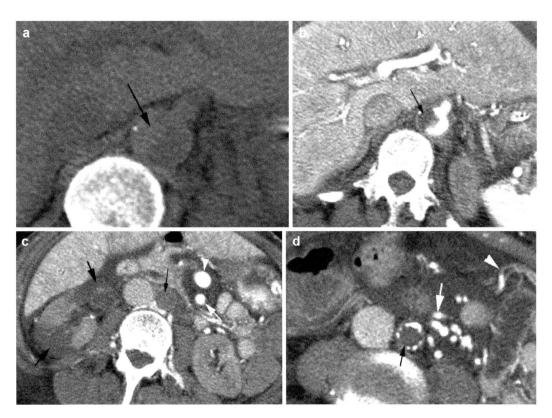

Fig. 2.28 Thrombus in the aorta with complete occlusion. Female patient with lung adenocarcinoma on chemo- and radiation therapy and low hemoglobin. No thrombus was seen in 2 months prior to CT study. (**a**) Noncontrast axial CT shows acute high-density thrombus (*arrow*) at the right side of the aorta, partially occluding the lumen. The density of thrombus is the same as the soft tissues due to anemic state. (**b**) Axial CECT shows filling defect in the aortic lumen (*arrow*) corresponding to the precontrast study. (**c–e**) Axial CT below level in (**a**) shows complete occlusion of the aorta and common iliac arteries by a thrombus (*thin black arrows*). Patchy areas of infarction in the right kidney (*thick black arrows*) and poor enhancement of the left kidney. Dilated SMA (*arrow*) and SMV (*arrowhead*) branches in mesentery providing collateral circulation. (**e**) Axial CT shows atherosclerotic aortic calcification (*thick black arrows*) of the distal aorta extending to the iliac arteries filled with thrombus (*thin arrows*). (**f**) Coronal reformatted image shows dilated SMA (*white arrow*), SMV (*black arrow*), and thrombosed aorta (*arrowhead*)

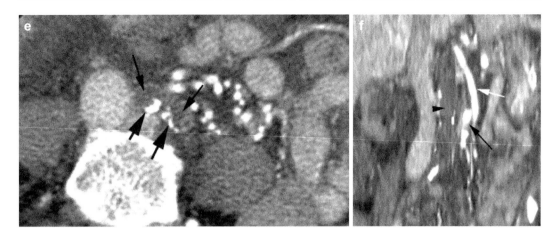

Fig. 2.28 (continued)

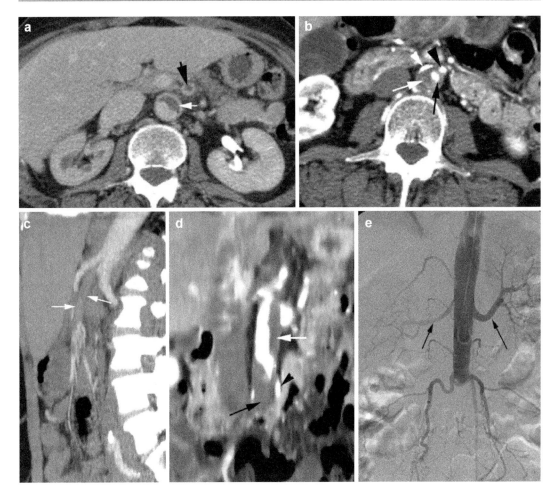

Fig. 2.29 Aortic thrombus partially occluding the lumen in a hyperthyroid female patient with minimal atherosclerotic calcification. Thrombus occluding the SMA, sparing the left renal artery, partially occluding the right renal artery, completely occluding the aorta distal to the IMA, and occluding bilateral iliac arteries. (**a**) Axial CECT shows central thrombus in the SMA (*black arrow*), eccentric thrombus in the aorta deforming contrast-filled aortic lumen (*white arrow*). (**b**) Axial CT at the level of the IMA shows contrast filling the IMA (*black arrowhead*) and aortic lumen (*black arrow*) narrowed by thrombus (*white arrow*). The aortic lumen distal to this is completely occluded. Atherosclerotic calcification of the anterior aortic wall (*white arrowhead*). (**c**) Sagittal reformatted image shows thrombus in proximal SMA (*arrows*). (**d**) Coronal reformatted CT shows thrombus compressing the aortic lumen (*thin white arrow*) up to the origin of the IMA (*black arrowhead*). Below this, the aorta is completely occluded by thrombus (*black arrow*). (**e**) Angiogram shows complete occlusion of the aorta below the IMA and poor enhancement of the right renal artery (*arrows*)

Diagnosis

Atherosclerotic Aortoiliac Occlusive Disease

Imaging Features

1. Atherosclerotic calcification of the abdominal aorta and iliac arteries
2. Thrombus occluding the aorta extending to the common iliac arteries with collateral blood flow

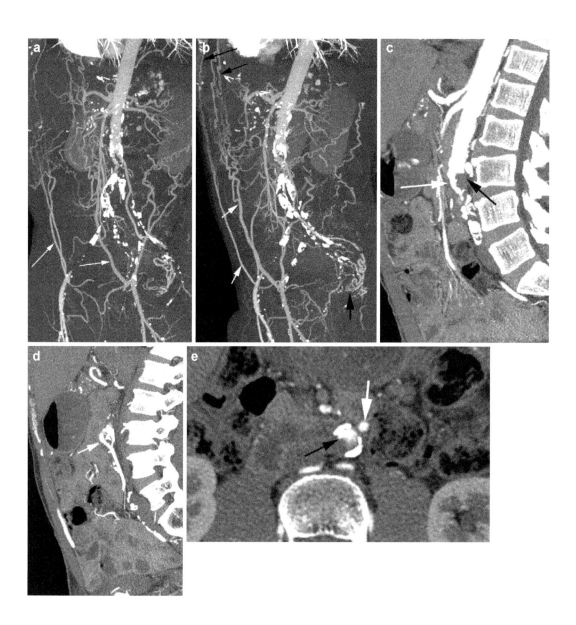

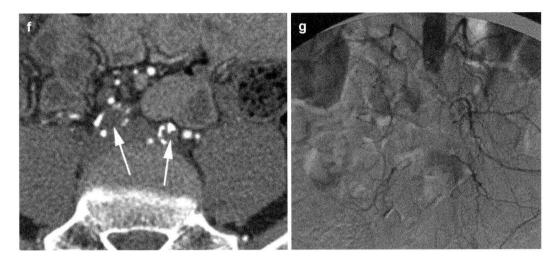

Fig. 2.30 (continued)

Fig. 2.30 Leriche's syndrome. (**a**, **b**) MIP images show extensive atherosclerotic calcification of the aorta which is occluded by thrombus from distal to origin of IMA and involving the bilateral common iliac arteries with extensive collateral circulation with dilated inferior epigastric arteries (*white arrows*), superior epigastric/internal thoracic arteries (*thin black arrows*), bilaterally, and dilated hemorrhoidal arteries (*thick black arrow*). (**c**, **d**) Sagittal reformatted images show thrombus (*black arrow*) occlud-ing the aorta from distal to origin of IMA (*white arrow*) which is dilated and patent. (**e**) Axial CT shows small contrast (*black arrow*) in the aortic lumen adjacent to the origin of the dilated IMA (*white arrow*). (**f**) Axial CT shows thrombosed atherosclerotic bilateral common iliac arteries. (**g**) Angiogram of the abdominal aorta on different patients shows complete occlusion of the infrarenal aorta and prominent collateral vessels

Vascular Dissection

3

Contents

R. Agarwala, *Atlas of Emergency Radiology:*   59
Vascular System, Chest, Abdomen and Pelvis, and Reproductive System,
DOI 10.1007/978-3-319-13042-2_3, © Springer International Publishing Switzerland 2015

Pulmonary Artery Dissection

Diagnosis
Dissection of the Pulmonary Artery

Imaging Features
1. Linear dissection flap traversing the main pulmonary artery and extending to the right pulmonary artery

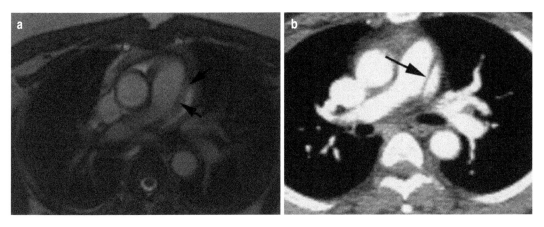

Fig. 3.1 Pulmonary artery dissection. (**a**) Axial FIESTA cardiac MRI and (**b**) axial CT show dissection of the main pulmonary artery (*arrows*). History of hypertension and COPD

Acute Aortic Syndrome

Aortic dissection, intramural hematoma, penetrating atherosclerotic ulcer, and aortic aneurysm rupture

Aortic Dissection

Diagnosis
Acute Aortic Dissection

Imaging Features

1. Intimal flap separating true and false lumen
2. Increased attenuation of acute thrombus in false lumen or intramural hematoma in pre-contrast study
3. False lumen almost always larger than true lumen
4. Internal displacement of intimal calcification
5. Mediastinal, pleural, and pericardial hematoma
6. Impaired perfusion of end organ either by static obstruction with intimal flap entering origin of the feeding artery or by dynamic obstruction with dissection flap prolapsing and covering the branch vessel ostium

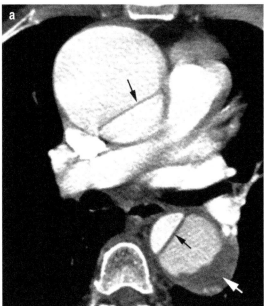
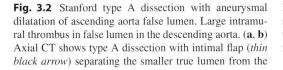
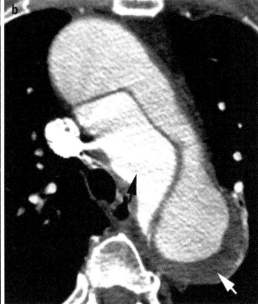

Fig. 3.2 Stanford type A dissection with aneurysmal dilatation of ascending aorta false lumen. Large intramural thrombus in false lumen in the descending aorta. (**a, b**) Axial CT shows type A dissection with intimal flap (*thin black arrow*) separating the smaller true lumen from the larger false lumen. In the ascending aorta the false lumen shows aneurysmal dilatation. The descending aorta has thrombus (*white arrow*) at the periphery of contrast-filled false lumen. True lumen smaller (*thick black arrow*)

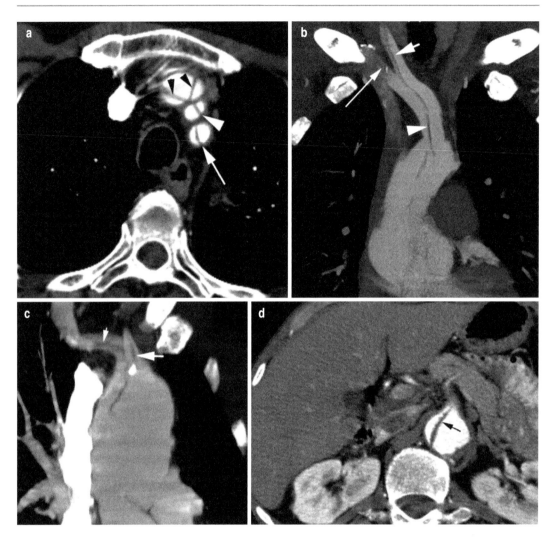

Fig. 3.3 Aortic dissection involving branch vessels. (**a**) Axial CT of Stanford type A dissection involving left subclavian (*arrow*), left common carotid (*white arrowhead*), and brachiocephalic arteries (*black arrowheads*). Three-channel dissection in the brachiocephalic artery with Mercedes-Benz sign. (**b**) Coronal MIP image of different patients. Dissection flap (*arrowhead*) in brachiocephalic artery extending to the right common carotid artery (*short arrow*) and right subclavian artery (*long arrow*). (**c**) Coronal reformatted image of another patient shows dissection flap in the right innominate artery (*thin white arrow*) and left carotid artery (*thick white arrow*). (**d**) Axial CT shows dissection flap extending into the celiac trunk (*arrow*)

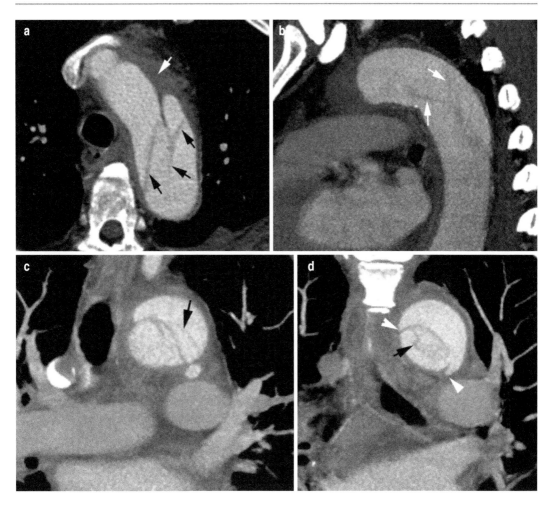

Fig. 3.4 Cobweb and beak sign of false lumen. (**a**) Axial, (**b**) sagittal, and (**c**) coronal reformatted CTs in this type B dissection show thin linear strands of low attenuation in false lumen (*black arrows*) due to incomplete shearing of the media. Surrounding mediastinal hematoma is seen (*white arrow*). (**d**) Coronal reformatted image shows beak sign of false lumen (*arrowheads*), collagenous medial remnants, and the cobwebs (*black arrow*)

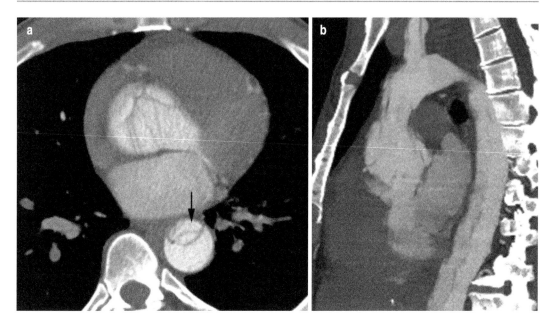

Fig. 3.5 Stanford type A dissection with aneurysm aortic root. History of hypertension and cocaine abuse. At surgery a cyanotic aneurysm was seen of the aortic root with blood in the adventitia and hematoma in the right atrium extending to the right ventricle. (**a**, **b**) Axial and coronal reformatted CTs show complex linear low-density intimal tear at root of the aorta from around the annulus. The true lumen is very compressed in the descending aorta (*arrow*). Aneurysm of the aortic root is best seen at sagittal view

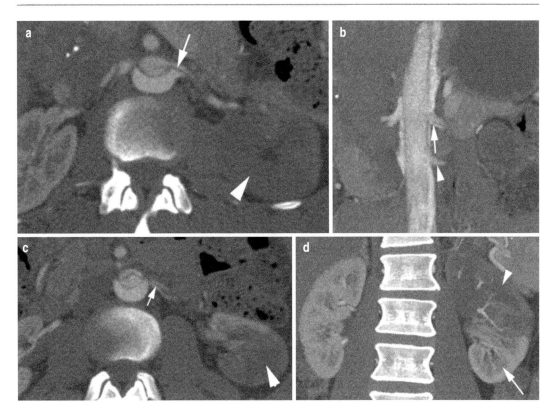

Fig. 3.6 Dissection with static obstruction of the left renal artery. (**a**, **b**) Axial CT and coronal reformatted images show intimal flap entering the left renal artery (*arrow*) with infarction of the upper pole left kidney (*large arrowhead*). The accessory renal artery (*small arrowhead*) shows no dissection. (**c**, **d**) Axial CT and coronal reformatted images show early branching with good contrast flow in both branches and no dissection of accessory renal artery (*short arrow*), being connected to the true lumen, supplying the well-perfused lower renal pole (*long arrow*)

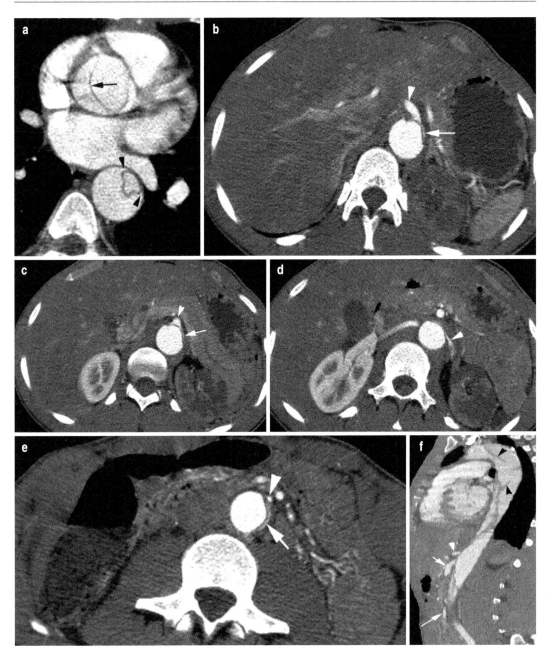

Fig. 3.7 Dynamic obstruction of major branch vessels of the abdominal aorta with ischemia of the liver, bowel, and left renal infarction in Stanford type A dissection. (**a**) Axial CT shows type A dissection involving root of the aorta. Dissection flap (*arrow*) in the ascending and descending aorta. Beak sign of false lumen (*arrowheads*). (**b–e**) Axial CT images show the celiac trunk, SMA, left renal artery, and IMA (*arrowheads*) originate from the slit-like true lumen (*white arrow*) with the origin of these vessels being covered by the dissection flap causing pressure deficit in the true lumen resulting in ischemia of the liver, bowel loops, and frank infarction of the left kidney. (**f**) Sagittal reformatted image shows wide false lumen with cobwebs (*black arrowheads*) with the celiac trunk (*white arrowhead*), SMA (*short arrow*), and IMA (*long arrow*) arising from narrow true lumen

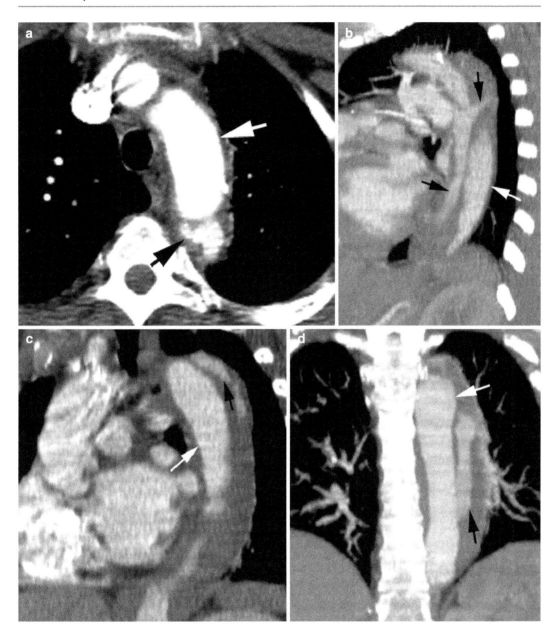

Fig. 3.8 Stanford type B dissection with contrast and thrombus in false lumen. CECT (**a**) axial and (**b**) sagittal reformatted images show contrast in false lumen (*black arrow*) with surrounding thrombus in the descending thoracic aorta spiraling around the true lumen (*white arrow*). (**c**, **d**) Sagittal and coronal reformatted images at different plane show false lumen with central contrast (*black arrow*) parallel to the true lumen (*white arrow*)

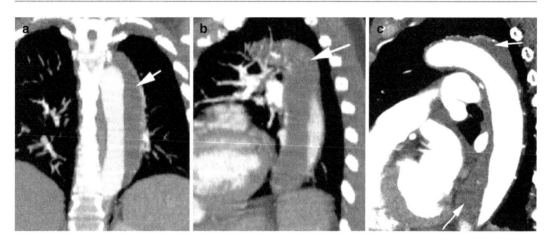

Fig. 3.9 Complete thrombosis of false lumen. Same patient as in Fig. 3.8, CT done 3 years later. (**a**) Coronal and (**b**, **c**) sagittal reformatted images show complete obliteration of false lumen (*arrow*) by thrombus, giving the appearance of large intramural hematoma

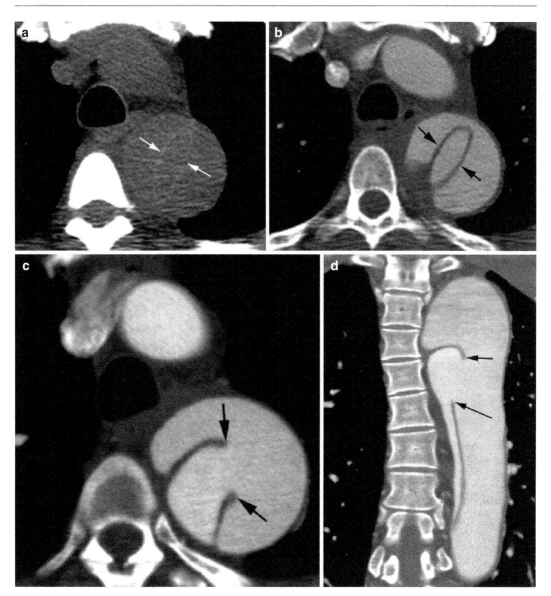

Fig. 3.10 Acute Stanford type B dissection. (**a**) Precontrast axial CT shows increased attenuation of dissected flap (*white arrows*). (**b**) Postcontrast axial CT shows intimal flap (*arrows*) with similar appearance to precontrast study with central small true lumen surrounded by larger false lumen. (**c, d**) Axial and coronal reformatted CTs show site of tear (*arrows*) with smaller true lumen with higher-density contrast

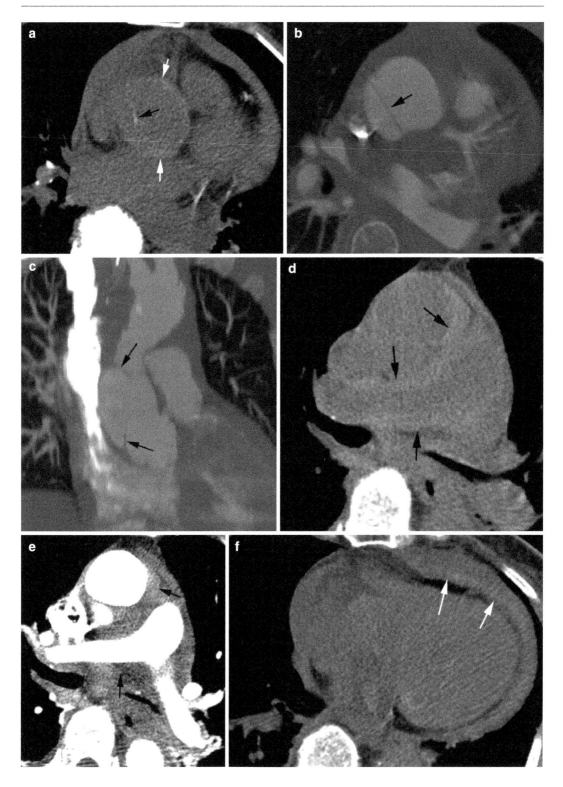

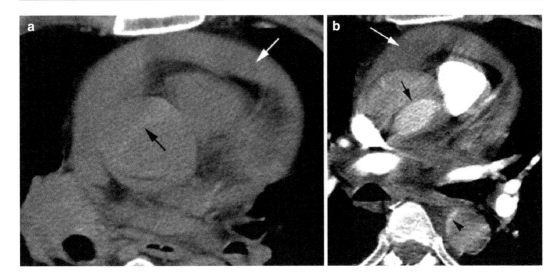

Fig. 3.12 Dissection of the aortic root with hemopericardium. (**a**) Axial precontrast CT shows acute dissection with high attenuation of intimal flap (*black arrow*) and high-density hemorrhagic fluid in the pericardium (*white arrow*). (**b**) Postcontrast axial study shows the intimal flap (*black arrow*) separating high-density smaller true lumen from false lumen. Compressed true lumen is seen in the descending aorta with contrast (*arrowhead*) and also the hemopericardium (*white arrow*)

Fig. 3.11 Dissection of the aortic root with displaced intimal calcification. Surgically proven focal Stanford type A dissection of the greater curvature of the ascending aorta near the pulmonary artery with tear into the pericardium. (**a**) Axial precontrast CT shows faint calcified plaque in the internally displaced flap (*black arrow*) and faint high attenuation in the aortic rim (*white arrow*). (**b**) Intimal flap better seen in postcontrast study, but the calcification is obscured by the contrast (*arrow*). (**c**) Coronal reformatted image shows the focal dissection which was about 1.5 cm long at surgery (*arrows*). (**d**) Precontrast axial study at higher level than (**a**) shows high-density hemomediastinum surrounding the aorta and pulmonary artery due to rupture of dissection posteriorly close to the pulmonary artery (*arrows*). (**e**) Postcontrast axial CT at same level shows the hematoma (*arrow*) which is better seen in precontrast CT. (**f**) Precontrast study shows thin layer of high-density hemorrhagic fluid (*arrows*) in the pericardium posterior to the low density pericardial fluid. At surgery blood was present at the posterior layers of the pericardium, but the pericardial fluid was serous

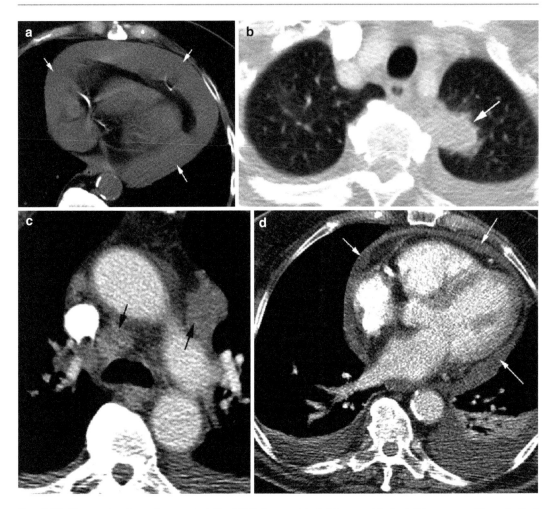

Fig. 3.13 Hemopericardium from metastatic NSCLC. History of hypertension and right upper quadrant pain in an 80-year-old person. (**a**) Noncontrast axial CT showed high-density hemopericardium (*arrows*). Pericardiocentesis of more than a liter of hemorrhagic fluid showed adenocarcinoma. (**b**, **c**) Contrast-enhanced axial CT shows NSCLC as nodule (*white arrow*) in the left lung apex with mediastinal lymphadenopathy (*black arrows*) and bilateral small pleural effusion. (**d**) Post-pericardiocentesis axial CT shows residual pericardial fluid (*arrows*) with no pericardial enhancement or nodularity and increase in bilateral small effusion with adjacent atelectasis

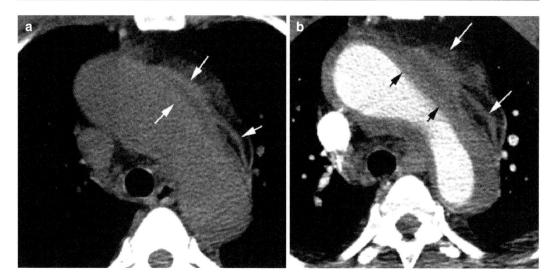

Fig. 3.14 Hemomediastinum from type A dissection. Acute hematoma in the periaortic mediastinum and wall of aorta. Type A dissection flap was seen 1 cm above the right coronary artery at surgery. (**a**) Noncontrast axial CT shows high attenuating hemorrhage in the wall of the greater curvature of the aortic arch and high attenuating stranding of mediastinal fat (*white arrows*). (**b**) Postcontrast axial CT shows hematoma in the outer wall of arch (*black arrows*) and hemorrhage in the mediastinum (*white arrows*) as irregular stranding

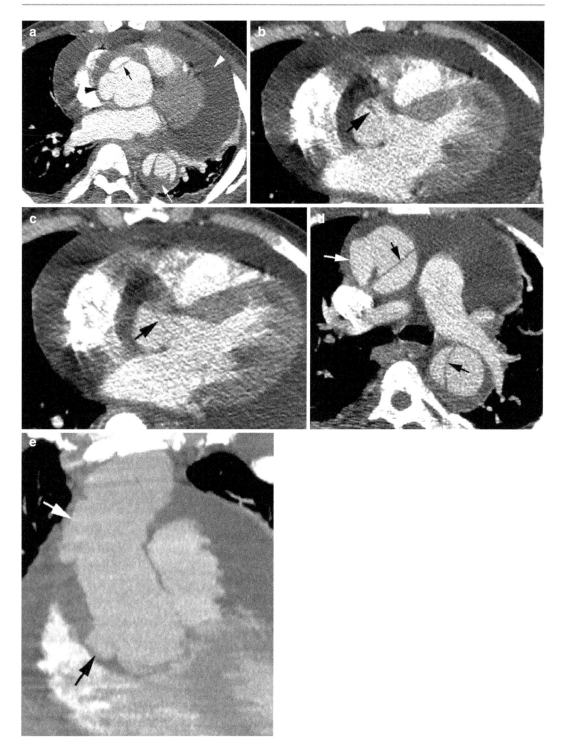

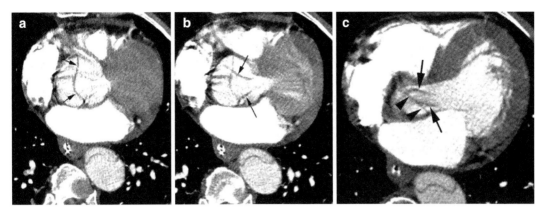

Fig. 3.16 Stanford type A dissection with intimointimal intussusception. At surgery there was complete circumferential tear of the intima just above the left coronary artery and below the sinotubular junction toward the noncoronary sinus side. (**a**) Axial CT shows the dissection flap (*arrows*). (**b**) Axial CT shows portion of prolapsing flap (*arrows*). (**c**) Prolapse of the flap (*arrows*) through the aortic annulus (*arrowheads*). Preoperative echocardiogram showed the back and forth prolapse of the flap through the aortic valve

Fig. 3.15 Stanford type A dissection from the aortic root with aneurysm of the sinus of Valsalva and large hemopericardium. (**a**) Postcontrast axial CT shows focal-dilated aortic root and saccular aneurysms at the sinus of Valsalva (*black arrowhead*), dissection flap at aortic root (*black arrow*) and large hemopericardium (*white arrowhead*). (1,000 cc of clotted blood was removed from pericardium at surgery.) The descending aorta shows partial thrombus in false lumen (*white arrow*). (**b, c**) Axial CT shows dissecting flap extending inferiorly to the annulus (*black arrow*). (**d**) Axial CT of the mid-ascending aorta shows saccular aneurysm (*white arrow*) and the dissecting flap (*black arrow*). (**e**) Coronal reformatted image shows saccular aneurysm at the sinus of Valsalva (*black arrow*) and ascending aorta (*white arrow*). At surgery the dissection was seen to involve the root of the aorta extending below the coronary arteries to the annulus with thrombus

Intramural Hematoma

Imaging Findings
Acute IMH
1. Crescentic, eccentric, hyperattenuating region of thickening of the aortic wall in unenhanced images.
2. No communication with true lumen.
3. In enhanced CT the intramural hematoma is nonenhancing and smooth, and crescentic wall thickening of the aorta extends partially or entirely around the opacified lumen with no spiraling of intimal flap.
4. Pericardial effusion and mediastinal hematoma may be present.

5. Type A IMH involves the ascending aorta, and early surgical repair considered.
6. Type B IMH, not complicated, treated with medical therapy.

Chronic IMH
1. Can have peripheral calcification which has a circular or semilunar configuration.
2. Hematoma may decrease in thickness or completely resolve.
3. Intimal tear may occur presenting as ulcer-like projection and can cause aortic dissection.
4. Saccular or fusiform aneurysm can form at site of hematoma and can lead to aortic rupture and pseudoaneurysm formation.

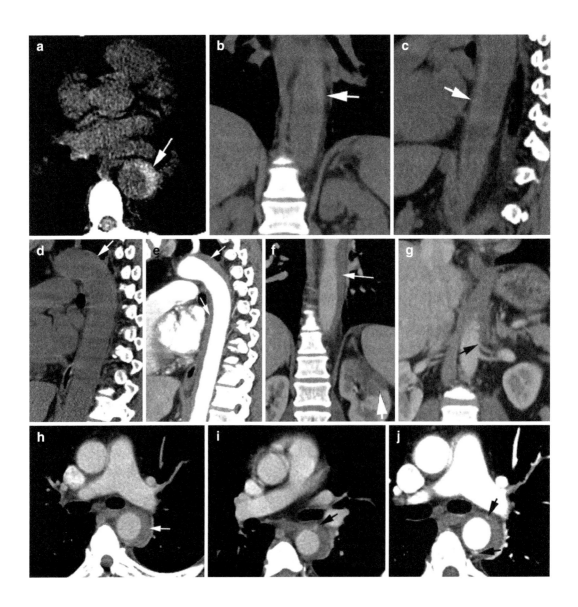

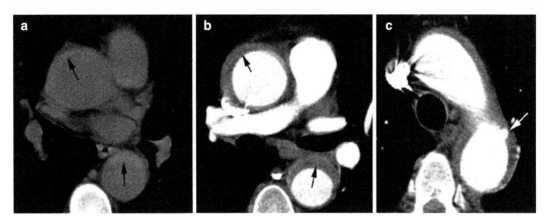

Fig. 3.18 Acute intramural hematoma in the ascending aorta. (**a**) Precontrast axial view shows high-density crescentic wall thickening of the ascending and descending aorta (*arrow*). (**b**) Axial postcontrast study shows wall thickening of the aorta. (**c**) Axial CECT shows ulcer-like projection (*arrow*) at the proximal descending aorta with surrounding IMH

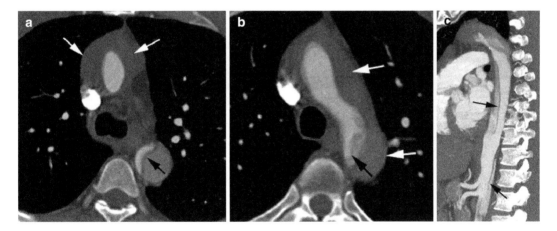

Fig. 3.19 Large IMH at the ascending and arch aorta confirmed at surgery. Type B dissection flap descending aorta. History of aortic insufficiency, malperfusion syndrome, and hypertension. (**a**) Axial CT shows large IMH (*white arrows*) compressing the contrast-filled aortic lumen. Type B intimal flap in the descending aorta (*black arrow*) compressing the true lumen. (**b**) Axial image shows large IMH at arch (*white arrows*) and origin of dissection flap at distal arch (*black arrow*). (**c**) Sagittal reformatted image shows the dissection flap spiraling around the true lumen (*arrows*)

Fig. 3.17 Acute IMH. Patient with high blood pressure and left flank pain. Precontrast axial (**a**), coronal (**b**), and sagittal (**c**, **d**) reformatted images show high-density intramural thrombus (*arrow*) extending up to the left subclavian artery. (**e**) Postcontrast sagittal reformatted image shows IMH (*arrows*) distal to the left subclavian artery. (**f**, **g**) Coronal reformatted images show IMH paralleling the contrast-filled lumen with no dissection flap (*thin arrows*). The hematoma extends up to the proximal of the two left renal arteries (*arrow* in **g**) resulting in infarction of upper pole of the left kidney (*thick white arrow* in **f**). (**h**) Axial CT shows crescentic hematoma around contrast-filled aortic lumen (*arrow*). (**i**, **j**) Axial CT shows focal contrast enhancement in IMH (*arrows*) and not communicating with the lumen

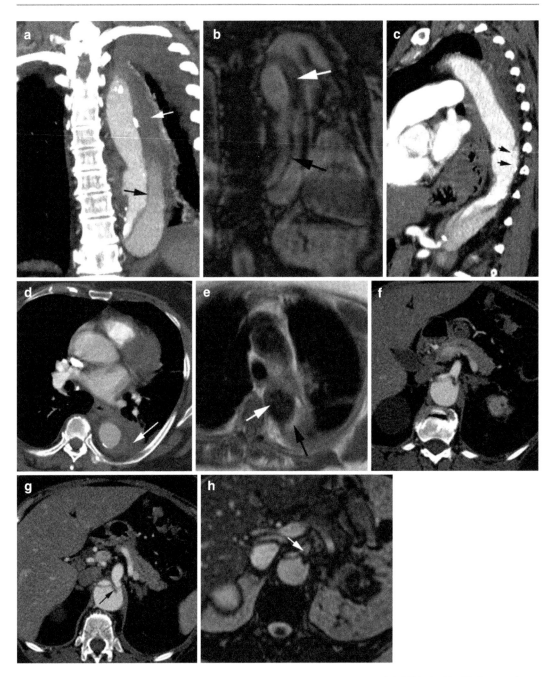

Fig. 3.20 Intramural hematoma and dissection flap of the descending aorta. (**a**, **b**) Coronal reformatted image and coronal MRI FIESTA image show large IMH (*white arrow*) in the proximal descending aorta which continues with the intimal flap (*black arrow*). (**c**) Sagittal reformatted CT shows site of tear of the intima (*arrows*). (**d**) Axial CT shows heterogeneous density of intramural hematoma (*white arrow*). (**e**) Axial MRI double IR image shows high-signal IMH (*black arrow*) and black blood (*white arrow*) in the aortic lumen. (**f**, **g**) Axial CT shows dynamic obstruction of celiac trunk and SMA by dissection flap. (**h**) Axial MRI FIESTA image shows dynamic obstruction with prolapse of flap into the lumen of SMA (*arrow*)

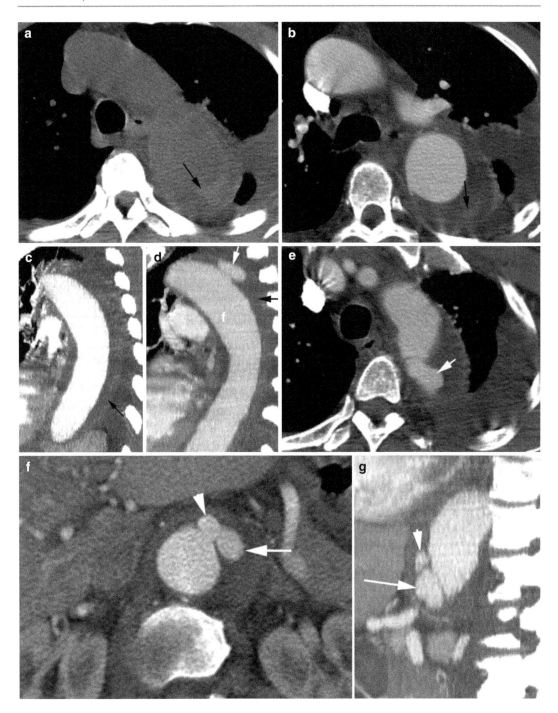

Fig. 3.21 Stanford type B acute or chronic IMH. (**a**, **b**) Axial pre- and postcontrast CTs show high-density acute thrombus (*arrow*) at posterior arch of the aorta better appreciated in precontrast image. (**c**) Sagittal reformatted image shows diffuse low-density chronic thrombus surrounding the descending aorta (*arrows*). (**d**, **e**) Sagittal reformatted and axial CTs show small saccular aneurysm in posterior arch (*white arrow*) with surrounding chronic low-density hematoma (*black arrow*) distal to the acute IMH. (**f**, **g**) Axial and sagittal reformatted images show small saccular aneurysm (*arrow*) adjacent to celiac trunk (*arrowhead*)

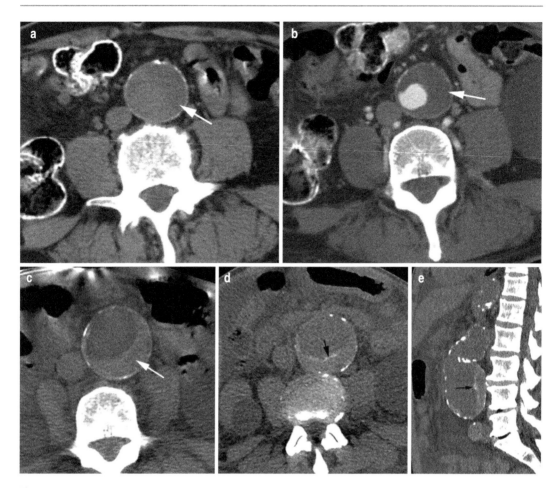

Fig. 3.22 Acute on chronic intramural thrombus within tortuous aorta with fusiform aneurysm. (**a**, **b**) Axial pre- and postcontrast CTs show aneurysmal dilatation of abdominal aorta with atherosclerotic calcification and large low-density intramural thrombus surrounding the contrast-filled lumen (*arrow*). (**c**) Axial precontrast CT 5 years later shows high-density acute intramural thrombus in the previous chronic thrombus (*arrow*) with increase in size of the aneurysm. (**d**, **e**) Axial and sagittal reformatted CTs 1 year later show acute thrombus had decreased in size and walled off by calcification (*arrow*) with no change in aneurysm size. High density is probably rebleed within walled-off thrombus

Arterial Aneurysm

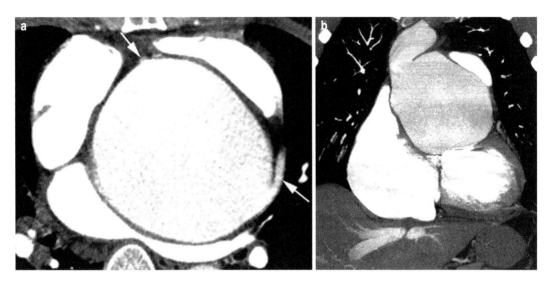

Fig. 3.23 Aneurysm of the aortic root. (**a**) Axial and (**b**) coronal reformatted CTs show large aneurysm at the root of the aorta involving right and left coronary sinuses (*arrows*)

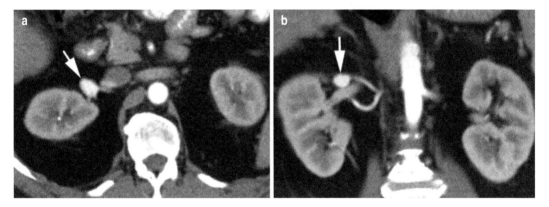

Fig. 3.24 Aneurysm of the right renal artery. Postcontrast axial (**a**) and coronal reformatted images (**b**) show focal aneurysm of the right main renal artery (*arrow*)

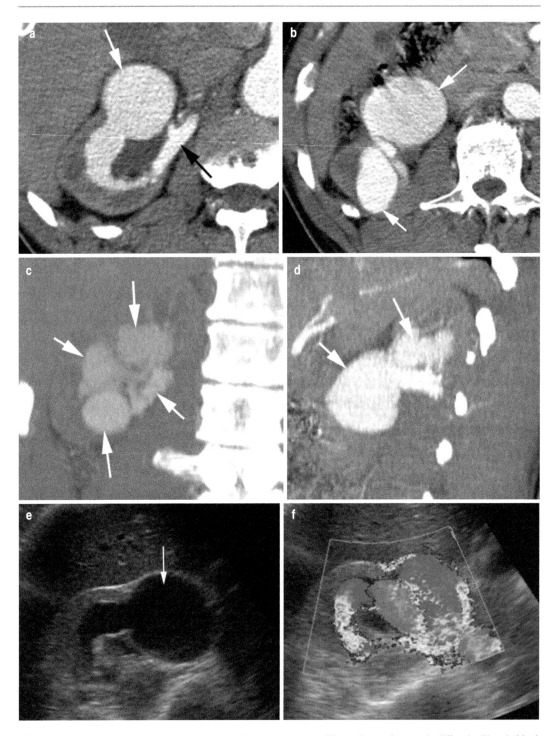

Fig. 3.25 Aneurysm of the right renal artery within the kidney. (**a**, **b**) Postcontrast axial CT, (**c**) coronal, and (**d**) sagittal reformatted views show multiple focal aneurysms of the intrarenal artery within the right kidney (*white arrows*). The main renal artery is diffusely dilated (*black arrow*). (**e**) Grayscale (**f**) color Doppler ultrasound shows large intrarenal aneurysm (*arrow* in **e**) similar to what is seen in axial CT in (**a**)

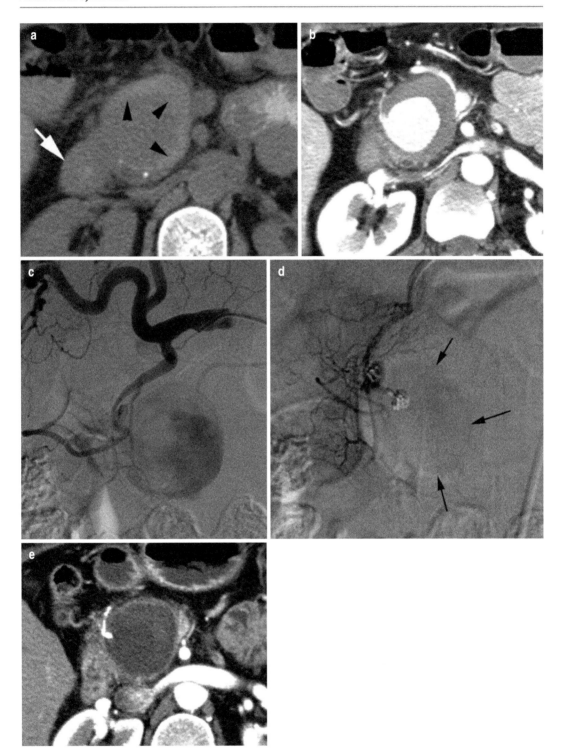

Fig. 3.26 Pseudoaneurysm of gastroduodenal artery in a patient with alcoholic pancreatitis. (**a**) Noncontrast axial CT shows large pseudoaneurysm medial to second part of duodenal sweep (*thick white arrow*). High-density thrombus (*arrowheads*) is seen surrounding the central low density of the aneurysm. (**b**) Axial CECT shows lumen of pseudoaneurysm filled with contrast with peripheral hematoma. (**c**) Celiac artery angiogram shows contrast flowing into lumen of pseudoaneurysm. (**d**) Post-coiled angiogram shows no filling of pseudoaneurysm (*arrows*). (**e**) Axial view of CT done few days later shows successful coiling with no contrast in pseudoaneurysm

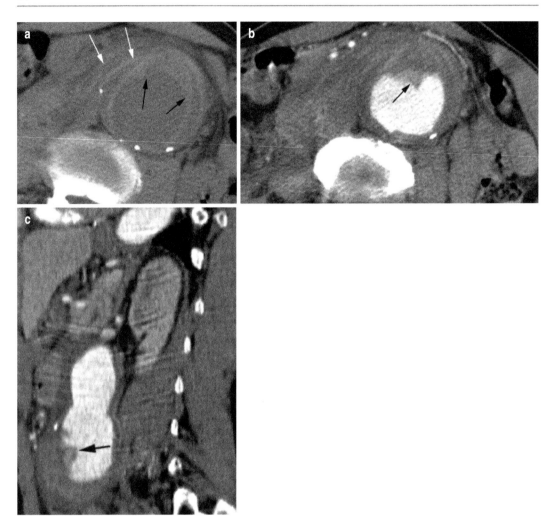

Fig. 3.27 Hyperattenuating crescent sign of acute rupture. (**a**) Precontrast axial CT shows curvilinear high-density hematoma within anterior wall (*black arrows*) of AAA. Surrounding periaortic region mostly on the right side shows streaky high density from acute hemorrhage (*white arrows*). (**b**, **c**). Axial and sagittal contrast-enhanced CTs show site of intimal tear with "V"-shaped defect in anterior wall of aorta plugged with thrombus (*arrow*)

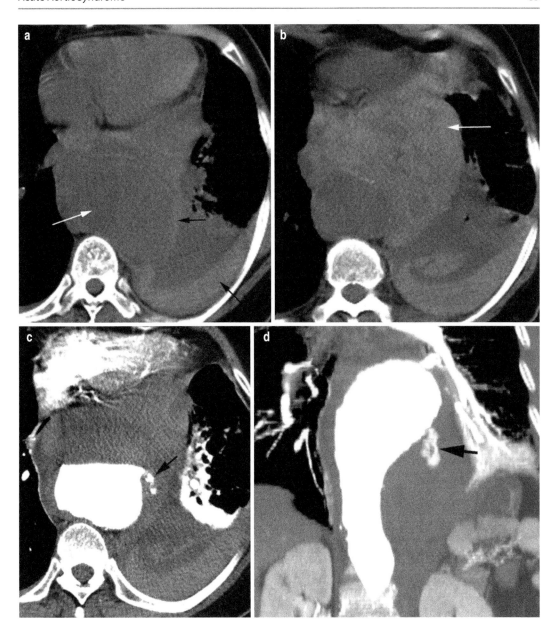

Fig. 3.28 Rupture of descending thoracic aortic aneurysm with active extravasation of contrast. (**a**) Axial nonenhanced CT shows large low-density distal thoracic aortic aneurysm (*white arrow*) with high-density hemothorax (*black arrows*). (**b**) Axial nonenhanced CT at a lower plane shows high-density hematoma (*arrow*) in mediastinum surrounding the aneurysm. (**c**, **d**) Contrast-enhanced axial and coronal reformatted CTs show active extravasation of contrast from aneurysm (*arrow*)

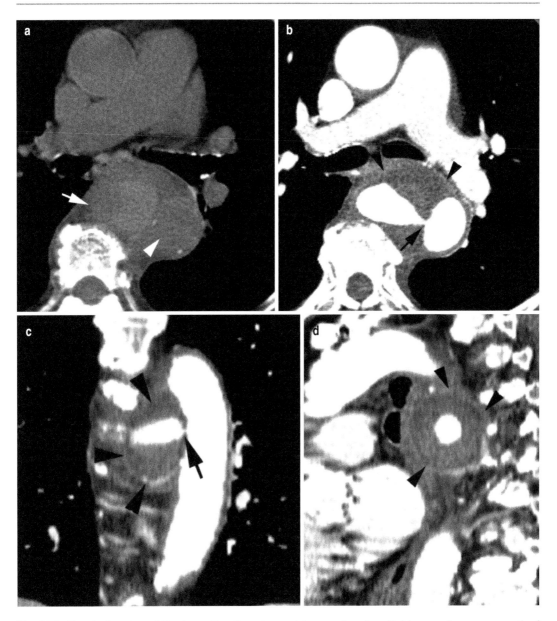

Fig. 3.29 Contained rupture of the descending thoracic aorta with pseudoaneurysm formation. (**a**) Precontrast image shows high-density hematoma (*arrow*) medial to the descending thoracic aorta (*arrowhead*). (**b–d**) CECT axial, coronal, and sagittal images show narrow neck of the pseudoaneurysm (*arrow*) with surrounding hematoma (*arrowhead*)

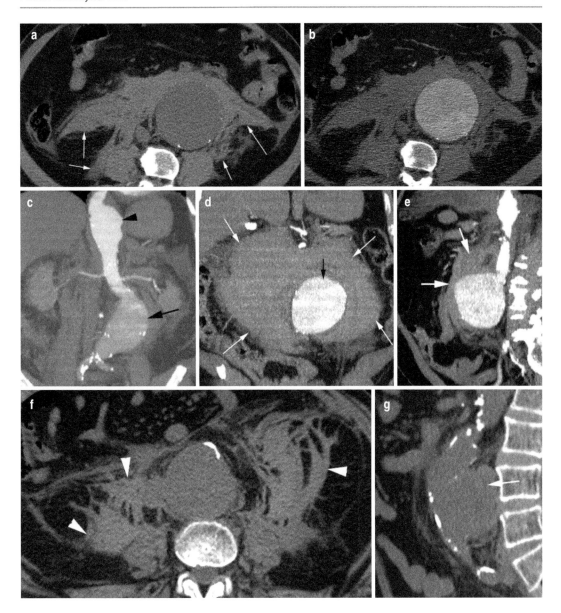

Fig. 3.30 Acute rupture of abdominal aortic aneurysm. (a–e) Patient 1: (a) Precontrast axial, (b) postcontrast axial, (c, d) coronal, and (e) sagittal reformatted images show bilateral spillage of fresh hemorrhage into the para-aortic and perirenal spaces (*arrows*) but no active contrast extravasation from the larger lower AAA (*black arrow*). The smaller aneurysm is seen in the proximal abdominal aorta (*arrowhead*). (f–h) Patient 2: Precontrast (f) axial, (g) sagittal, and (h) coronal reformatted images show spillage of fresh hemorrhage (*arrowhead*) into the retroperitoneum from a saccular aneurysm arising from posterior wall of AA (*arrow*). (i) Patient 3: Axial precontrast image shows rupture of fusiform AAA aneurysm on the left side (*arrow*)

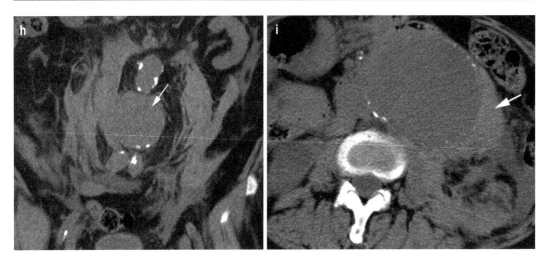

Fig. 3.30 (continued)

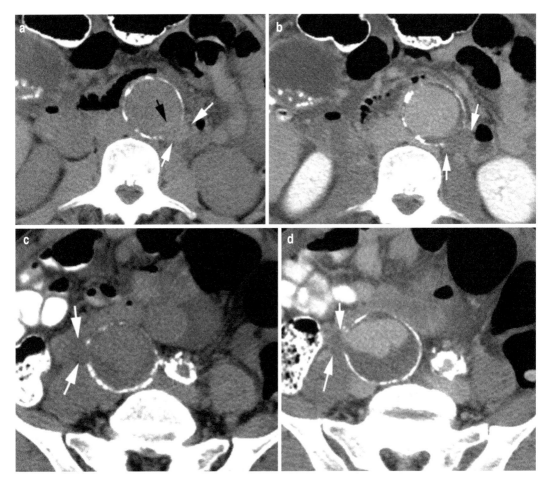

Fig. 3.31 Contained rupture of aortic aneurysm and right common iliac artery aneurysms. (**a**) Axial precontrast image shows small high-density thrombus extending outside the calcified rim of the abdominal aorta (*white arrows*) with crescent sign of acute IMH (*black arrow*). (**b**) CECT shows no extension of contrast into the thrombus (*arrow*).

(**c**) Precontrast axial image of the right common iliac artery aneurysm shows low-density thrombus outside the lumen (*arrows*). (**d**) Axial CECT of the right common iliac artery shows low-density thrombus extending outside the lumen (*arrow*) with small bulging of contrast from true lumen outside the wall forming a pseudoaneurysm

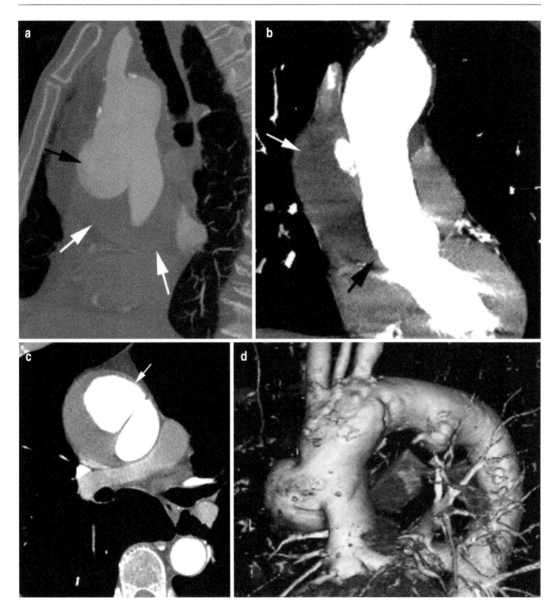

Fig. 3.32 Large saccular aneurysm of the proximal ascending aorta with intramural hematoma extending to sinotubular junction. (**a**) Sagittal and (**b**) coronal reformatted images show large saccular aneurysm at proximal ascending aorta (*black arrow*) with surrounding IMH (*white arrows*). Low-density intramural hematoma extending low to sinotubular junction (*thick black arrow* in **b**). (**c**) Axial contrast-enhanced CT shows saccular aneurysm (*arrow*) with surrounding low-density intramural hematoma. (**d**) 3D volume-rendered image shows the saccular aneurysm ascending aorta

Aortic Ulcers

Diagnosis
Ulcer-Like Projection

Imaging Findings

1. Focal   intimal   projection   into   intramural
   hematoma
2. More common with type A hematoma
3. Can   develop   into   fusiform   or   saccular
   aneurysm
4. Can convert into aortic dissection

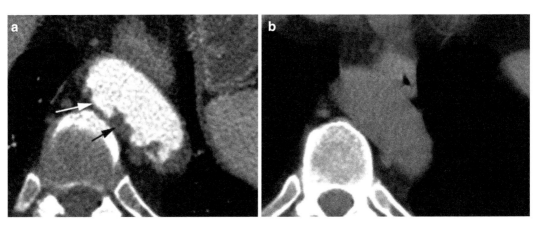

Fig. 3.33 Ulcer-like projection descending thoracic aorta. (**a**) CECT shows multiple lobulated projections of the distal descending thoracic aorta wall due to multiple ulcer-like projections (*white arrow*) with surrounding intramural hematoma (*black arrow*). (**b**) Noncontrast study shows no evidence of calcified atherosclerosis or any acute intramural hematoma

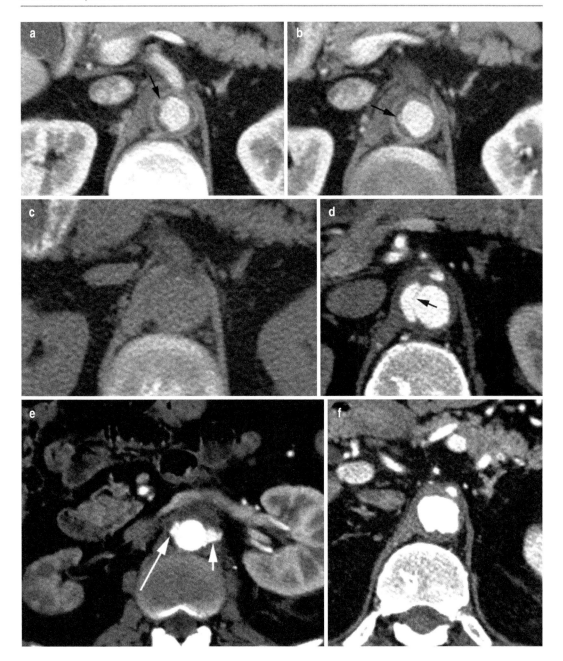

Fig. 3.34 Ulcer-like projection progressing to saccular aneurysm. Patient 1: (**a**, **b**). CECT axial shows two ulcer-like projections (*arrow*) at level of celiac artery with small surrounding IMH. (**c**) Precontrast axial image shows no calcified atherosclerosis or high-density acute hemorrhage. (**d**) Axial CT 5 months later shows saccular aneurysm (*arrow*) has developed at the same level. Patient 2:

(**e**) Ulcer-like projections are also seen at the origins of renal arteries (*arrows*) partially obstructing the right renal artery causing decreased perfusion and atrophy of the right kidney. (**f**, **g**) Axial and coronal reformatted CTs 7 years later show focal AA at level of celiac artery and diffuse irregular ulceration of the aorta. (**h**) Axial CT shows increased atrophic changes of the right kidney

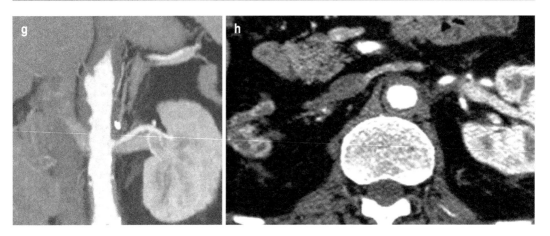

Fig. 3.34 (continued)

Diagnosis

Penetrating Atherosclerotic Aortic Ulcer

Imaging Features

1. Seen with atherosclerosis
2. Other features as ulcer-like projection

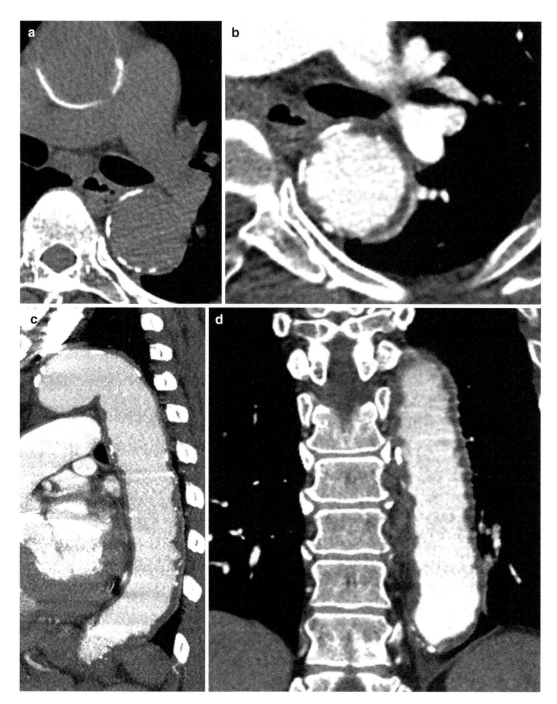

Fig. 3.35 Penetrating aortic ulcer with atherosclerotic calcification. (**a**) Noncontrast axial CT shows the atherosclerotic calcification in the ascending and descending thoracic aorta. (**b–d**) Postcontrast axial, sagittal, and coronal reformatted images show multiple contrast-filled ulcer outpouchings through the intima into the thrombus of the media

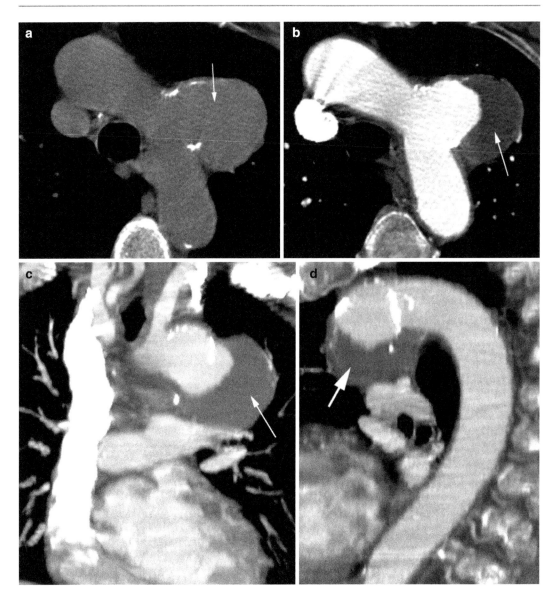

Fig. 3.36 Large saccular aneurysm arising from atherosclerotic aortic arch. (**a**) Axial precontrast CT shows large saccular aneurysm (*arrow*) at the arch with atherosclerotic change. Postcontrast axial, (**b**) coronal, (**c**) and sagittal (**d**) reformatted images show large saccular aneurysm with surrounding hematoma (*arrow*) and atherosclerotic calcification

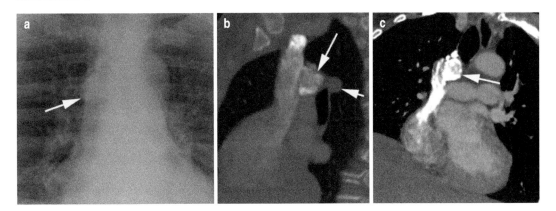

Fig. 3.37 Azygos diverticulum. (**a**) Frontal chest X-ray shows a mediastinal mass as an incidental finding. (**b**, **c**) CECT sagittal and rotated coronal reformatted images show contrast-filled aneurysmal dilatation (*long arrow*) of the distal azygos vein (*short arrow*)

Traumatic Injury to Vessels

4

Contents

R. Agarwala, *Atlas of Emergency Radiology:*
Vascular System, Chest, Abdomen and Pelvis, and Reproductive System,
DOI 10.1007/978-3-319-13042-2_4, © Springer International Publishing Switzerland 2015

Aorta

Diagnosis
Complete Aortic Rupture

Imaging Features
1. Periaortic hematoma in direct continuity with the aortic wall
2. Rupture at isthmus (commonest site)
3. Intimal flap, traumatic pseudoaneurysm, intramural thrombus, abnormal aortic contour, and active extravasation of contrast

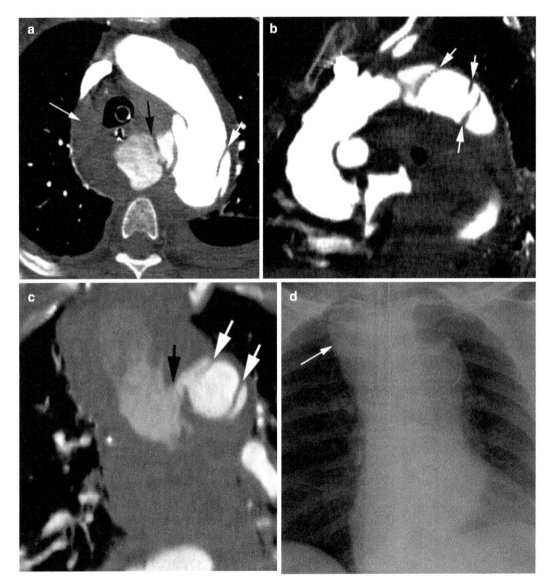

Fig. 4.1 Aortic transection. (**a**) Axial, (**b**) oblique sagittal, and (**c**) coronal reformatted CECT shows aortic transection at the isthmus (*thick white arrows*) with active hemorrhage into the mediastinum (*black arrow*), large hemomediastinum (*long thin arrow*) and left hemothorax. Multiple intimal flaps are seen (*short white arrow*). (**d**) Frontal chest X-ray shows hematoma widening the superior mediastinum (*arrow*)

Diagnosis
Incomplete Aortic Rupture

Imaging Features
1. Saccular outpouching of the aortic lumen at anteromedial aspect of the isthmus by a collar
2. Surrounding hemomediastinum

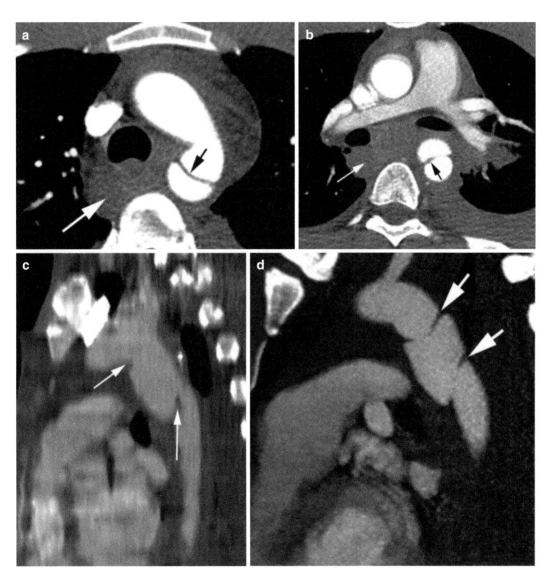

Fig. 4.2 Traumatic pseudoaneurysm of the aorta. (**a, b**) Axial CECT shows upper and lower end of the pseudoaneurysm at the isthmus (*black arrows*) with large hemomediastinum and hemothorax (*white arrow*). (**c, d**) Sagittal reformatted image in 2 patients shows pseudoaneurysm at the isthmus with dissection flaps at the neck (*arrows*).

(**e, f**) Coronal reformatted images of patient in (**d**) show the upper and lower end of the tears (*black arrows*) with mediastinal hematoma (*white arrow*). (**g**) 3D volume-rendered image of the pseudoaneurysm. At surgery 90 % of the aorta was torn

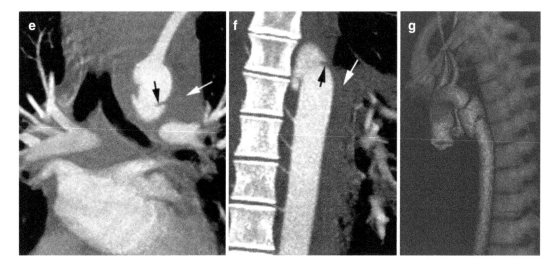

Fig. 4.2 (continued)

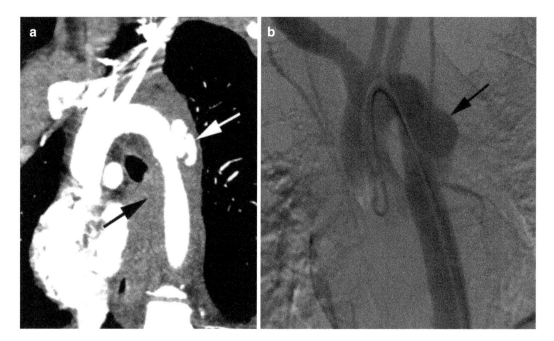

Fig. 4.3 Pseudoaneurysmic aorta following motor vehicle accident. (**a**) Sagittal reformatted image of lobulated saccular outpouching of pseudoaneurysm at anterolateral aortic isthmus (*white arrow*) with surrounding mediastinal hematoma (*black arrow*). (**b**) Angiogram showing pseudoaneurysm (*arrow*) with no extravasation of contrast

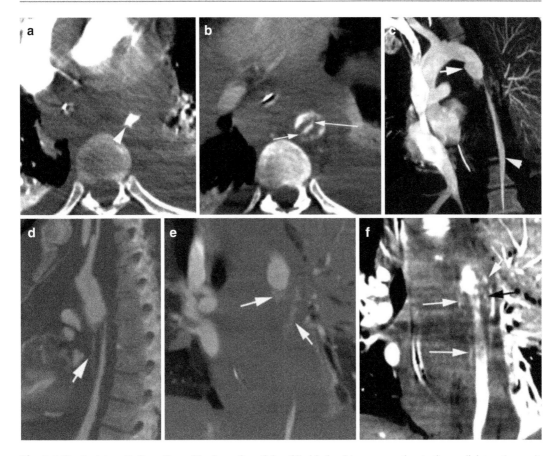

Fig. 4.4 Stanford type B dissection with circumferential intimomedial tear. High-speed MVA. Axial CT (**a**) early arterial phase shows narrowed contrast-filled descending thoracic aorta (*arrow head*). (**b**) Delayed arterial phase shows hematoma surrounding the true lumen with contrast filling the media at the periphery. Thin strands of contrast-filled intimal tear connecting to the medial tear (*arrows*). (**c**) Oblique coronal reformatted view shows pseudoaneurysm (*arrow*) at the aortic isthmus with constricted true lumen distal to it (*arrow head*). (**d**) Sagittal, (**e, f**) coronal reformatted images show irregular linear contrast filling the media from the pseudoaneurysm (*arrows*)

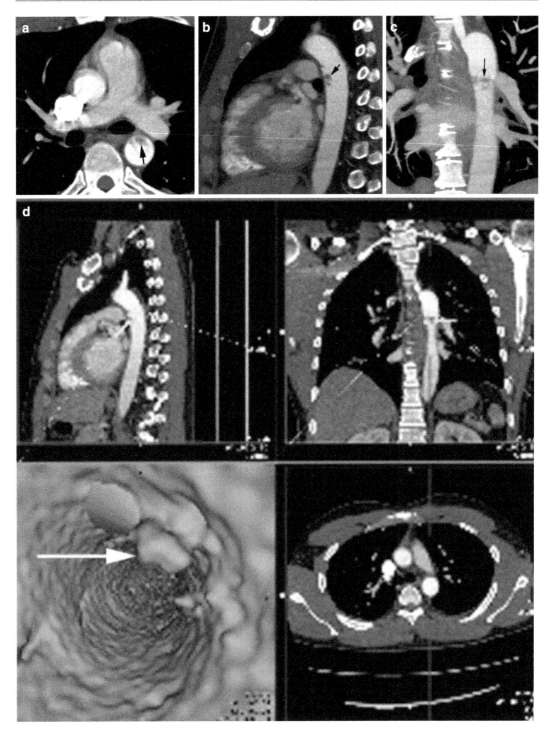

Fig. 4.5 Acute traumatic intramural hematoma at the aortic isthmus from deceleration MVA injury. (**a**) Axial, (**b**) sagittal, and (**c**) coronal reformatted images show irregular hematoma (*arrow*) in tunica media with no intimal flap and no significant mediastinal hematoma. (**d**) Flythrough endovascular postprocessed image shows protrusion of the intima into the lumen due to medial hematoma (*arrow*) with no intimal tear. The green patch represents the marking of *arrow* in the coronal and sagittal reformatted images

Pulmonary Artery

Diagnosis
Pseudoaneurysm of Left Pulmonary Artery

Imaging Features
1. Focal saccular outpouching of contrast in left main pulmonary artery

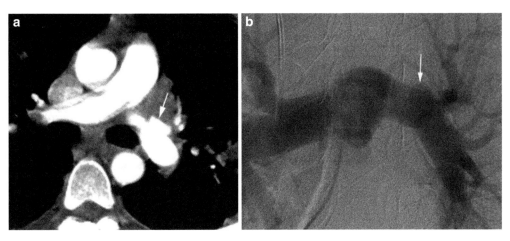

Fig. 4.6 Pseudoaneurysm of the left main pulmonary artery post MVA. (**a**) Axial CECT shows pseudoaneurysm of the left main pulmonary artery (*arrow*). (**b**) Pulmonary angiogram shows pseudoaneurysm (*arrow*) just proximal to the origin of the left upper lobe branch

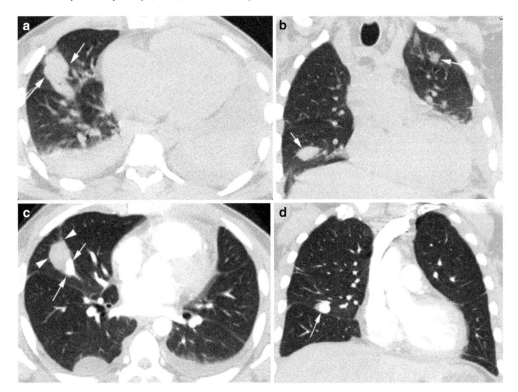

Fig. 4.7 Pulmonary artery pseudoaneurysm. History of penetrating injury. (**a, b**) Axial and coronal reformatted noncontrast CT chest shows elongated solid density at the right middle lobe (*arrows*), bilateral pleural effusion, and other patchy solid pulmonary densities (*arrows*) no different from contusion/consolidation. (**c, d**) CECT axial and coronal reformatted images 5 days later show density in the middle lobe (*arrows*) to be a pulmonary pseudoaneurysm which is partially thrombosed (*arrowheads*) and smaller in size than the noncontrast study. This resolved in later CT studies

Inferior Vena Cava

Diagnosis
Laceration of IVC

Imaging Features

1. Extravasation of contrast-enhanced blood from infrahepatic IVC
2. Large amount of high-density hemorrhagic fluid in the subhepatic space and subphrenic spaces bilaterally

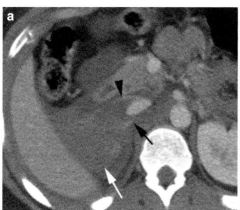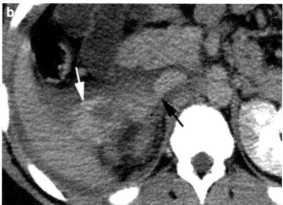

Fig. 4.8 Laceration of infrahepatic IVC post MVA trauma. (**a**) Axial CT in portal venous phase shows extravasated contrast (*black arrow*) from subhepatic IVC just below the inferior margin of caudate lobe of the liver (*black arrowhead*). Large amount of hemorrhagic fluid in the adjacent subhepatic space (*white arrow*). (**b**) Axial CT delayed phase shows pooling of high-density extravasated contrast-mixed blood in the subhepatic space (*white arrow*). Site of IVC tear is again seen (*black arrow*)

Diagnosis

IVC Pseudoaneurysm

Imaging Features

1. Well-marginated focal outpouching from IVC just proximal to the right renal vein
2. Surrounding hemorrhagic fluid extending to the adjacent perirenal space

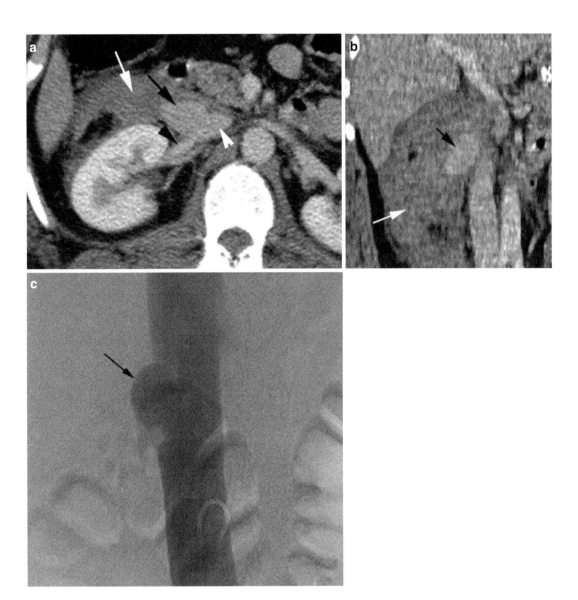

Fig. 4.9 Pseudoaneurysm of IVC in patient post MVA trauma. (**a**) Axial postcontrast CT shows saccular pseudoaneurysm (*black arrow*) of IVC (*white arrowhead*) just above the right renal vein (*black arrowhead*) with hemorrhagic fluid surrounding the aneurysm and in the right perirenal space (*white arrow*). (**b**) Coronal reformatted image shows pseudoaneurysm (*black arrow*) with surrounding hemorrhage (*white arrow*). (**c**) Angiogram shows the pseudoaneurysm (*arrow*) with no active extravasation of contrast

Diagnosis
Bullet in IVC

Imaging Features
1. Metallic bullet in the right paravertebral region on chest X-ray
2. CT shows the bullet to be within the contrast-enhanced IVC

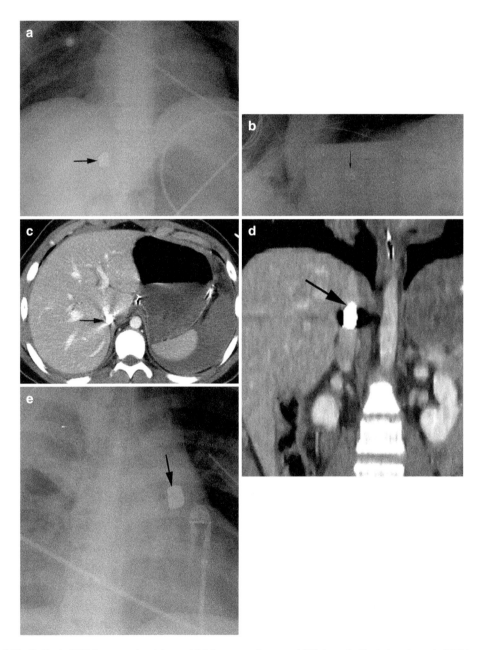

Fig. 4.10 Bullet in IVC from gunshot injury which later migrated to the left pulmonary artery. (**a**, **b**) AP portable and cross-stable lateral X-ray views of the upper abdomen show bullet in IVC in the right paravertebral region of T11-T12 (*arrow*). (**c**, **d**) CECT axial and coronal reformatted CT shows bullet in intrahepatic IVC (*arrow*). (**e**) Portable AP chest shows same bullet migrated to the left pulmonary artery (*arrow*) (en route to surgery) which was surgically removed

Diagnosis
Broken IVC Filter

Imaging Features

1. IVC filter prong extending into the right renal vein
2. Broken fragment in the kidney parenchyma

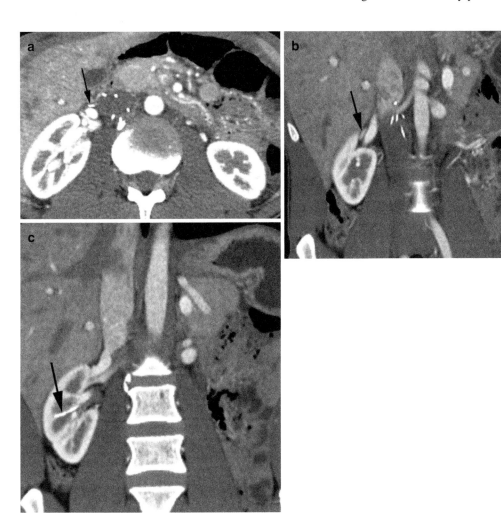

Fig. 4.11 Patient with hematuria. IVC filter placed during old trauma to prevent clot migration. (**a**, **b**) Axial and coronal reformatted CT shows IVC filter prong in the right renal vein (*arrow*). (**c**) Coronal reformatted image shows another broken prong in midpole right renal parenchyma (*arrow*)

Pseudoaneurysm

Imaging Features
1. Focal saccular outpouching from one wall of a vein or artery.
2. Color Doppler shows flow swirling with forward and backward flow through the neck.
3. Spectral waves show to-and-fro flow with waves above and below the base line.

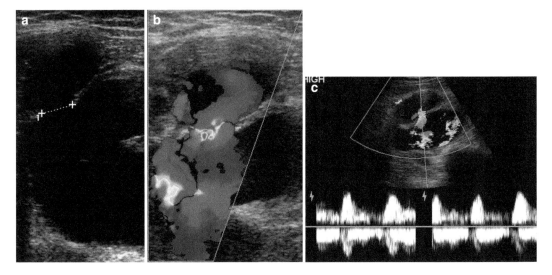

Fig. 4.12 Pseudoaneurysm of the femoral vein. History of stab wound. (**a**) Gray scale shows focal outpouching from the femoral vein with a wide neck (*calipers*). (**b**) Color Doppler shows the "yin-yang sign" of forward and backward flow (*blue and red color*) with blood flowing toward and away from the transducer within the aneurysm and the adjacent femoral vein. (**c**) Spectral study shows bidirectional flow at the neck

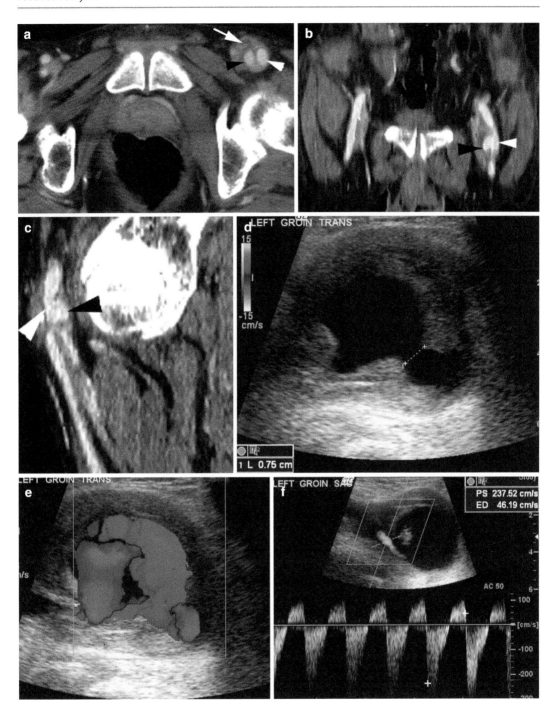

Fig. 4.13 Pseudoaneurysm of the left femoral artery. CECT axial (**a**), coronal (**b**), and sagittal (**c**) reformatted CT shows pseudoaneurysm (*black arrowhead*) arising from the femoral artery (*white arrowhead*) with surrounding hematoma (*arrow*). (**d**) Grayscale US shows large pseudoaneurysm from the femoral artery with a wide neck (*calipers*) and surrounding hematoma. (**e**) Color Doppler shows yin and yang flow in the aneurysm. (**f**) Spectral waves show to-and-fro arterial flow at the neck

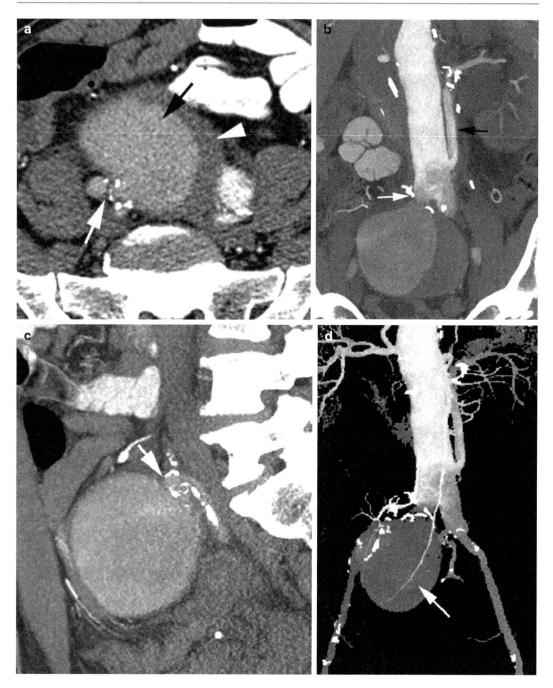

Fig. 4.14 Pseudoaneurysm from the right iliac artery with surrounding hematoma. History of previous vascular surgery. (**a**) Axial CECT shows pseudoaneurysm (*black arrow*) with the small neck (*white arrow*) arising from the right common iliac artery and with surrounding hematoma (*white arrowhead*). (**b**, **c**) Coronal and sagittal reformatted CT shows multiple surgical clips around the neck of the pseudoaneurysm (*white arrow*) and surrounding the aorta and with reconstituted left renal artery (*black arrow*). (**d**, **e**) Volume-rendered oblique image again shows aneurysm (*arrow*) with surgical clips at the neck (*arrowhead*). (**f**) Grayscale US shows sonolucent aneurysm (*white arrow*) with layered hematoma (*arrowhead*) with low-level echogenicity posterior to the lumen of the pseudoaneurysm

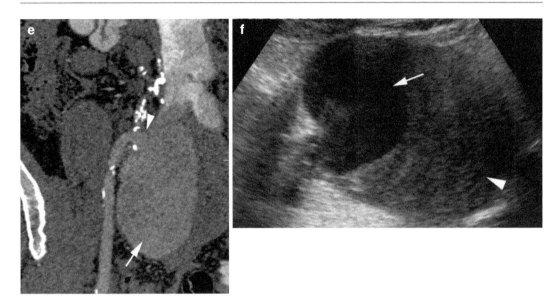

Fig. 4.14 (continued)

Endoleak

Imaging Features
1. Persistent perfusion of excluded aorta post endograft placement.

2. Graft can be for aortic aneurysm or acute aortic syndrome or injury.

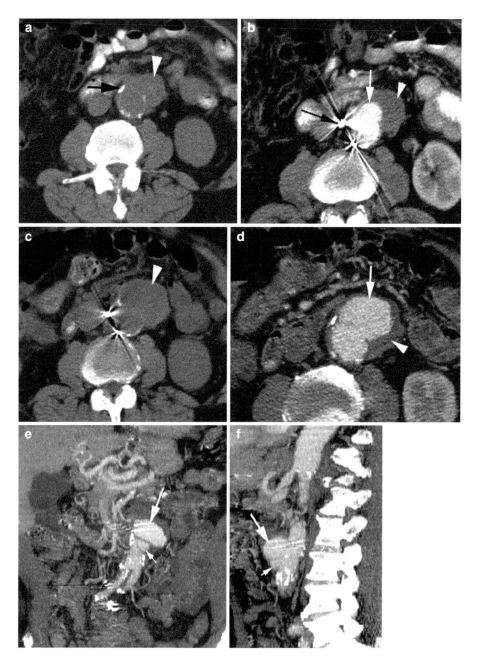

Fig. 4.15 Type 1 endoleak. (**a**, **b**) Axial pre- and postcontrast CT shows focal saccular aneurysm (*thin white arrow*) of the aorta above the aortofemoral graft (*black arrow*) with surrounding thrombus (*arrowhead*). Two years later (**c**, **d**) axial pre- and postcontrast CT shows increase in size of the previous saccular aneurysm (*thin white arrow*) with decrease in surrounding hematoma (*arrowhead*). (**e**, **f**) Coronal and sagittal reformatted images show a smaller saccular aneurysm (*small arrow*) just below the larger aneurysm (*large arrow*)

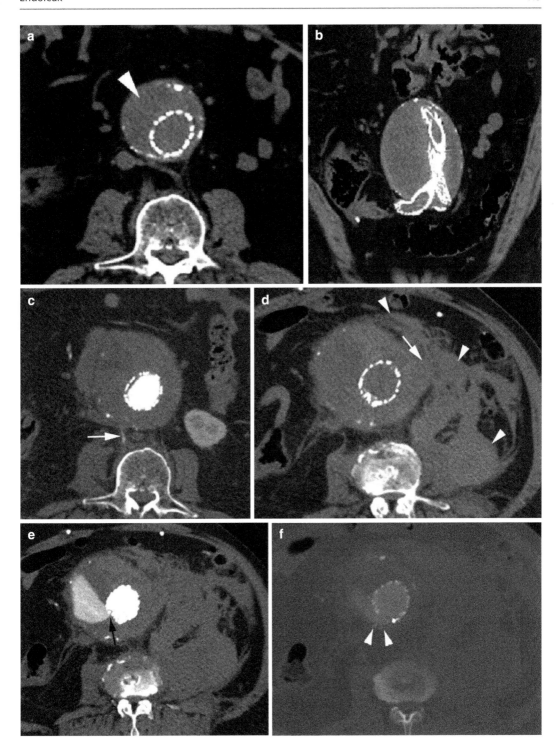

Fig. 4.16 Endoleak type II and III. (**a**, **b**) Axial and coronal reformatted noncontrast CT of post aortobifemoral endograft placement in AAA (*arrowhead*). One and a half year later, patient comes in with lower back pain. (**c**) Axial CECT shows increased size of the aneurysm with heterogeneous density and no extravasated contrast. Feeding lumbar vessel is seen entering the aneurysm (*arrow*). Six months later (**d**) axial noncontrast CT shows retroperitoneal rupture of the aneurysm (*arrowheads*), and *arrow* shows site of rupture. (**e**) Axial CECT at this time shows active spillage of contrast into the aneurysm from graft lumen (*arrow*). (**f**) Axial CT shows disruption of graft at site of contrast extravasation with posterior displacement of graft wall (*arrow heads*)

Vasculitis

5

Contents

R. Agarwala, *Atlas of Emergency Radiology:*
Vascular System, Chest, Abdomen and Pelvis, and Reproductive System,
DOI 10.1007/978-3-319-13042-2_5, © Springer International Publishing Switzerland 2015

Noninfectious Aortitis

Diagnosis
Takayasu Vasculitis

Imaging Features
1. Affects large vessels with predilection for the aorta and its branch vessels and young or middle-aged females.
2. Noncontrast study shows high attenuation of aortic or pulmonary artery wall, CECT shows concentric thickening of the vessel wall and double ring of the aorta in early disease.
3. Stenosis is common, also occlusion, thrombosis, ectasia, aneurysms, and ulcers.
4. Arterial wall calcification in chronic cases.

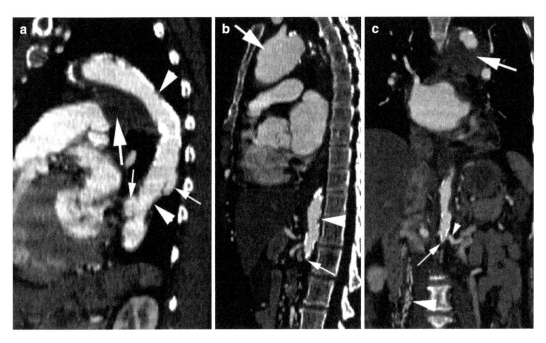

Fig. 5.1 Takayasu arteritis—late phase. (**a**) Sagittal reformatted CT shows stenosis of mid-arch of the aorta and proximal descending aorta (*arrowheads*) with large chronic intramural thrombus (*thick arrow*) at the arch. The proximal descending aorta shows two saccular aneurysms (*thin arrows*). (**b**) Sagittal reformatted CT shows aneurysm of the ascending aorta (*thick arrow*), focal stenosis of the proximal abdominal aorta (*arrowhead*), and complete occlusion of the aorta distal to renal arteries (*thin arrow*). (**c**) Coronal reformatted images show complete occlusion of the aorta (*thin arrow*) distal to the origin of renal arteries (*thin arrowhead*) and dilated collateral arteries mostly medial to the right kidney (*thick arrowhead*). Mural thrombus is again seen around proximal arch of the aorta (*thick arrow*). (**d**) Coronal reformatted image shows concentric stenosis of distal thoracic aorta (*black arrow*). Large intramural thrombus at arch (*white arrow*) and collateral vessels adjacent to the right kidney (*arrowhead*) are again seen. (**e**, **f**) Pre- and postcontrast axial images show aneurysm of the ascending aorta (caliper) and thick, rough transmural degenerative atherosclerotic calcification (*thick arrowhead*) and thin dystrophic calcification (*thin white arrow*) and large focal chronic intramural hematoma in posterior arch (*thick arrow*)

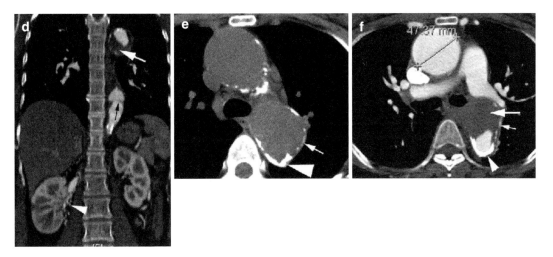

Fig. 5.1 (continued)

Diagnosis
Giant Cell Arteritis

Imaging Features

1. Affects large- and medium-sized vessels in individuals over 50 years
2. Predominantly affects extracranial carotid branches especially the temporal arteries, aorta, and rarely central pulmonary arteries
3. Similar to Takayasu arteritis with wall thickening, stenosis, and aneurysm formation
4. Aneurysms more frequent in the thoracic aorta and prone to dissection

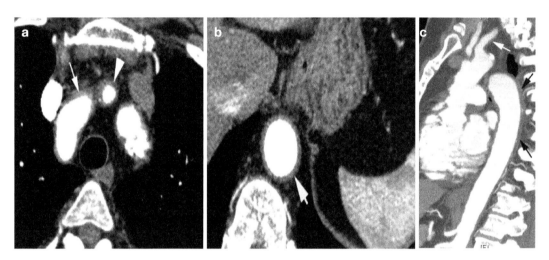

Fig. 5.2 Giant cell arteritis in a 70-year-old woman. (**a**, **b**) Axial CT angiogram shows diffuse wall thickening of anterior arch (*arrow*), origin of left common carotid (*arrowhead*) and distal thoracic aorta (*short arrow*). (**c**) Sagittal reformatted image shows diffuse wall thickening of the left subclavian artery (*white arrow*) and descending thoracic aorta (*black arrows*). (**d**, **e**) Angiogram shows stenosis of left subclavian artery (*black arrow*), mild narrowing at origin of right vertebral artery (*arrowhead*), and stenosis of distal arch of the aorta (*white arrow*). (**f**) Sagittal reformatted CT angiogram shows stenosis of distal arch of the aorta (*arrow*)

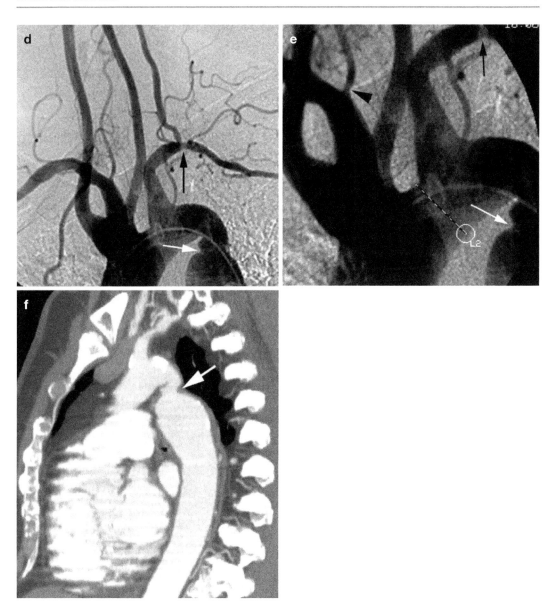

Fig. 5.2 (continued)

Diagnosis

Granulomatosis with Polyangiitis (Wegener Granulomatosis)

Imaging Features

1. Vasculitis primarily of small- to medium-sized vessels can also have aortitis and periaortitis.
2. Granulomatous inflammation of upper and lower respiratory tracts and glomerulonephritis.
3. Pulmonary nodules, multiple, bilateral, and tend to cavitation.
4. Pulmonary infiltrates (waxing and waning), hemorrhage or edema, and hilar lymphadenopathy.

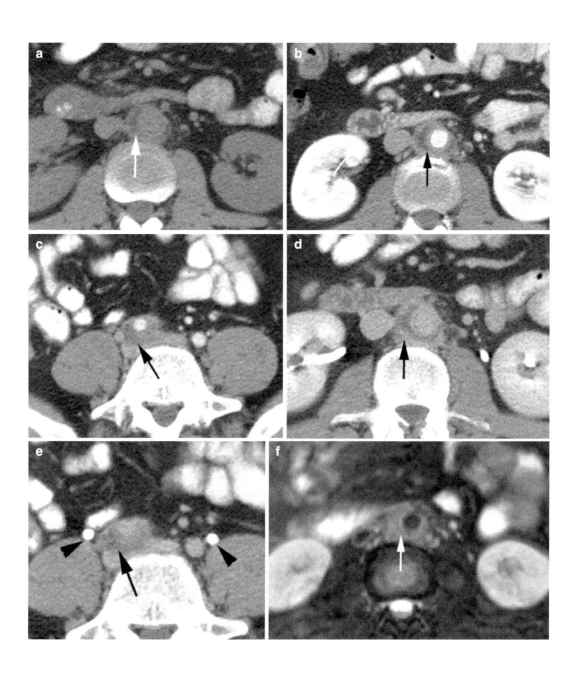

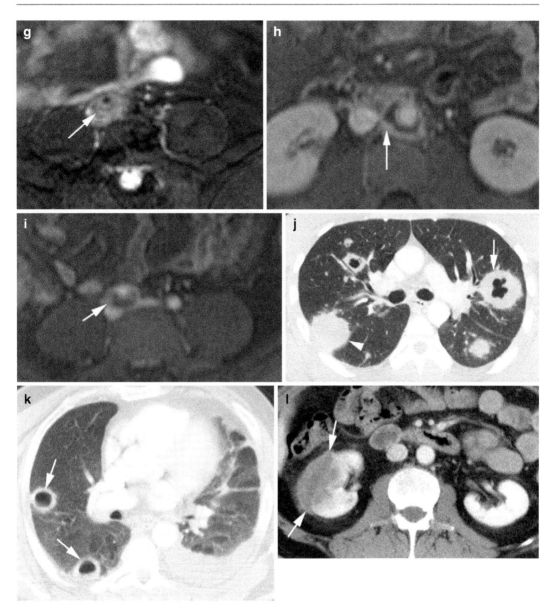

Fig. 5.3 (continued)

Fig. 5.3 Granulomatosis with polyangiitis (**a**) precontrast axial CT shows layered soft tissue around infrarenal aorta with central lower density (*arrow*). (**b**, **c**) Postcontrast axial CT again shows layered soft tissue around the infrarenal aorta and right common iliac artery with no significant enhancement of the peripheral rind (*arrow*). (**d**) Delayed phase axial CT shows mild enhancement of the peripheral rim of inflammatory tissue around the abdominal aorta (*arrow*). (**e**) Delayed-phase axial CT shows the ureters in their usual location (*arrowheads*) and separate from the inflammatory tissue around the common iliac artery (*arrow*). (**f**, **g**) T2 fat-sat axial MRI of the infrarenal aorta and right common iliac artery shows high signal intensity in soft tissue around the vessels (*arrow*). (**h**, **i**) Post-gad axial MRI shows appreciable enhancement of the rind surrounding the necrotic tissue around the vessels (*arrow*). (**j**, **k**) Axial CT of two patients with known Wegener granulomatosis show multiple bilateral pulmonary nodules. (**j**) Thick-walled cavitating nodules (*arrow*) and solid nodules (*arrowhead*). (**k**) Thinner-walled cavitating nodules (*arrows*). (**l**) Axial CT of the same patient in (**k**) shows focal glomerulonephritis of the right kidney showing low-density mass with poor enhancement (*arrows*). (**m–o**) Axial and coronal reformatted CT and chest X-ray of a known case of Wagner granulomatosis showing bilateral diffuse pulmonary hemorrhage with ground-glass densities and consolidations

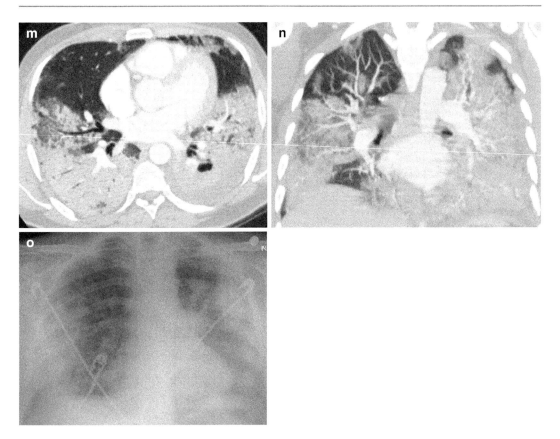

Fig. 5.3 (continued)

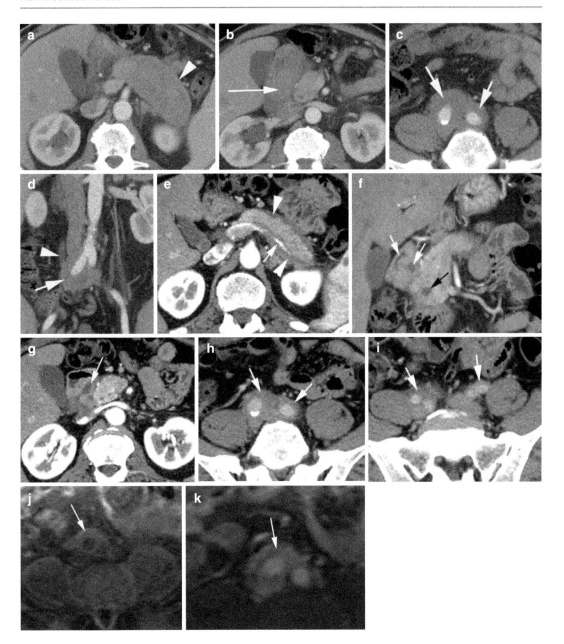

Fig. 5.4 Antiphospholipid syndrome. History of abdominal pain for few months with clinical evidence of pancreatitis and with positive antiphospholipid antibody. Axial CECT (**a**) shows diffuse enlargement of body and tail of the pancreas with loss of lobular contour, thick rim, and linear irregular lucencies (*arrowhead*) and decreased enhancement. (**b**) Head of the pancreas not enlarged, but the second part of duodenum is very edematous and thickened (*arrow*). The right kidney shows hydronephrosis. (**c**, **d**) Axial CT lower abdomen and coronal reformatted CT show periaortitis with large thick soft tissue around the aortic bifurcation and the common iliac arteries (*arrows*). The right ureter is obstructed by the periaortitis (*arrowhead*). (**e**) Axial CECT 3 months later shows decreased size of the pancreas with return of lobulations, increased enhancement, and with thin capsule-like rim of low attenuation halo around pancreatic body and tail (*arrowhead*). The splenic vein is narrowed by the halo but patent (*arrow*). (**f**, **g**) Coronal reformatted and axial CT shows small cyst at uncinate process (*black arrow*) and in the thickened wall of second portion of the duodenum (*white arrow*). (**h**, **i**) Axial CT shows decrease in periaortitis (*arrows*) with resolution of hydronephrosis (as seen in **g**). (**j**, **k**) Axial MRI with predynamic T1W shows intermediate signal in the inflammatory tissue around the right common iliac artery and enhancement in postdynamic T1W images (*arrow*)

Diagnosis

Idiopathic Inflammatory Aortic Aneurysm

Imaging Features

1. Hypoattenuating aortic wall thickening
2. Sparing the posterior wall of the aorta

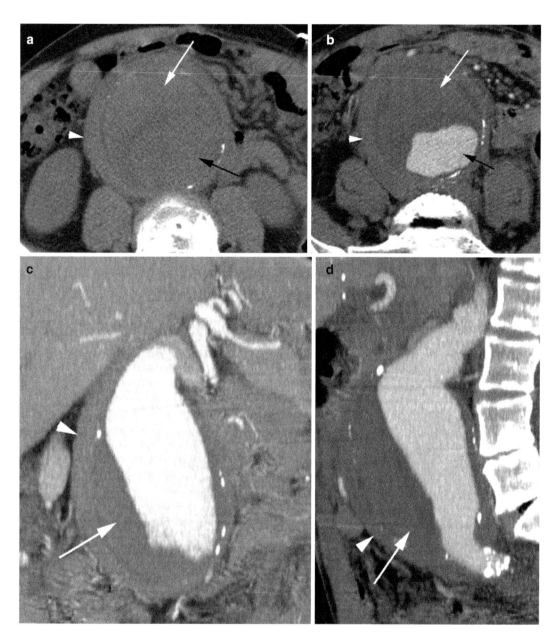

Fig. 5.5 Idiopathic inflammatory aortic aneurysm. Axial pre-contrast CT (**a**) and CECT (**b**) reformatted images in coronal (**c**) and sagittal (**d**) planes show fusiform aneu- rysm (*black arrow*) with large intramural thrombus (*white arrow*). The aorta shows diffuse wall thickening (*arrow- head*) with sparing of the posterior aspect

Diagnosis
Idiopathic Inflammatory Aortic Aneurysm with Aortoduodenal Fistula

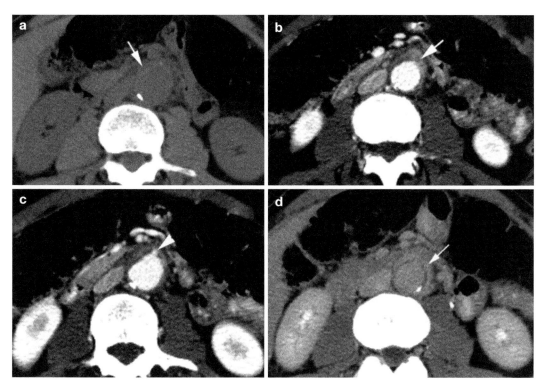

Fig. 5.6 Ruptured aortic aneurysm with aortoduodenal fistula confirmed at surgery. (**a**) Axial CT shows periaortitis with periaortic wall thickening of infrarenal aorta sparing the posterior wall (*arrow*). (**b, c**) Postcontrast axial CT shows the thick wall to have mild enhancement in arterial phase (*arrow*) and small ulcer-like projection (*arrowhead*). (**d**) Axial CT in delayed phase shows increased enhancement of the wall (*arrow*). Five months later. (**e**) Precontrast axial CT shows high-density hemorrhage (*white arrow*) surrounding the infrarenal aorta which now shows aneurysmal dilatation (*black arrow*). The surrounding small bowel loops show high-density hemorrhagic fluid (*arrowheads*) filling the lumen. (**f**) Postcontrast axial CT shows irregularity of the intima at the site of rupture with surrounding low-density mural thrombus (*arrow*). (**g**) Sagittal reformatted image shows low-density thrombus (*thin arrow*) surrounding the irregular intima. SMV (*thick arrow*) and SMA (*arrowhead*) are draping over the aneurysm

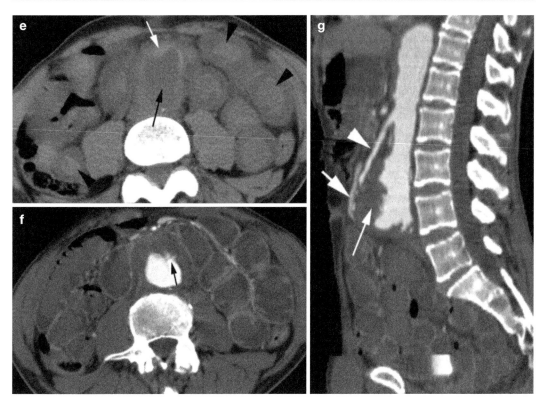

Fig. 5.6 (continued)

Diagnosis

Retroperitoneal Fibrosis (Chronic Periaortitis)

Imaging Features

1. Soft tissue around the aorta and inferior vena cava with no aortic displacement
2. Ureters can be deviated medially with varying degree of obstruction
3. Varying degree of enhancement depending of the stage of the disease

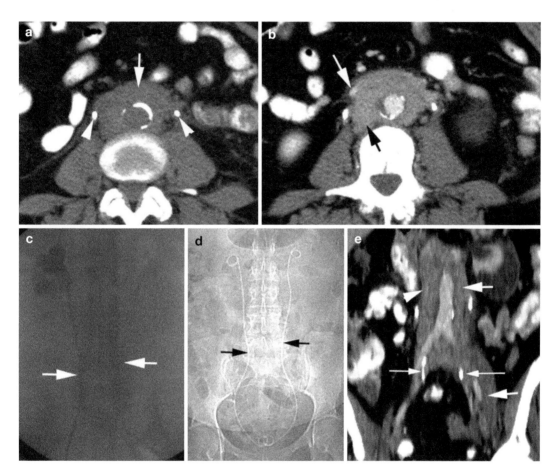

Fig. 5.7 Retroperitoneal fibrosis—idiopathic. (**a**) Precontrast axial CT shows soft tissue surrounding the atherosclerotic aorta (*white arrow*) and bilateral ureteral stents (*arrowheads*). (**b**) CECT shows enhancement of the periaortic soft tissue which is encasing the gonadal veins (*white arrow*) and IVC (*black arrow*). (**c**) Retrograde cystogram shows medial deviation of both ureters (*arrows*) and bilateral hydronephrosis. (**d**) Scanogram shows medial deviation of the ureteral stents (*arrows*). (**e**) Coronal reformatted image shows the fibrosis around the aorta and extending along the common iliac arteries (*thick white arrow*) and around the stents (*thin white arrows*) and IVC (*arrowhead*)

Infectious Aortitis

Diagnosis

H. influenzae Aortitis

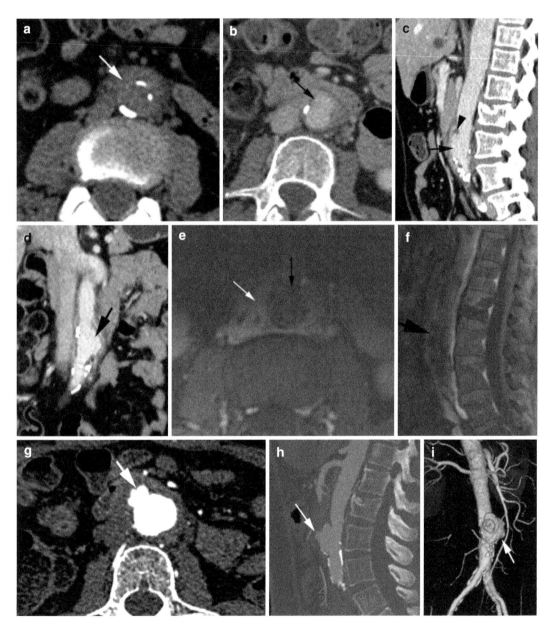

Fig. 5.8 Infectious aortitis by *H. influenzae*. Patient with back pain. (**a**) Axial precontrast shows soft tissue thickening around the atherosclerotic aortic wall and sparing the posterior wall (*arrow*). (**b–d**) CECT axial, sagittal, and coronal reformatted images show enhancement of the aortic wall thick soft tissue with small saccular aneurysm (*black arrow*) and intramural thrombus at the superior and inferior aspect of the aneurysm (*arrowhead*). (**e, f**) Axial and sagittal post-MRI with fat-sat done for lumbar vertebrae shows enhancing soft tissue around the aorta (*white arrow*) at the same level as the CT with saccular aneurysm (*black arrow*). (**g–i**) Postcontrast axial CT, MIP image, and 3D volume-rendered image done 1 week later show enlargement of mushroom-shaped mycotic aneurysm with increasing periaortitis (*arrow*). This was surgically treated

Diagnosis
HIV Aortitis

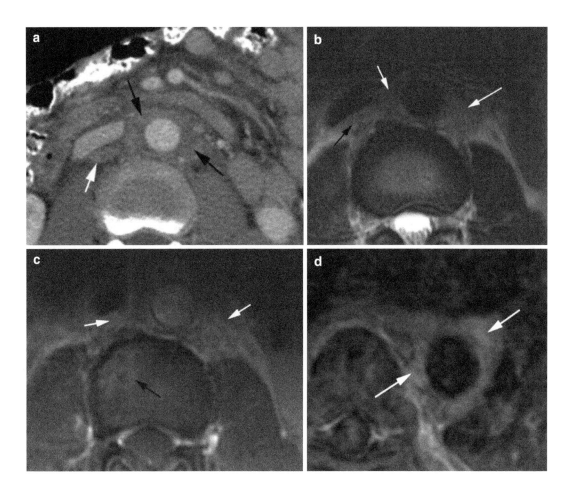

Fig. 5.9 HIV aortitis. Patient with Kaposi's Sarcoma. (**a**) Postcontrast axial CT shows periaortitis with soft tissue surrounding the aorta (*black arrows*) and enlarged retrocaval lymph node (*white arrow*). (**b**) T2W MRI study shows soft tissue surrounding the aorta (*white arrows*) and in retrocaval region (*black arrow*). (**c**) Post-gad T1W axial MRI shows enhancement of periaortic and retrocaval soft tissue (*white arrow*) and metastasis of vertebral body (*black arrow*). (**d**) Post-gad MRI on a different date shows enhancement of periaortic soft tissue around the descending thoracic aorta (*arrows*)

Diagnosis

Mycotic Aneurysm with Aortocaval Fistula and
Sigmoid Colon Diverticular Abscess

Imaging Features

1. Atherosclerosis, graft, and catheter are predisposing factors.
2. Mostly infrarenal aorta affected.
3. Mostly saccular aneurysms.
4. Early stage is periaortic soft tissue mass with or without rim enhancement.

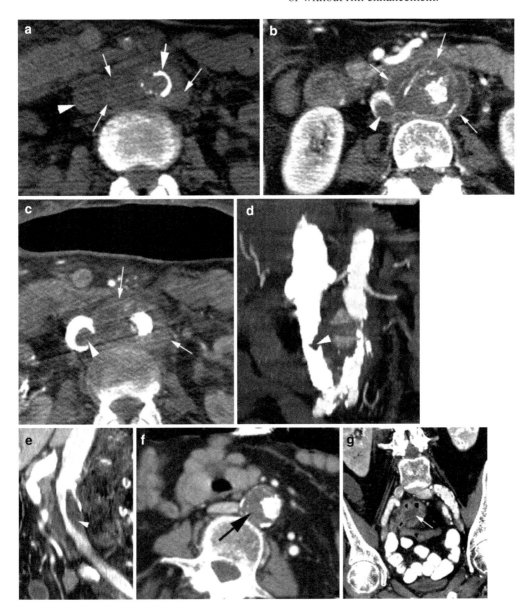

Fig. 5.10 Mycotic aneurysm from diverticulitis sigmoid colon and with aortocaval fistula formation. At surgery the diverticular abscess extended to the aneurysm. (**a**) Precontrast axial CT abdomen shows large periaortic soft tissue (*thin arrows*) extending to IVC (*arrowhead*). Atherosclerotic calcification is also seen of the involved aorta (*thick arrow*). CECT (**b**, **c**) axial, (**d**) coronal, and (**e**) sagittal reformatted images show peripheral enhancement of the periaortic necrotic soft tissue proximally (*white arrows* in **b**) but not enhancing distally (*arrows* in **c**). Thrombus in IVC continuous with the periaortic soft tissue (*arrowhead*). (**f**, **g**) One week prior CT, axial and coronal reformatted images show thrombus in aortic aneurysm (*black arrow*) and sigmoid diverticular abscess (*white arrow*) with no periaortic soft tissues or IVC thrombus

Vascular Stenosis

Contents

R. Agarwala, *Atlas of Emergency Radiology:*
Vascular System, Chest, Abdomen and Pelvis, and Reproductive System,
DOI 10.1007/978-3-319-13042-2_6, © Springer International Publishing Switzerland 2015

Kommerell Diverticulum

Diagnosis
Stenosis of Origin of Anomalous Left Subclavian
Artery with Kommerell Diverticulum

Imaging Features
1. Right-sided arch of the aorta
2. Stenosis of aberrant left subclavian artery
   with post stenotic dilatation
3. Kommerell diverticulum of the aorta at origin
   of the subclavian artery

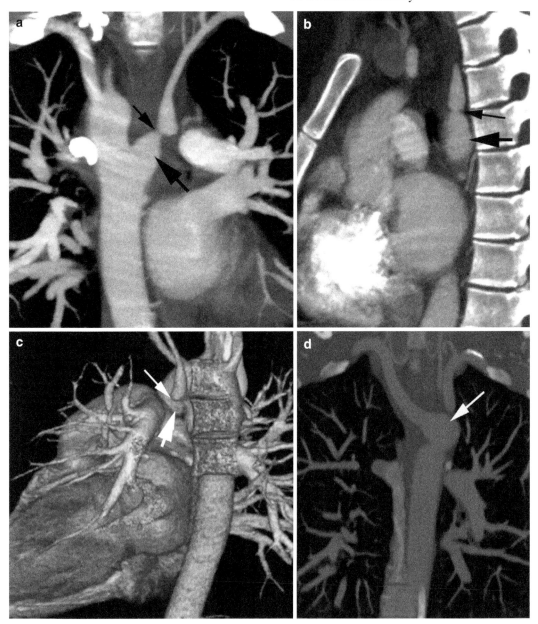

Fig. 6.1 Stenosis of the subclavian artery. Aberrant origin of left subclavian artery from right-sided arch of the aorta with Kommerell diverticulum at its origin and stenosis distal to the diverticulum presenting with subclavian steal syndrome. (**a**) Coronal reformatted image shows Kommerell diverticulum (*thick arrow*) at origin of the aberrant subclavian artery and marked stenosis distal to the diverticulum (*thin arrow*) with post stenotic dilatation. (**b, c**) Oblique sagittal reformatted image and 3D volume-rendered images show stenosis of left subclavian artery (*thin arrows*) and the Kommerell diverticulum (*thick arrows*). (**d**) Coronal reformatted image in different patients shows Kommerell diverticulum (*arrow*) at left-sided descending thoracic aorta at the origin of aberrant right subclavian artery

Coarctation of Aorta

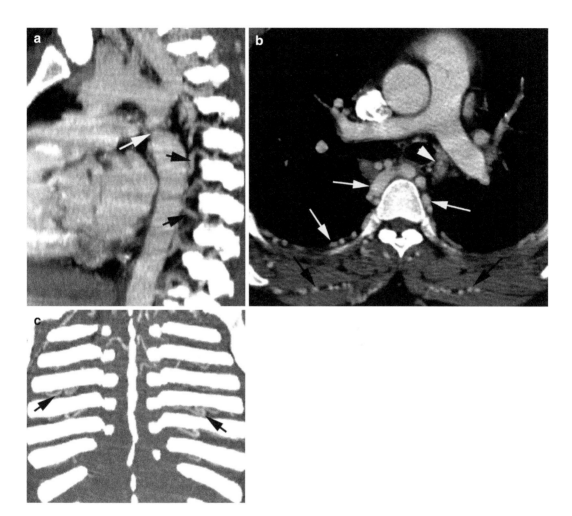

Fig. 6.2 Coarctation of the aorta in adult. (**a**) Sagittal reformatted image shows short segment of stenosis of the aorta in the region of the ductus (*white arrow*) with dilated intercostal arteries (*black arrows*). (**b**) Axial CT shows narrowed segment of the aorta (*arrowhead*), dilated intercostal arteries (*white arrows*), and also dilated intermuscular arteries. (**c**) Coronal reformatted image shows dilated intercostal arteries (*arrows*)

Renal Artery Stenosis

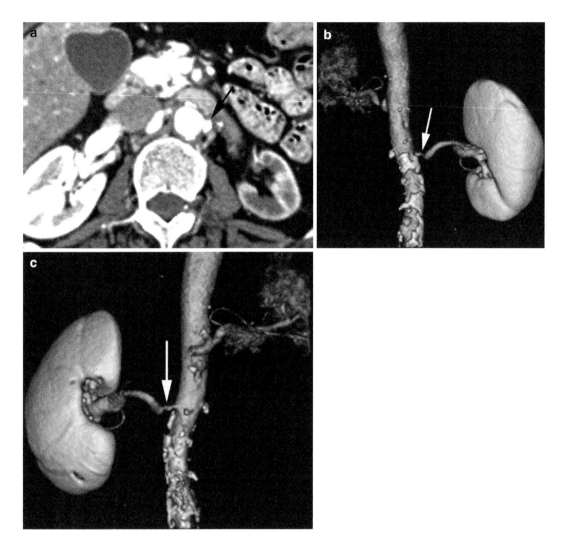

Fig. 6.3 Stenosis of the renal artery. Atherosclerosis with stenosis of the left renal artery. Contrast-enhanced axial CT (**a**) shows large calcification at origin of the left renal artery (*arrow*). The left kidney is atrophic with decreased perfusion. 3D volume-rendered images, (**b**) frontal view, and (**c**) posterior view show narrowing of origin of the left renal artery (*arrow*)

Mediastinal Fibrosis

Diagnosis
SVC Obstruction by Mediastinal Fibrosis

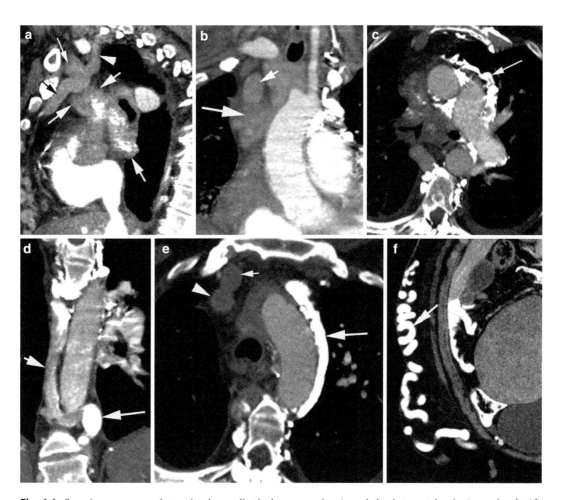

Fig. 6.4 Superior vena cava obstruction by mediastinal fibrosis confirmed by biopsy. Urine *Blastomyces* antigen was positive. CECT (**a**, **b**) sagittal, coronal reformatted, and (**c**) axial images show large mediastinal mass (*thick arrows*) with areas of calcification (*long thin arrow* in **c**) obstructing the SVC (*short arrow* in **b**) with dilatation of the internal thoracic vein (*black arrow*), IJ vein (*thin arrow* in **a**), and the intercostal vein (*arrowhead*). (**d**) Coronal reformatted CT shows dilated azygos (*short arrow*) and hemiazygos vein (*long arrow*). (**e**) Axial CT shows dilated left superior intercostal vein (*long arrow*), internal thoracic vein (*short arrow*), and SVC (*arrowhead*). (**f**) Dilated veins in the right abdominal wall subcutaneous tissue which drain into the femoral vein (*arrow*)

IVC Stenosis

Diagnosis
Tumor Compression of IVC and Hepatic Veins

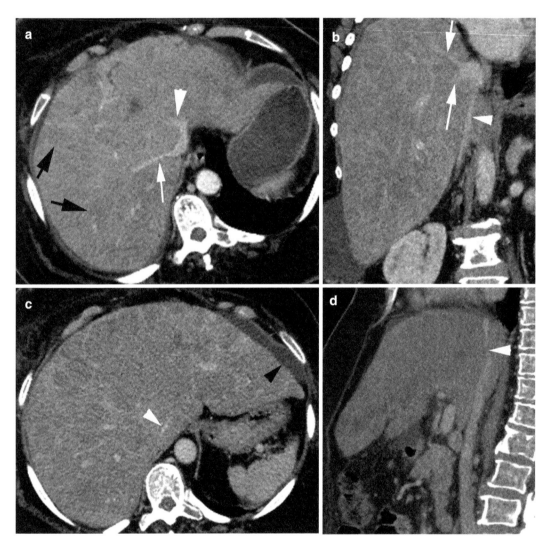

Fig. 6.5 Intrahepatic IVC and hepatic vein compression by tumor. Patient with infiltrating ductal breast cancer with diffuse liver metastasis. CECT (**a**) axial shows markedly compressed IVC, narrowed right (*white arrow*) and left hepatic veins (*arrowhead*) and absent middle hepatic vein (*long arrow* in **b**), and diffuse low-density metastasis (*black arrows*). (**b, c, d**) Coronal reformatted, axial, and sagittal reformatted CT show markedly narrowed IVC (*white arrowhead*) and small ascites (*black arrowhead*)

Diagnosis
Hypoplastic IVC

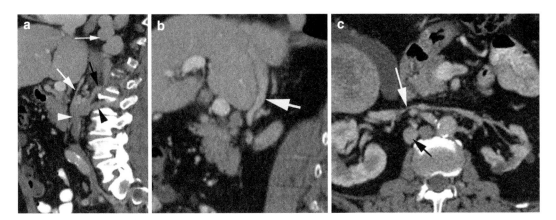

Fig. 6.6 Hypoplastic infrahepatic IVC, incidental finding. (**a**) Sagittal reformatted image shows narrow caliber of IVC (*thick white arrow*). The IVC below the renal veins is normal in size (*arrowhead*). Collateral flow is seen through the dilated ascending lumbar vein (*black arrow*) draining into the dilated azygos vein (*thin white arrow*) and the lumbar vein (*black arrowhead*). (**b**) Sagittal reformatted CT shows normal IVC (*arrow*) within the liver. (**c**) Axial CT shows very narrow IVC (*white arrow*) between the renal veins and dilated ascending lumbar vein (*black arrow*)

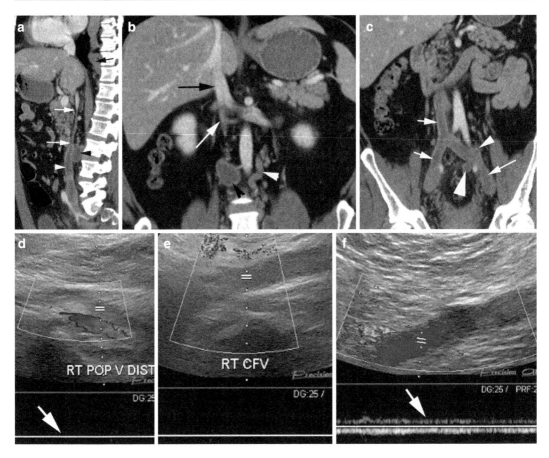

Fig. 6.7 Hypoplastic IVC with thrombus. (**a**) Sagittal reformatted image shows a very narrow segment of IVC (*arrows*) below the renal veins. Thrombus distending the IVC below the stenotic region (*white arrowhead*) and thrombus in a lumbar vein (*black arrowhead*). (**b**) Coronal reformatted CT shows normal size of IVC at the renal veins and with thin median septa (*black arrow*). IVC narrow below the renal veins (*white arrow*). The left ascending lumbar vein (*white arrowhead*) is dilated and there is thrombus in a right lumbar vein (*black arrowhead*). (**c**) Coronal reformatted CT shows thrombus in IVC, iliac veins (*white arrows*), in the origin of ascending left lumbar vein (*thin arrowhead*), and median sacral vein (*thick arrowhead*). (**d**, **e**) Duplex and spectral Doppler imaging of the right leg shows thrombus in the right popliteal vein extending to CFV with absent spectral flow (*arrow* in **d**). (**f**) Left common femoral vein is patent but shows lack of respiratory variation due to proximal occlusion (*arrow*)

Bibliography

1. Agarwal PP, Chughtai A, Matzinger FRK, et al. Multidetector CT of thoracic aortic aneurysm. Radiographics. 2009;29:537–52.
2. Alkadhi H, Wildermuth S, Desbiolles L, et al. Vascular emergencies of the thorax after blunt and iatrogenic trauma: multi-detector row CT and three-dimensional imaging. Radiographics. 2004;24:1239–55.
3. Araoz PA, Gotway MB, Harrington JR, et al. Pulmonary embolism: prognostic CT findings. Radiology. 2007;242:889–97.
4. Arita T, Matsunaga M, Takano K, et al. Abdominal aortic aneurysm: rupture associated with the high-attenuating crescent sign. Radiology. 1997;204:765–8.
5. Batra P, Bigoni B, Manning J, et al. Pitfalls in the diagnosis of thoracic aortic dissection at CT angiography. Radiographics. 2000;20:309–20.
6. Bluemke DA. Definitive diagnosis of intramural hematoma of the thoracic aorta with MR imaging. Radiology. 1997;204:319–23.
7. Castaner E, Gallardo X, Ballesteros E, et al. CT diagnosis of chronic pulmonary thromboembolism. Radiographics. 2009;29:31–53.
8. Castaner E, Alguersuari A, Gallardo X, et al. When to suspect pulmonary vasculitis: radiologic and clinical clues. Radiographics. 2010;30:33–53.
9. Chao CP, Walker TG, Kalva SP. Natural history and CT appearances of aortic intramural hematoma. Radiographics. 2009;29:791–804.
10. Chhabra A, Batra K, Mulhern CB, et al. Pulmonary embolism in segmental and subsegmental arteries: optimal technique, imaging appearances, and potential pitfalls in multidetector CT. Appl Radiol. 2007;36:34–40.
11. Chung JW, Park JH, Im JG, et al. Spiral CT angiography of the thoracic aorta. Radiographics. 1996;16:811–24.
12. Chung MP, Yi CA, Lee HY, et al. Imaging pulmonary vasculitis. Radiology. 2010;255:322–41.
13. Creasy JD, Chiles C, Routh WD, et al. Overview of traumatic injury of the thoracic aorta. Radiographics. 1997;17:27–45.
14. de Monye W, Murphy M, Hodgson R, et al. Acute aortic syndromes: pathology and imaging. Imaging. 2004;16(3):230–9.
15. Dogan J, Kroft LJM, Huisman MV, et al. Right ventricular function in patients with acute pulmonary embolism: analysis with electrocardiography-synchronized multi-detector row CT. Radiology. 2007;242:78–84.
16. Elliott RJ, McGrath LT. Calcification of the human thoracic aorta during aging. Calcif Tissue Int. 1994;54(4):268–73. PMID: 8062142.
17. Engelke C, Rummeny EJ, Marten K. Pulmonary embolism at multi-detector row CT of chest: one year survival of treated and untreated patients. Radiology. 2006;239:563–75.
18. Fisher ER, Stern EJ, Godwin II JD, et al. Acute aortic dissection: typical and atypical imaging features. Radiographics. 1994;14:1263–71.
19. Frazier AA, Galvin JR, Franks TJ, et al. Pulmonary vasculature: hypertension and infarction. Radiographics. 2000;20:491–524.
20. Frazier AA, Franks TJ, Mohammed TLH, et al. Pulmonary veno-occlusive disease and pulmonary capillary hemangiomatosis. Radiographics. 2007;27:867–82.
21. Ghaye B, Ghuysen A, Bruyere PJ, et al. Can CT pulmonary angiography allow assessment of severity and prognosis in patients presenting with pulmonary embolism? What the radiologist needs to know. Radiographics. 2006;26:23–40.
22. Ghaye B, Ghuysen A, Willems V, et al. Severe pulmonary embolism: pulmonary artery clot load scores and cardiovascular parameters as predictors of mortality. Radiology. 2006;239:884–91.
23. Glatard AS, Hillare S, d'Assignies G. Obliterative portal venopathy: findings at CT imaging. Radiology. 2012;263(3):741–50.
24. Gonsalves CF. The hyperattenuating crescent sign. Radiology. 1999;211:37–8.
25. Gorich J, Rilinger N, Sokiranski R, et al. Leakages after endovascular repair of aortic aneurysms: classification based on findings at CT, angiography, and radiography. Radiology. 1999;213:767–72.
26. Gotway MB, Yee J. Helical CT pulmonary angiography for acute pulmonary embolism. Appl Radiol. 2002;31:21–9.
27. Halliday KE, Al-Kutoubi A. Draped aorta: CT sign of contained leak of aortic aneurysms. Radiology. 1996;199:41–3.
28. Han D, Lee KS, Franquet T, et al. Thrombotic and non-thrombotic pulmonary arterial embolism: spectrum of imaging findings. Radiographics. 2003;23:1521–39.
29. Inoue D, Zen Y, Abo H, et al. Immunoglobulin G4-related periaortitis and periarteritis: CT findings in 17 patients. Radiology. 2011;261:625–33.
30. Kalva SP, Jagannathan JP, Hahn PF, et al. Venous thromboembolism: indirect CT venography during CT pulmonary angiography—should the pelvis be imaged? Radiology. 2008;246:605–11.
31. Kandpal H, Sharma R, Gamangatti S, et al. Imaging the inferior vena cava: a road less traveled. Radiographics. 2008;28:669–89.
32. Kapur S, Paik E, Rezaei A, et al. Where there is blood there is a way: unusual collateral vessels in superior and inferior cava obstruction. Radiographics. 2010;30:67–78.
33. Kaushik S, Federle MP, Shur PH, et al. Abdominal thrombotic and ischemic manifestation of antiphospholipid syndrome: CT findings in 42 patients. Radiology. 2001;218:768–71.
34. Konen E, Merchant N, Gutierrez C, et al. True versus false left ventricular aneurysm: differentiation with MR imaging – initial experience. Radiology. 2005;236:65–70.
35. LaBerge JM, Kerlan RK, Reilly LM, et al. Mycotic pseudoaneurysm of the abdominal aorta in association with mycobacterial psoas abscess-a complication of BCG therapy. Radiology. 1999;211:81–5.

36. LePage MA, Quint LE, Sonnad SS, et al. Aortic dissection: CT features that distinguish true lumen from false lumen. AJR Am J Roentgenol. 2001;177:207–11.

37. Liu Q, Lu JP, Wand F, et al. Three-dimensional contrast-enhanced MR angiography of the aortic dissection: a pictorial essay. Ragiographics. 2007;27:1311–21.

38. Matsunaga N, Hayashi K, Sakamoto I, et al. Takayasu arteritis: protean radiologic manifestations and diagnosis. Radiographics. 1997;17:579–94.

39. McMahon MA, Squirrell CA. Multidetector CT of aortic dissection: a pictorial review. Radiographics. 2010;30:445–60.

40. Morita S, Ueno E, Masukawa A, et al. Hyperattenuating signs of unenhanced CT indicating acute vascular disease. Radiographics. 2010;30:111–25.

41. Murray JD, Manisali M, Flamm SD, et al. Intramural hematoma of the thoracic aorta: MR image findings and their prognostic implications. Radiology. 1997;204:349–55.

42. Nastri MV, Baptisia LPS, Baroni RH, et al. Gadolinium-enhanced three –dimensional MR angiography of Takayasu arteritis. Radiographics. 2004;24:773–86.

43. Park GM, Ahn JM, Kim DH, et al. Distal aortic intramural hematoma: clinical importance of focal contrast enhancement on CT images. Radiology. 2011;259:100–8.

44. Patel NH, Stephens Jr KE, Mirvis SE, et al. Imaging of acute thoracic aortic injury due to blunt trauma: a review. Radiology. 1998;209:335–48.

45. Pena E, Dennie C, Veinot J, et al. Pulmonary hypertension: how the radiologist can help. Radiographics. 2012;32:9–32.

46. Quint LE, Francis IR, Williams DM, et al. Synthetic interposition grafts of the thoracic aorta: postoperative appearance on serial CT studies. Radiology. 1999;211:317–24.

47. Quint LE, Williams DM, Francis IR, et al. Ulcerlike lesion of the aorta: imaging features and natural history. Radiology. 2001;218:719–23.

48. Rakita D, Newatia A, Hines JJ, et al. Spectrum of CT findings in rupture and impending rupture of abdominal aortic aneurysms. Radiographics. 2007;27:497–507.

49. Remy-Jardin M, Remy J. Spiral CT angiography of the pulmonary circulation. Radiology. 1999;212:615–36.

50. Remy-Jardin M, Duhamel A, Deken V, et al. Systemic collateral supply in patients with chronic thromboembolic and primary pulmonary hypertension: assessment with multi-detector row helical CT angiography. Radiology. 2005;235:274–81.

51. Resten A, Maitre S, Humbert M, et al. Pulmonary arterial hypertension: thin-section CT predictors of epoprostenol therapy failure. Radiology. 2002;222:782–8.

52. Restrepo CS, Carrillo JA, Martinez S, et al. Pulmonary complications from cocaine and cocaine-based substances: imaging manifestations. Radiographics. 2007;27:941–56.

53. Restrepo CS, Ocazionez D, Suri R, et al. Aortitis: imaging spectrum of the infectious and inflammatory conditions of the aorta. Radiographics. 2011;31:435–51.

54. Santiago I, Vilgrain V, Cipriano MA, et al. Obliterative portal venopathy. Radiology. 2012;264(1):297–302.

55. Sebastia C, Pallisa E, Quiroga S, et al. Aortic dissection: diagnosis and follow-up with helical CT. Radiographics. 1999;19:45–60.

56. Shiau MC, Godoy MCB, de Groot PM, et al. Thoracic aorta: acute syndromes. Appl Radiol. 2010;39:1.

57. Stavropoulos SW, Charagundla SR. Imaging techniques for detection and management of endoleaks after endovascular aortic aneurysm repair. Radiology. 2007;243:641–55.

58. Steenburg SD, Ravenel JG, Ikonomidis JS, et al. Acute traumatic aortic injury: imaging evaluation and management. Radiology. 2008;248:748–62.

59. Sueyoshi E, Matsuoka Y, Imada T, et al. New development of an ulcerlike projection in aortic intramural hematoma: CT evaluation. Radiology. 2002;224:536–41.

60. Thurnher SA, Dorffner R, Thurnher MM, et al. Evaluation of abdominal aortic aneurysm for stent-graft placement: comparison of gadolinium-enhanced MR angiography versus helical CT angiography and digital subtraction angiography. Radiology. 1997;205:341–52.

61. Tolia AJ, Landis R, Lamparello P, et al. Type II endoleaks after endovascular repair of abdominal aortic aneurysms: natural history. Radiology. 2005;235:683–6.

62. Vaglio A, Salvarani C, Buzio C. Retroperitoneal fibrosis. Lancet. 2006;367(9506):241–51.

63. Williams DM, Lee DY, Hamilton BH, et al. The dissected aorta. Part III. Anatomy and radiologic diagnosis of branch-vessel compromise. Radiology. 1997;203:37–44.

64. Wittram C, Maher MM, Yoo AJ, et al. CT angiography of pulmonary embolism: diagnostic criteria and causes of misdiagnosis. Radiographics. 2004;24:1219–38.

65. Yoshida S, Akiba H, Tamakawa M, et al. Thoracic involvement of Type A aortic dissection and intramural hematoma: diagnostic accuracy—comparison of emergency helical CT and surgical findings. Radiology. 2003;228:430–5.

Part II

Chest

Trauma

Contents

R. Agarwala, *Atlas of Emergency Radiology:*
Vascular System, Chest, Abdomen and Pelvis, and Reproductive System,
DOI 10.1007/978-3-319-13042-2_7, © Springer International Publishing Switzerland 2015

Chest Wall Injury

Diagnosis
Flail Chest

Imaging Findings
1. Fracture of the ribs at two or more sites of two or more contiguous ribs
2. Parallel rows of the ribs in chest radiograph
3. Adjacent pulmonary contusion, pneumothorax, and chest wall emphysema

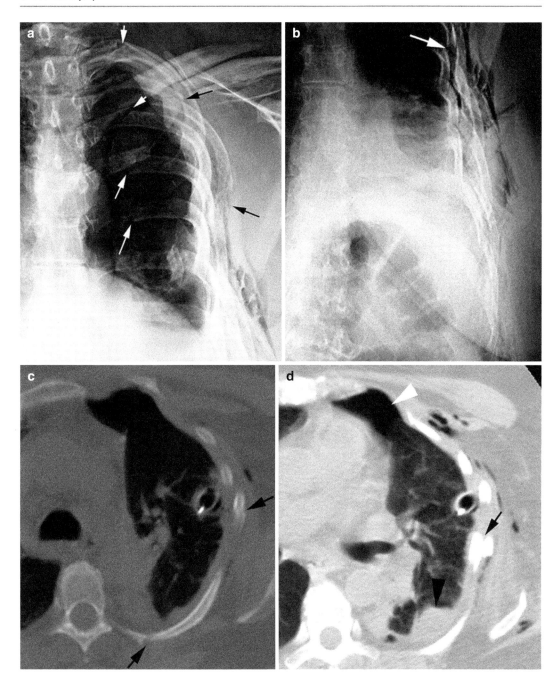

Fig. 7.1 Flail chest with history of local trauma. (**a**, **b**) PA Chest x-rays show segmental fractures (*white arrows* show posterior fractures, *black arrows* show lateral fractures in **a**) of multiple ribs with displaced fractured segments forming two parallel rows of the ribs (*arrow* in **b**). (**c**) Axial CT shows two fractures of the same rib (*arrows*) and deformity of the thoracic wall due to the displacement of the segmental fractures. (**d**) Axial CT shows pneumothorax (*white arrowhead*), pulmonary contusion (*black arrowhead*), rib fracture (*arrow*), and emphysema of the thoracic wall

Mediastinal Injury

Diagnosis
Pneumomediastinum

Imaging Features
1. Linear air parallel to the heart border
2. Continuous diaphragm sign
3. Air around the pulmonary artery and main branches—ring around artery sign
4. Air outlining the major aortic branches—tubular artery sign
5. Air outlining the bronchial wall—double bronchial wall sign
6. Elevated thymus—thymic wing sign

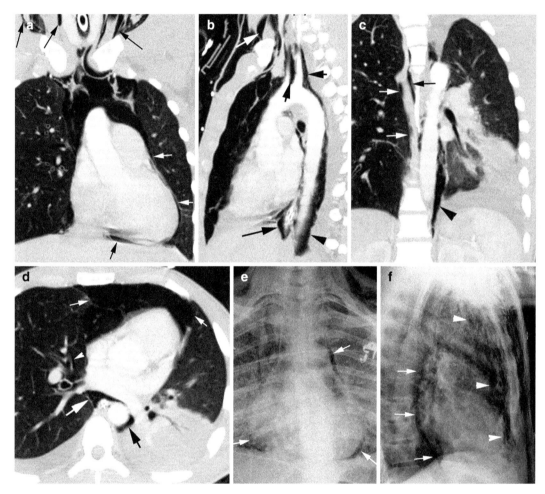

Fig. 7.2 Pneumomediastinum. History of trauma. (**a**) Coronal reformatted CT shows air parallel to the left heart border (*white arrows*) and diaphragmatic surface of the heart (*short black arrow*). Gas is also seen tracking from the superior mediastinum to the neck around the vessels (*long black arrows*). (**b**) Sagittal reformatted image shows air around the distal esophagus (*long black arrow*) and adjacent aorta (*black arrowhead*). Air tracking to the neck around the aortic branches (*short black arrows*) and fascial planes (*white arrow*). (**c**) Coronal reformatted image shows air around the azygos vein (*arrows*) and around the descending aorta (*arrowhead*). (**d**) Axial CT shows air in the anterior mediastinum causing mild compression of the surrounding lung (*thick white arrows*). Air is seen surrounding the right lower lobe pulmonary artery (*thin white arrow*) and bronchus (*arrowhead*). Air is also surrounding the esophagus and aorta (*black arrows*). (**e**) PA chest x-ray shows linear air surrounding the heart and extending above the arch of the aorta (*arrows*). (**f**) Lateral chest x-ray shows air in the anterior mediastinum (*arrowheads*) and around the esophagus (*arrows*)

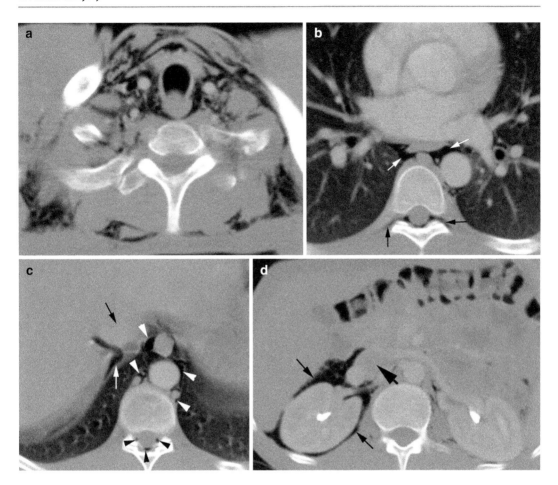

Fig. 7.3 Pneumomediastinum with gas tracking to the retroperitoneum, the spinal canal, and neck tracking along the blood vessels and nerve roots. History of traumatic asphyxia syndrome. (**a**) Axial CT at thoracic inlet shows gas around the vessels, trachea, adjacent muscle planes, and posteriorly air is in the paraspinal muscle planes. (**b**) Axial CT shows gas tracking along nerve roots through neural foramen into the spinal canal (*black arrows*) and air around the esophagus and aorta (*white arrows*). (**c**) Axial CT shows gas tracking into the retroperitoneum in between the IVC (*black arrow*) and diaphragm (*white arrow*) and through both esophageal and aortic hiatus, around the azygos and hemiazygos veins (*arrowheads*). Air is also seen in the spinal canal (*black arrowheads*). (**d**) Axial CT shows air in the perirenal space (*thin black arrows*) and around the IVC (*thick black arrow*)

Diagnosis

Hemopneumomediastinum

Imaging Features

1. Loculated high-density hemorrhagic fluid and
    gas collection in the anterior mediastinum

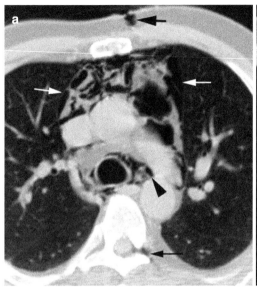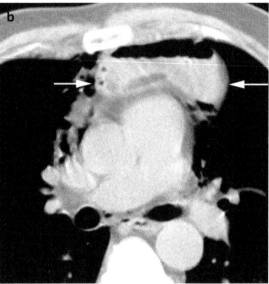

Fig. 7.4 Hemopneumomediastinum post gunshot injury.
(**a**) Axial CT shows gas and patchy soft tissue density in
the anterior mediastinum (*white arrows*) and around the
trachea (*arrowhead*). Gas is seen in the spinal canal along
the nerve root through the left intervertebral foramina

(*thin black arrow*). Bullet tract is seen in the anterior chest
wall (*thick black arrow*). (**b**) Axial CT a week later shows
loculated hemopneumomediastinum in the anterior mediastinum (*arrows*) with layered gas and high-density
hemorrhage

Diagnosis

Pneumopericardium

Imaging Features

1. Gas collection in the pericardial cavity restricted below arch of the aorta
2. The gas crosses the midline

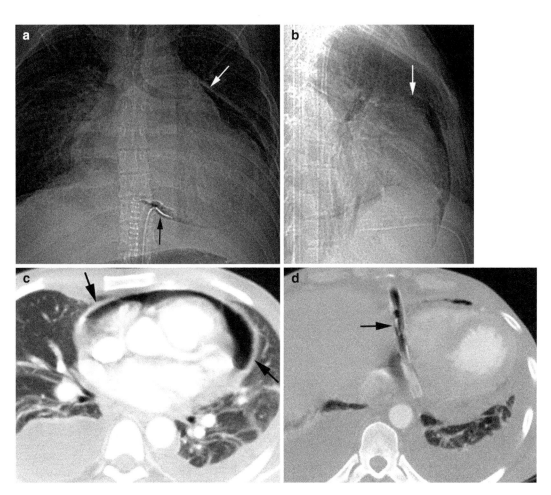

Fig. 7.5 Iatrogenic pneumopericardium as a result of catheter placement for bacterial pericarditis. (**a**, **b**) Topogram of two views of the chest for CT chest shows air in the pericardium which stops below the arch of the aorta (*white arrow*). Catheter with surrounding gas is at the inferior surface of the heart (*black arrow*). (**c**) Axial CT shows pericardial gas displacing the thick pericardium (*arrows*) and outlining the cardiac border. (**d**) Axial CT shows catheter (*arrow*) in the pericardium with pneumopericardium

Diagnosis
Traumatic Pneumothorax, Pneumomediastinum,
and Tension Pneumopericardium

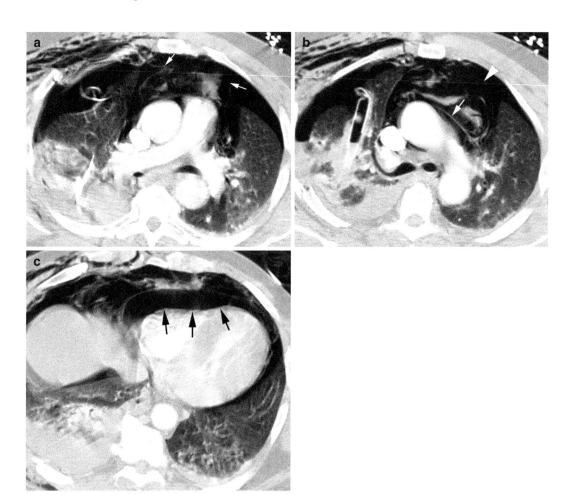

Fig. 7.6 Pneumothorax, pneumomediastinum, and tension pneumopericardium. History of polysubstance abuse and fall from ladder. (**a**) Axial CT shows hemorrhagic pneumomediastinum contained by the mediastinal parietal pleura (*arrows*) and pneumothorax in pleural space displacing lungs bilaterally. (**b**) Axial CT shows pneumopericardium displacing the pericardium (*arrow*) and pneumomediastinum surrounded by parietal pleura (*arrow head*). (**c**) Axial CT shows compression of the right heart by pneumopericardium (*black arrows*). Patient had tachycardia

Pleural Injury

Diagnosis
Hemothorax

Imaging Features
1. Heterogeneous high density hemorrhagic fluid
   in the pleural space

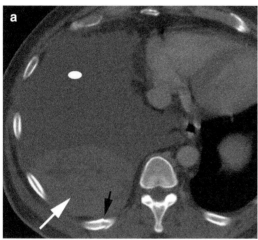 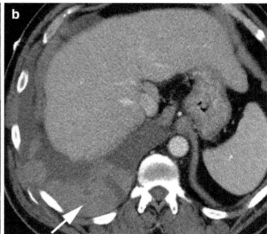

Fig. 7.7 Hemothorax. History of trauma. (**a, b**) Axial CT chest shows high-density hematoma (*white arrows*) in the pleural space in dependent pleural cavity extending to the posterior costophrenic angle and surrounded by large low-density pleural fluid (*ellipse*) and with rib fracture (*black arrow*)

Diagnosis

Hemopneumothorax

Imaging Features

1. High-density hemorrhagic fluid in the pleural cavity
2. Gas in the pleural cavity
3. Partial lung collapse

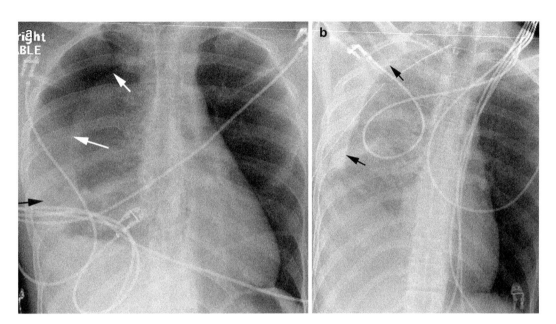

Fig. 7.8 Hemopneumothorax. History of stab wound. (**a**) Portable chest x-ray shows partial collapse of the right lung (*white arrows*) by lucent pneumothorax in the upper thorax and high-density hemorrhage (*black arrow*) in the lower pleural cavity. (**b**) Chest x-ray after chest tube placement shows partial re-expansion of the right lung with no pneumothorax. Hemorrhagic high-density pleural fluid (*arrows*) is filling the pleural space

Diagnosis
Tension Hemopneumothorax

Imaging Features
1. High-density hemothorax in the right lateral pleural cavity

2. Pneumothorax protruding into the mediastinum to the left
3. Collapse of the right lung
4. Mediastinal shift

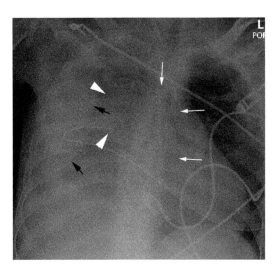

Fig. 7.9 Tension hemopneumothorax. Complication of misplaced IJ catheter. After removal of malpositioned catheter, the patient developed shortness of breath.
Supine chest x-ray shows:
1. Hemothorax as high-density fluid with sharp medial border in lateral right hemithorax (*black arrows*) marginated inferiorly by low-density pneumothorax and superiorly by the less dense collapsed lung (*arrowheads*).
2. Right tension pneumothorax protruding into the left side of the mediastinum (*arrows*) and mediastinal shift to the left side.
3. The tip of the right chest tube very anterior and adjacent to the collapsed lung and possibly is obstructed by the lung parenchyma; hence pneumothorax is not relieved. Tension was relieved following surgery

Acute Lung Parenchymal Changes

8

Contents

R. Agarwala, *Atlas of Emergency Radiology:*
Vascular System, Chest, Abdomen and Pelvis, and Reproductive System,
DOI 10.1007/978-3-319-13042-2_8, © Springer International Publishing Switzerland 2015

Miliary Nodules

Imaging Features
1. Innumerable, tiny, both sharply and poorly defined noncalcified nodules, 1–4 mm throughout both lungs, and generally of uniform size
2. Diffuse random distribution in both lungs

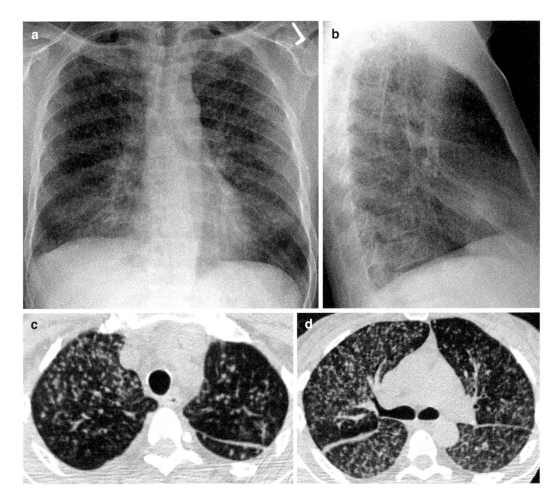

Fig. 8.1 Miliary nodules. History of TB infection presented with cough, fever, and night sweats. (**a**, **b**) PA and lateral chest x-ray (**c**, **d**) and axial CT of the chest show miliary nodules in random distribution with lower lobe predominance

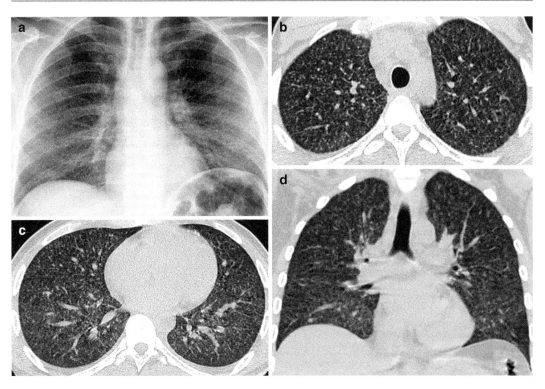

Fig. 8.2 Coccidiomycosis. (**a**) PA chest x-ray, (**b**, **c**) axial CT, and (**d**) coronal reformatted CT images show miliary nodules in random distribution and mild basilar predominance

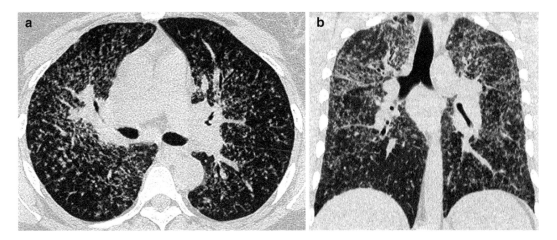

Fig. 8.3 Patient with history of sarcoidosis. (**a**, **b**) Axial and coronal reformatted CT show miliary nodules with upper lobe predominance and bilateral hilar lymphadenopathy. Nodules involving pleural surface and septa

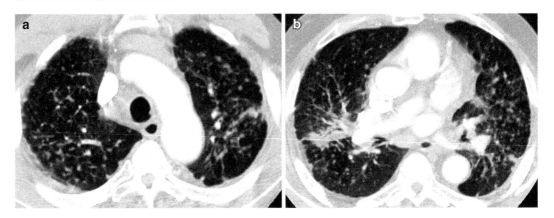

Fig. 8.4 Silicosis. (**a**, **b**) Axial CT shows miliary nodule with fibrosis more in the upper lungs involving the septa and pleural surface

Centrilobular Nodules

Imaging Features

1. Nodules separate from the pleural surface, fissures, and interlobular septa.
2. May be dense or ground glass in attenuation.
3. May be a few millimeters to a centimeter in size.
4. May be a single or a rosette of nodules.
5. May be patchy or diffuse in distribution.

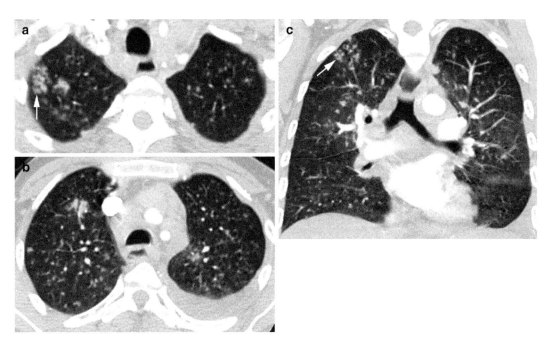

Fig. 8.5 Active TB. History of immune-compromised syndrome with active TB infection. (**a, b**) Axial and (**c**) coronal reformatted CT of the chest show centrilobular micronodules sparing the pleural surfaces and fissures and are of varying sizes. Some nodules in the right upper lobe are arranged in rosette, best seen in coronal reformatted image (*arrow* in **a, c**), and small left effusion (**b, c**)

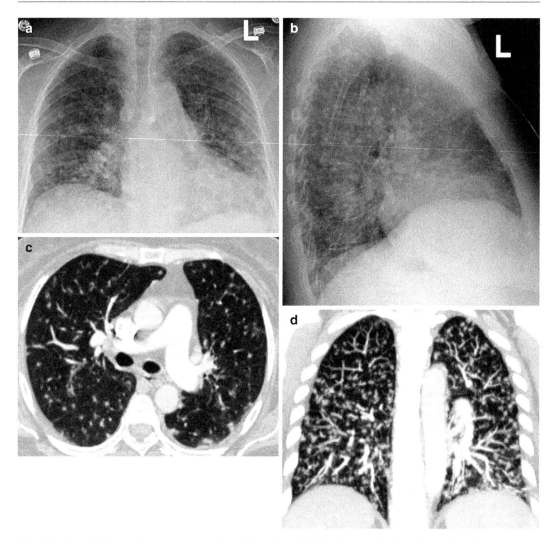

Fig. 8.6 Centrilobular nodules in a patient with ALL and candida infection. (**a**, **b**) Chest PA and lateral views, (**c**, **d**) axial CT, and coronal reformatted image show micronodules sparing the pleural surface and fissures

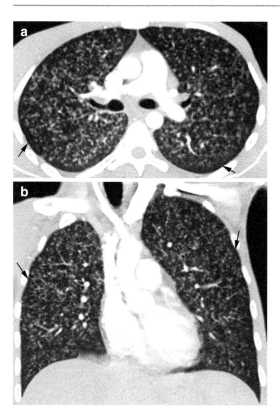

Fig. 8.7 Centrilobular distribution of histoplasma infection in an HIV-positive patient. Urine was positive for histoplasma antigen. (**a**, **b**) Axial and coronal reformatted images show diffuse micronodules in both lungs, sparing the pleural surface and subpleural region (*arrows*)

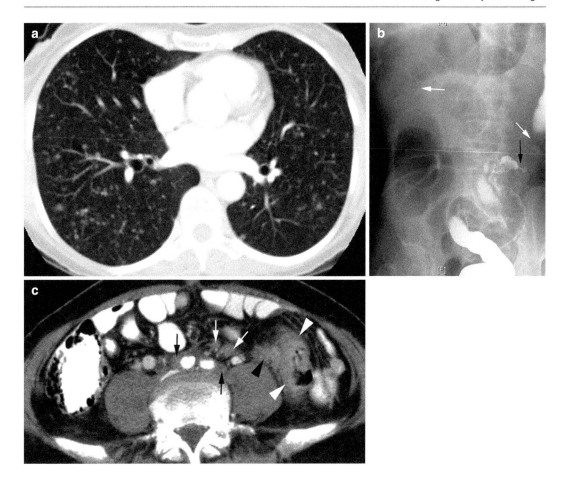

Fig. 8.8 Metastasis with centrilobular nodules from colon cancer. (**a**) Axial CT of the chest shows centrilobular lung nodules of varying size not involving fissures and abutting the pleura. (**b**) Double-contrast barium enema shows focal constriction of the proximal sigmoid colon (*black arrow*) and dilatation of adjacent descending colon (*white arrows*). (**c**) Axial CT of the abdomen shows diffuse wall thickening of the sigmoid colon in the same area as seen in the enema study (*white arrowheads*) with extension of tumor medially outside the colon over the left psoas muscle (*black arrowhead*). Enlarged lymph nodes or tumor and linear strands extending to common iliac arteries (*thin white arrows*) and surrounding the iliac arteries (*thin black arrows*)

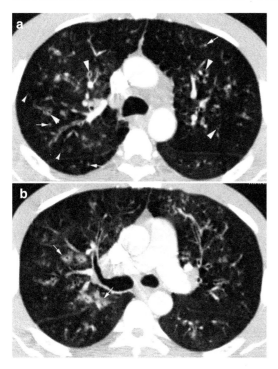

Fig. 8.9 Viral cellular bronchiolitis. (**a**) Axial CT shows diffuse thick-walled bronchi and bronchioles (*thick arrowheads*). Diffuse centrilobular nodules are seen, some of which are solid (*arrows*) and some are subsolid (*thin arrowheads*). (**b**) Axial CT at lower level shows some of the thick-walled bronchi to have surrounding ground-glass density (*arrows*)

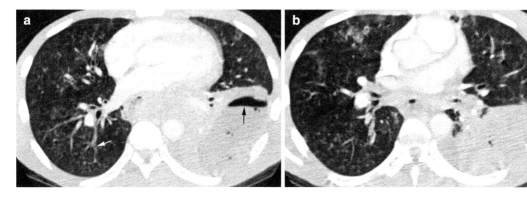

Fig. 8.10 Endobronchial abscess spreads with centrilobular nodules. (**a**, **b**) Axial CT shows centrilobular nodules in the middle lobe and right lower lobe from endobronchial spread of the left lower lobe abscess with air-fluid level (*black arrow*). A right lower lobe bronchus is filled with soft tissues (*white arrow*)

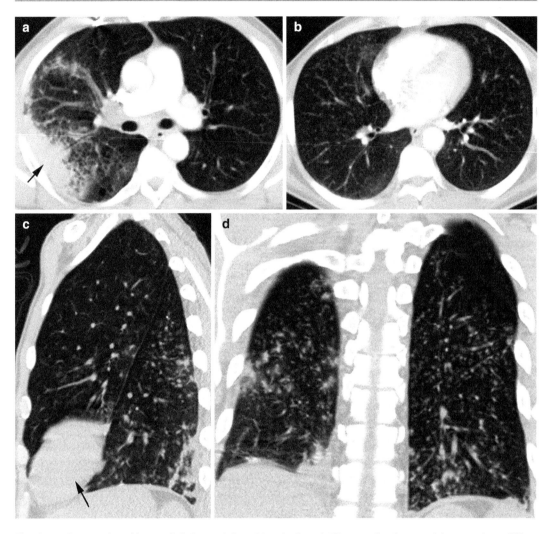

Fig. 8.11 Pneumonia with centrilobular nodules: (**a**) Axial CT shows consolidation RUL (*arrow* in **a**, **c**) with surrounding interstitial thickening. (**b**) Axial CT, (**c**) sagittal, and (**d**) coronal reformatted images show diffuse centrilobular nodules of the lower lobes bilaterally

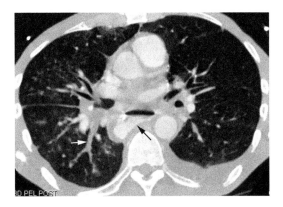

Fig. 8.12 Centrilobular nodules due to aspiration. Patient with achalasia. Axial CT shows multiple centrilobular nodules mainly of ground-glass density, distributed mostly in the middle and right lower lobes, fluid-filled right lower lobe bronchus (*white arrow*), and dilated esophagus (*black arrow*)

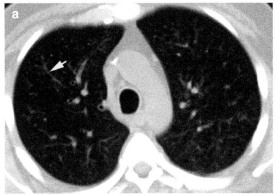

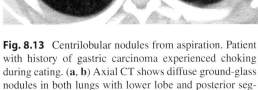
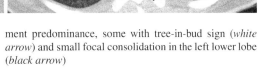

Fig. 8.13 Centrilobular nodules from aspiration. Patient with history of gastric carcinoma experienced choking during eating. (**a, b**) Axial CT shows diffuse ground-glass nodules in both lungs with lower lobe and posterior seg-ment predominance, some with tree-in-bud sign (*white arrow*) and small focal consolidation in the left lower lobe (*black arrow*)

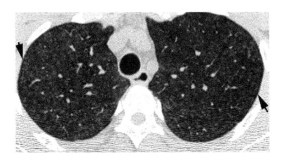

Fig. 8.14 Hypersensitivity pneumonitis in a bird breeder. Diffuse ground-glass centrilobular bilaterally with sub-pleural sparing (*arrows*)

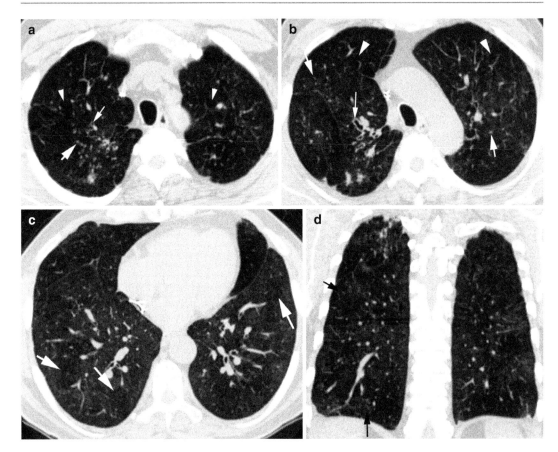

Fig. 8.15 Respiratory bronchiolitis. History of chronic cigarette smoking. (**a**, **b**) Axial CT shows bronchial wall thickening in RUL (*thin arrow*), centrilobular emphysema (*arrowheads*), and centrilobular nodules (*thick short arrows*). (**c**) Axial CT shows diffuse centrilobular nodules and mosaic attenuation (*white arrows*) from obstructive bronchiolitis. (**d**) Coronal reformatted image shows multiple ground-glass centrilobular nodules (*black arrows*) which appear more at the lower lung field due to emphysematous changes in the upper lungs

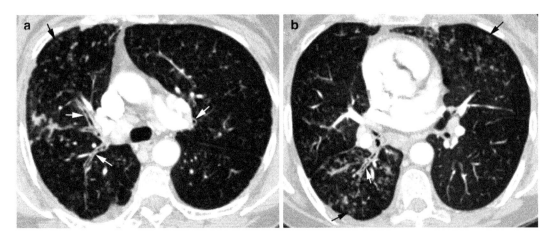

Fig. 8.16 Diffuse panbronchiolitis mimicking asthma. (**a**, **b**) Axial CT shows bronchial thickening (*white arrows*) with diffuse centrilobular nodules (*black arrows*) of both lungs

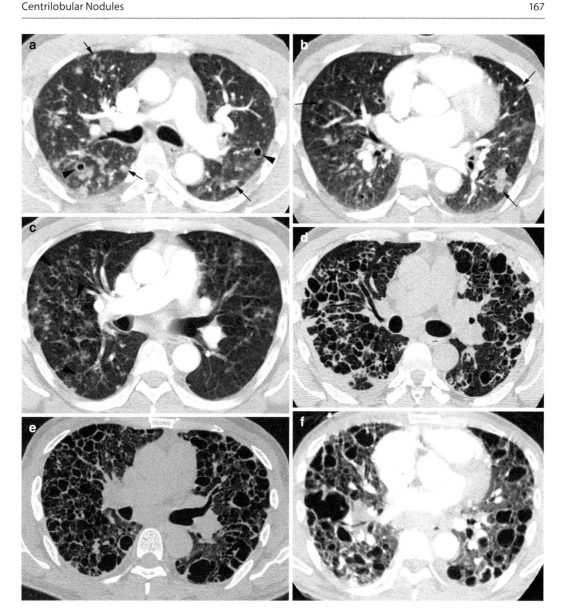

Fig. 8.17 Langerhans cell histiocytosis. Same patient in 2004, 2005, 2006, and 2008. Axial CT (**a**, **b**) in 2004 shows multiple mostly solid nodules (*arrows*) with upper lobe predominance and in centrilobular distribution. A few thick-walled cysts are also seen (*arrowheads*). (**c**) In 2005, the cystic spaces have increased (*arrowheads*) with decrease of solid nodules at same level as (**a**). (**d**) 2006, shows further increase in size and a number of the cystic spaces, some are thick walled and others are thin walled. (**e**, **f**) 2008, shows further progression in cystic spaces with upper lobe predominance and decrease in normal lung

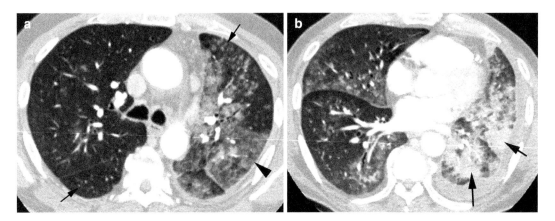

Fig. 8.18 Invasive mucinous adenocarcinoma. (**a**, **b**) Axial CT shows multicentric densities with solid (*thick arrows*) and subsolid areas (*arrowhead*) in the left lower lobe and lingula and diffuse solid and subsolid centrilobular nodules (*thin arrows*) bilaterally

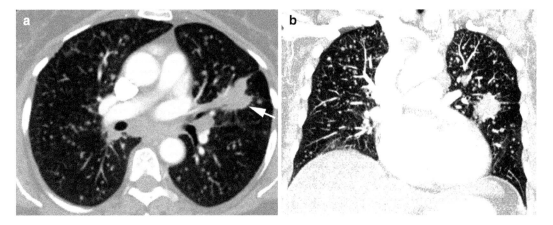

Fig. 8.19 Adenocarcinoma with metastasis. (**a**, **b**) Axial and coronal reformatted CT shows a solid invasive spiculated mass in the left perihilum with pleural tags, extension to left hilum (*arrow*), and diffuse bilateral centrilobular solid nodular metastasis

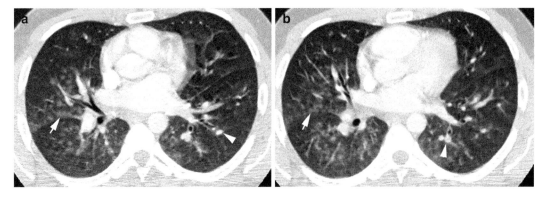

Fig. 8.20 Acute pulmonary edema, postoperative (angiocentric disease). (**a**, **b**) Axial CT shows centrilobular ground-glass nodules mostly in the medial and central lungs and more at the bases along the fissures but not involving them (*arrows*). Dilated arteries more at the lower lung field (*arrowhead*)

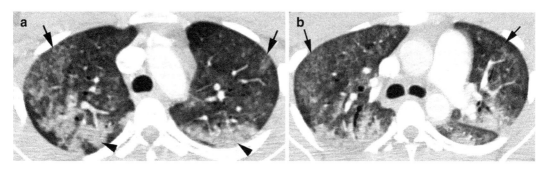

Fig. 8.21 Pulmonary hemorrhage (angiocentric disease) in a patient with SLE and hemoptysis. (**a**, **b**) Axial CT shows ground-glass centrilobular nodules bilaterally, sparing the pleural surface (*arrows*) and lobular consolidation (*arrowheads*)

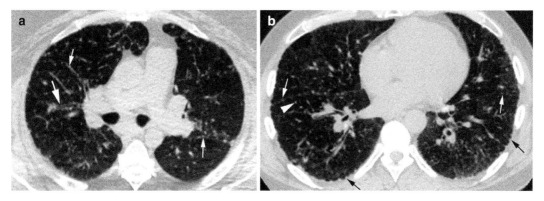

Fig. 8.22 Sarcoidosis, perilymphatic disease. Axial CT shows sharp nodules. (**a**) Nodules along the bronchial wall (*thick white arrow*) and vascular markings (*thin white arrow*). (**b**) Along fissures (*thin white arrow*) and centrilobular nodules (*thick arrowhead*) and nodular thickening of pleural surfaces (*black arrows*)

Tree-in-Bud Sign

Diagnosis
Centrilobular Nodules—Tree-in-Bud Sign

Imaging Features
1. Branching appearance with most peripheral nodules several millimeters from the pleural surface
2. Centrilobular clusters of nodules

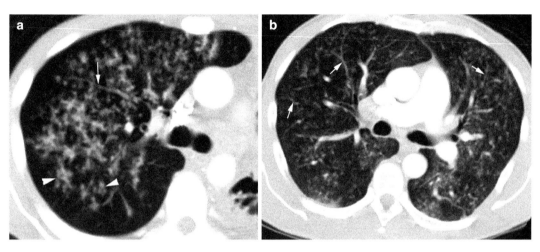

Fig. 8.23 TB in two patients. (**a**, **b**) Axial CT shows diffuse centrilobular nodules and with tree-in-bud pattern (*arrows*). Some of the nodules show centrilobular clustering (*arrowheads*)

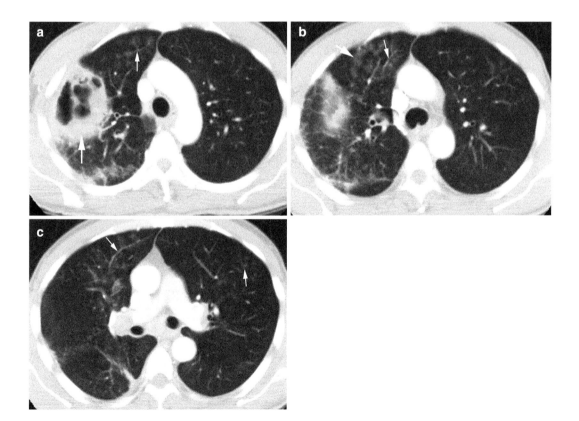

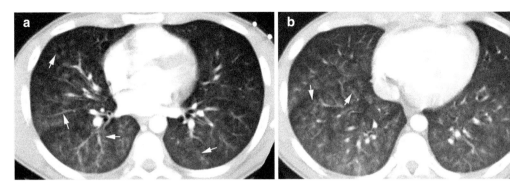

Fig. 8.25 Streptococcus mitis infection. Patient with pre-B-ALL and neutropenic fever. Axial CT of the chest (**a**, **b**) shows diffuse ground-glass nodules linearly arranged along the bronchovascular bundles, some showing tree-in-bud distribution (*arrows*)

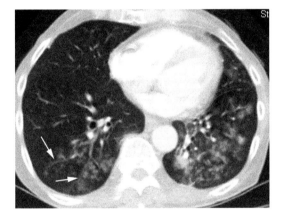

Fig. 8.26 Laryngeal carcinoma with endobronchial spread. Axial CT shows diffuse subsolid nodules, some with tree-in-bud arrangement (*white arrows*)

Fig. 8.24 Pseudomonas lung abscess with endobronchial spread. (**a**) Axial CT shows thick-walled abscess in RUL (*thick white arrow*) with ground-glass nodules at the end of the bronchi adjacent to it (*thin white arrow*). (**b**) Tree-in-bud distribution of ground-glass nodules (*thin white arrow*) and also linearly arranged ground-glass nodules in bronchovascular distribution (*thick white arrow*). (**c**) Axial CT of the chest at lower level shows bilateral centrilobular nodules, some with tree-in-bud arrangement (*arrow*)

Centrilobular Low Attenuation

Imaging Features
1. Abnormal areas of low attenuation of the secondary lobule.
2. Walls are imperceptible in emphysema.
3. Thick walls are seen in bronchiolectasis and cavitary nodules.

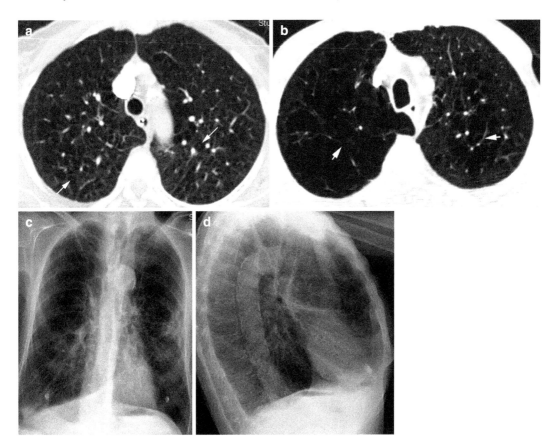

Fig. 8.27 (**a**, **b**) Centrilobular (centriacinar) emphysema. (**a**) Axial CT shows low-attenuation areas in the center of lobules with imperceptible walls. Centrilobular arteries (*arrows*) are seen in some of the low-attenuated areas. (**b**) Axial CT of different patients shows larger centrilobular emphysema. Thick visible walls (*arrows*) with prominent veins are due to fibrosis of the interlobular septa. (**c**, **d**) PA and lateral chest x-ray show hyperinflated lungs with flattened diaphragms and increased retrosternal space

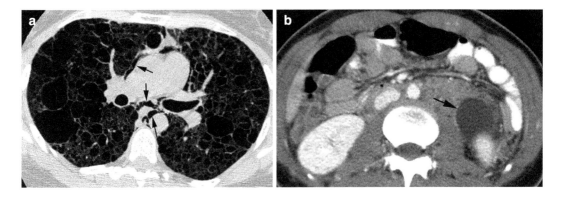

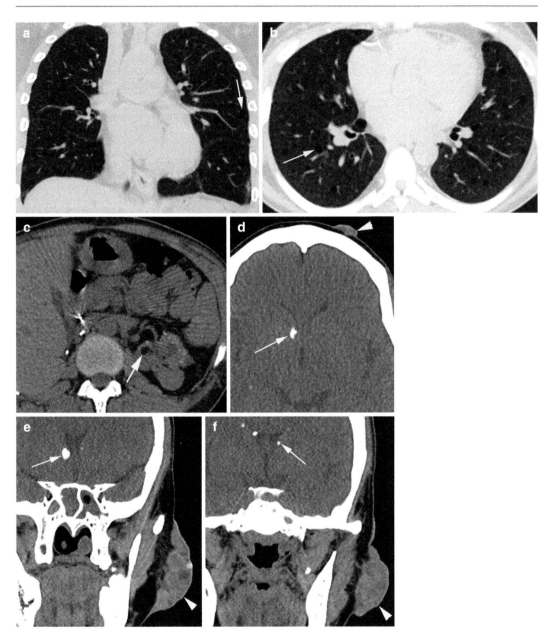

Fig. 8.29 TSC-associated LAM. (**a**, **b**) Coronal and sagittal reformatted CTs show diffuse cysts throughout both lungs (*arrow*). (**c**) Axial CT of the abdomen shows angiomyolipoma with fatty foci in the left kidney (*arrow*). (**d–f**) CT head, (**d**) axial, (**e**, **f**) and coronal reformatted images show subependymal hamartomas with calcification (*arrow*) and facial angiofibromas (adenoma sebaceum) (*arrowheads*)

Fig. 8.28 Lymphangioleiomyomatosis. (**a**) Axial CT of the chest shows diffuse cysts with well-defined walls with intervening normal lung parenchyma and with pneumo-mediastinum (*arrows*). (**b**) Axial CT of the upper abdomen shows retroperitoneal lymphangioma with a large fluid collection adjacent to the upper pole left kidney (*arrow*)

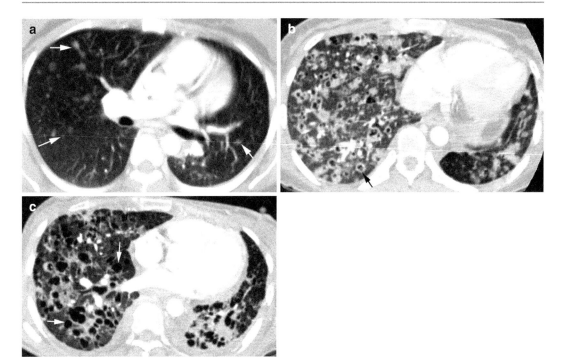

Fig. 8.30 Cavitating metastasis from adenocarcinoma of the lung with left upper lobectomy. Axial CT of the chest (**a**) shows multiple small nodules of various sizes in both lungs (*arrows*). (**b**) Two years later multiple cavitating nodules are seen, some with thick walls (*arrow*). (**c**) Five months later the nodules show increased cystic changes, some with very thin walls (*arrows*)

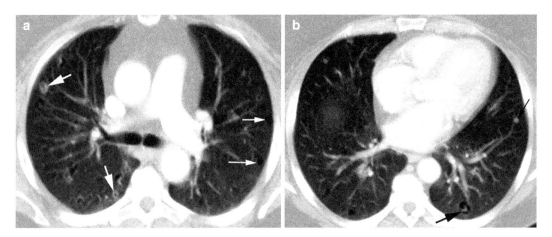

Fig. 8.31 Cystic changes in pulmonary metastases of endometrial carcinoma. (**a**, **b**) Axial CT shows the metastasis to range from solid (*thin black arrow*), thick-walled cavitary (*thick white arrow*), cystic with solid center (*thick black arrow*), and purely cystic lesions (*thin white arrow*)

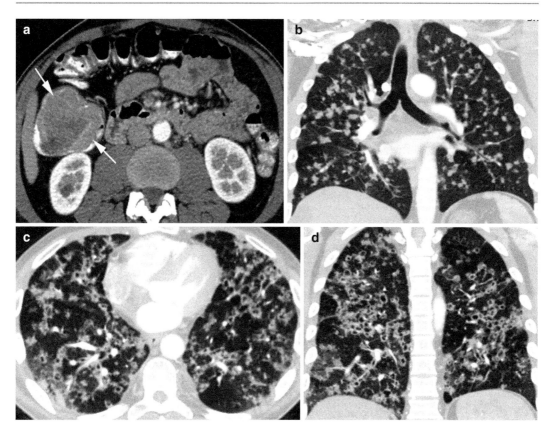

Fig. 8.32 Cavitating centrilobular lung metastasis from colon cancer. (**a**) Axial CT of the upper abdomen shows a large adenocarcinoma in the proximal ascending colon (*arrows*). (**b**) Coronal reformatted image of chest few months later shows diffuse solid centrilobular nodular metastasis bilaterally. (**c, d**) Axial and coronal reformatted images 1 year later show increase in pulmonary nodular metastasis which now show cavitation

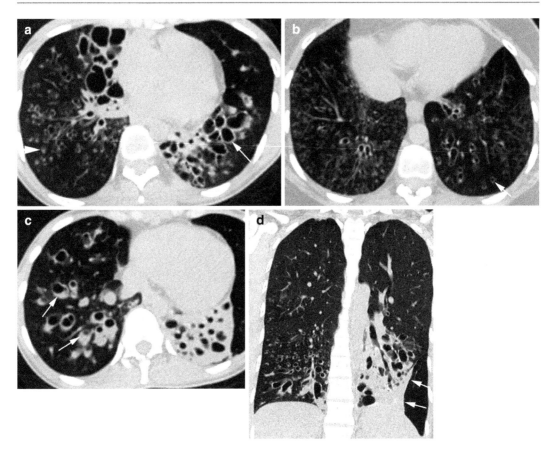

Fig. 8.33 Bronchiolectasis. Dilated bronchi and bronchioles mostly in the lung bases, in two patients. Patient 1: Axial CT (**a**, **b**) shows bronchiectasis (*thin long arrows*) with tree-in-bud centrilobular nodules, some of the latter have central lucencies due to dilated bronchioles (*thick white arrows*). Patient 2: (**c**) Some of the bronchi have fluid (*arrows*). (**d**) Coronal reformatted image shows the dilated bronchi in the left lower lobe are surrounded with fibrosis as seen by retraction (*arrows*)

Fig. 8.35 Fungal pneumonia with cavitating nodules. History of a 19-year-old patient with steroid-resistant ulcerative colitis. (**a**, **b**) Axial and coronal reformatted CTs show multiple thick-walled cavitary nodules, some with air-fluid level (*black arrow*) mostly in the mid-lung zone with small areas of consolidation (*white arrows*). (**c**) Axial CT several months later shows increase in consolidation areas (*arrows*) and decreased cavitary nodules

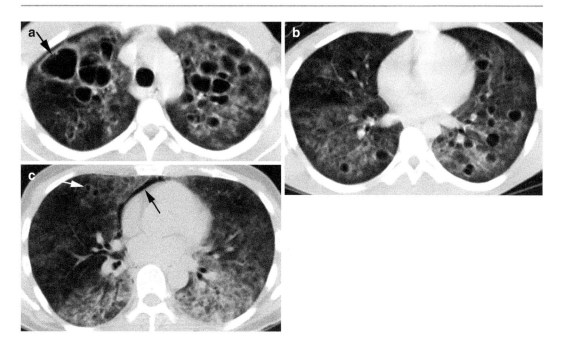

Fig. 8.34 Cystic pneumocystis infection. (**a**, **b**) Axial CT shows thick-walled cysts (*arrows*) in both lungs, with larger cysts in the upper lobes. The cysts are surrounded by diffuse ground-glass infiltration. (**c**) Axial CT of differ-ent patients shows pneumomediastinum (*black arrow*) in addition to bilateral ground-glass infiltrations and small cysts (*white arrow*)

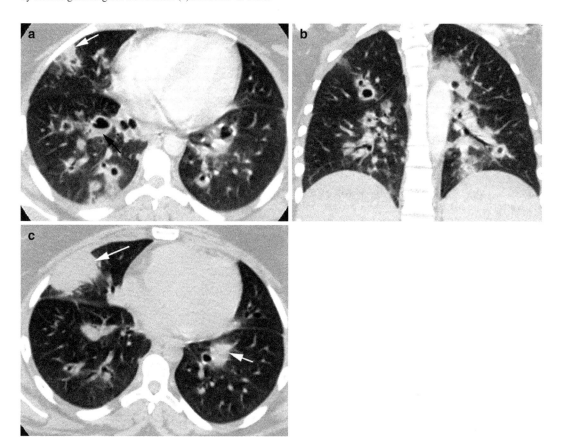

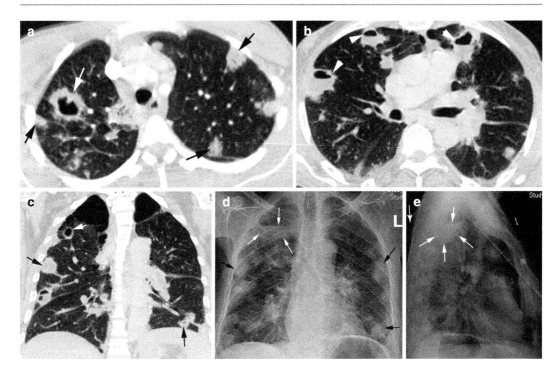

Fig. 8.36 Septic emboli. History of IV drug abuse. (**a**, **b**) Axial and (**c**) coronal reformatted CTs show multiple nodules in the periphery of the lungs and mostly pleural based. Some nodules are solid (*black arrows*), some show cavitation (*white arrow*), and some with air-fluid levels from abscess formation (*arrowheads*), and all with shaggy borders. (**d**, **e**) PA and lateral chest x-ray shows peripheral nodules, some showing cavitation (*black arrows*). A thin-walled infected bulla is also seen in the right lung apex with air-fluid level (*white arrow*)

Fig. 8.38 Lobular ground-glass opacity from pneumonia. (**a**, **b**) Axial CT in a patient with community-acquired pneumonia with groups of lobules involving the right lower and middle lobes. (**c**, **d**) Axial and coronal reformatted CTs in different patients with Legionella pneumonia show focal lobular peripheral consolidation in RUL (*arrow*) and ground-glass lobular involvement in the rest of the bilateral upper lobes

Panlobular Abnormalities

Imaging Features
1. Involvement of single or groups of lobules with normal-appearing adjacent lobules—mosaic attenuation

2. Lobular increased attenuation from consolidation or ground-glass density
3. Lobular low attenuation from decreased perfusion, air trapping, or lobular destruction

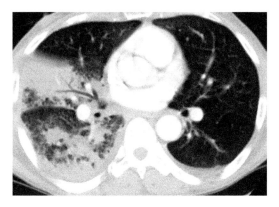

Fig. 8.37 Lobular consolidation from bronchopneumonia. Axial CT shows panlobular consolidation involving a large area of consolidation in RML and multiple small groups of lobules in RLL

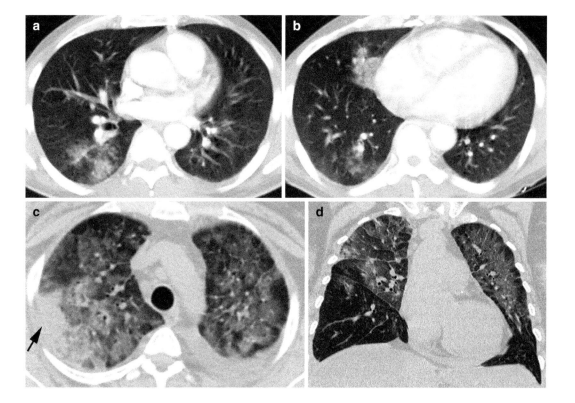

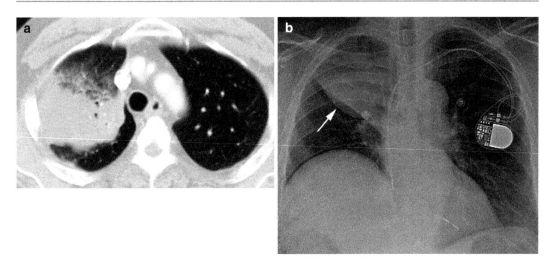

Fig. 8.39 Adenocarcinoma. Axial CT (**a**) shows large lobular consolidation of the right upper lobe. (**b**) PA chest x-ray shows Golden "S" sign formed by mass and partial collapse of RUL (*arrow*)

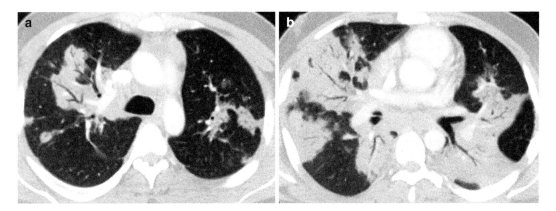

Fig. 8.40 Hodgkin's lymphoma biopsy proven. (**a**, **b**) Patient presented with night sweat and loss of weight. Axial CT shows multiple areas of lobular consolidation

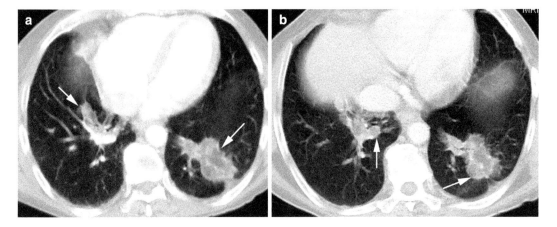

Fig. 8.41 Lipoid pneumonia. (**a**, **b**) Axial CT shows with well-marginated ground-glass focal densities in both lung bases (*arrows*) with density measurement of fatty tissue. Patient was a baker by trade

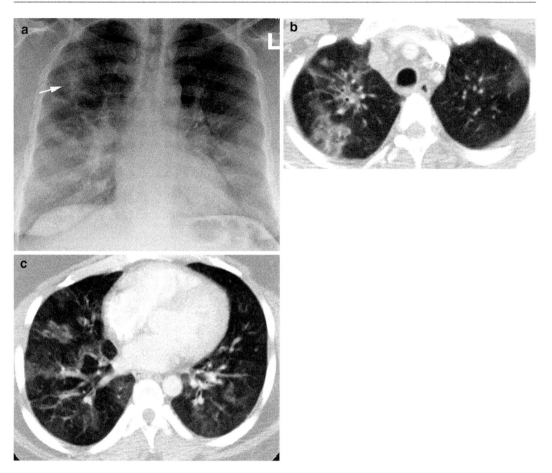

Fig. 8.42 Eosinophilic pneumonia in a patient with congenital erythropoietic porphyria. (**a**) Chest x ray shows patchy infiltration in the right upper lobe (*arrow*). (**b, c**) Axial CT shows lobular ground-glass densities bilaterally more at the bases

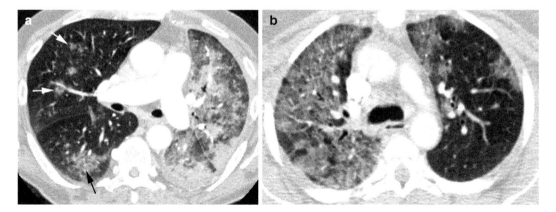

Fig. 8.43 Lung carcinoma. Axial CT shows (**a**) mucinous adenocarcinoma with multiple focal solid areas and panlobular ground-glass tumor infiltration on the left side, focal lobular infiltration of the right lower lobe (*black arrow*), and subsolid nodules in the middle lobe (*white arrows*). (**b**) Non-small cell carcinoma with panlobular infiltrate of the right lung and patchy lobular ground-glass infiltrate of the left side

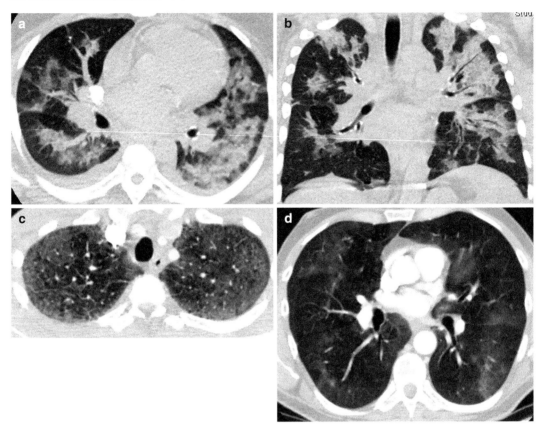

Fig. 8.44 Pneumocystis infection in three patients. (**a, b**) Axial and coronal reformatted CTs show lobular consolidation and ground-glass densities bilaterally. (**c, d**) Axial CTs in two different patients show diffuse lobular ground-glass opacities bilaterally

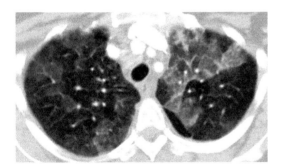

Fig. 8.45 Hypersensitivity pneumonitis. Axial CT shows lobular ground-glass opacities bilaterally

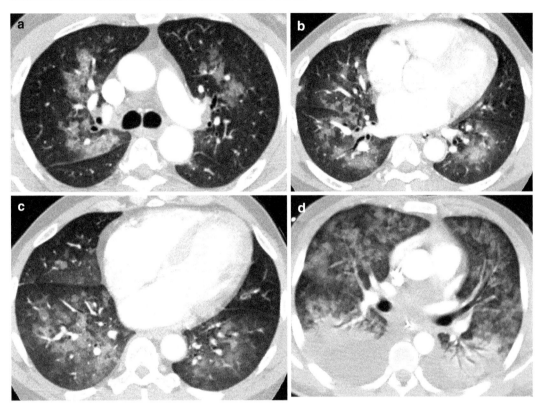

Fig. 8.46 Panlobular ground-glass opacities resulting from acute CHF with pulmonary edema in two patients. (**a–c**) Axial CT in a patient with mitral valve disease. (**d**) Axial CT in a patient with end-stage renal disease. There is also lobular consolidation of both lower lobes in this patient

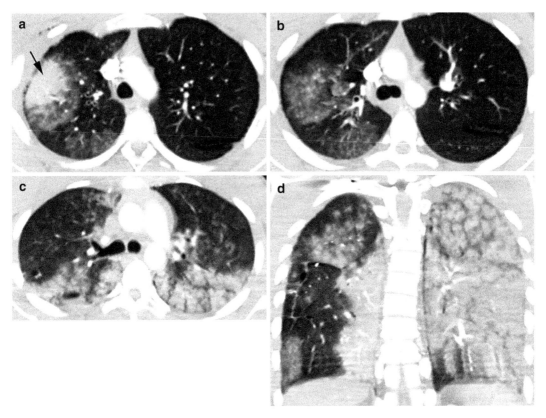

Fig. 8.47 Panlobular ground-glass opacity in pulmonary contusion from GSW in two patients. Patient 1: (**a, b**) Axial CT shows lobular consolidation (*black arrow*) with surrounding lobular ground-glass opacities in RUL. Patient 2: (**b, c**) Axial CT shows diffuse lobular ground-glass densities bilaterally

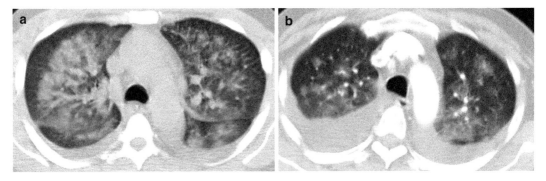

Fig. 8.48 Alveolar hemorrhage in two patients. Patient 1: (**a**) Hemorrhagic necrotizing pneumonia in a patient with acute renal failure with *E. coli* bacteremia and hemoptysis. Axial CT of the chest shows bilateral lobular ground-glass densities with small bilateral effusion. Patient 2: (**b**) Acute renal failure on anticoagulation and bronchoscopy confirmed alveolar hemorrhage. Axial CT of the chest shows bilateral lobular ground-glass densities and bilateral pleural effusion

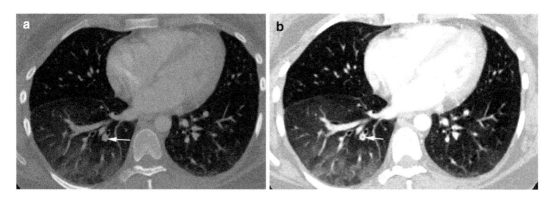

Fig. 8.49 Acute pulmonary infarction with lobular infarction with ground-glass density. (**a**, **b**) Axial CT of the chest shows thrombus in a right lower lobe branch of the pulmonary artery (*arrow*) with surrounding ground-glass lobular densities

Lobular Ground-Glass Opacity and Crazy Paving

Imaging Features
1. Ground-glass opacity with superimposition of septal thickening

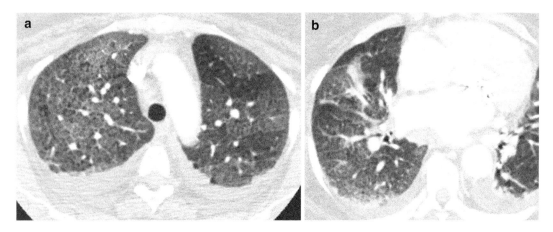

Fig. 8.50 CHF with cardiomegaly, pulmonary edema, and bilateral effusion. History of mitral and tricuspid valve repair and diastolic CHF. (**a**, **b**) Axial CT shows diffuse ground-glass density with increased reticular pattern especially in the right lung giving a crazy paving appearance

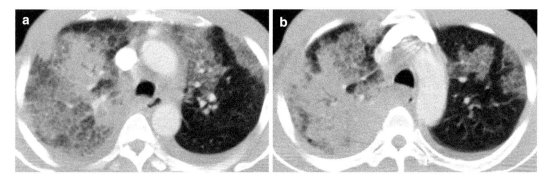

Fig. 8.51 Klebsiella pneumonia. (**a**, **b**) Axial CT of the chest shows lobular ground-glass opacities with crazy paving. There are also large areas of lobular consolidation in the right lung and bilateral small pleural effusion

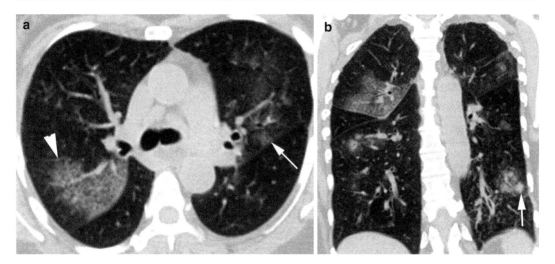

Fig. 8.52 Multilobar bronchopneumonia. (**a**, **b**) CT axial and coronal reformatted images show multiple lobular areas of ground-glass attenuation with crazy paving (*arrowhead*), smaller lobular ground-glass densities (*thin arrow*), and focal consolidation (*thick arrow*)

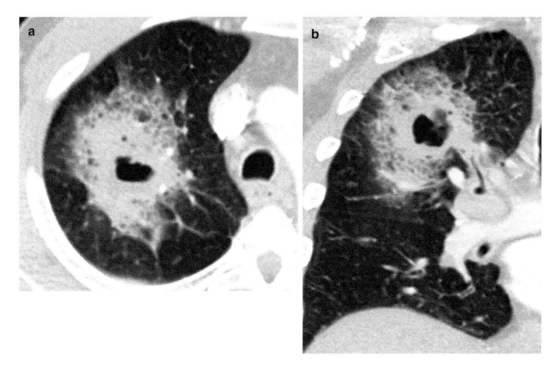

Fig. 8.53 Lung abscess. (**a–c**) Axial, coronal, and sagittal reformatted CTs show large lobular area of consolidation with central air-fluid collection of necrotic abscess. Reactive changes of the surrounding lung showing crazy paving. (**d**, **e**) Chest x-ray, PA, and lateral views showing same abscess (*arrows*)

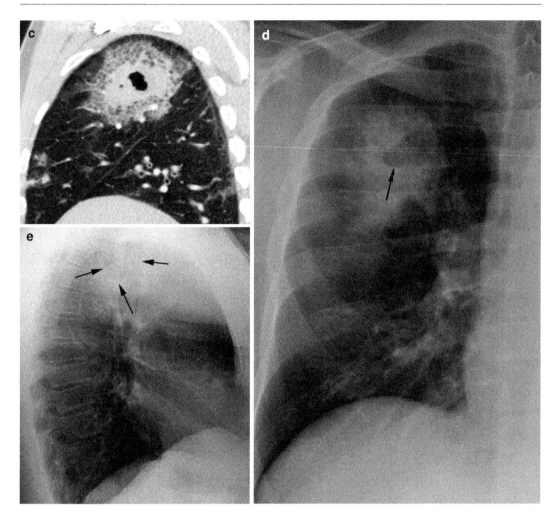

Fig. 8.53 (continued)

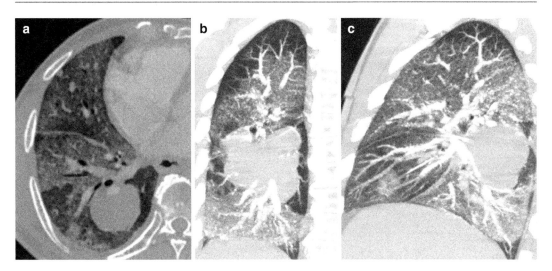

Fig. 8.54 Radiation pneumonitis with crazy paving surrounding stage IV adenocarcinoma. (**a–c**) Axial, coronal, and sagittal reformatted CTs show a large solid mass with surrounding diffuse panlobular ground-glass density with a crazy paving appearance

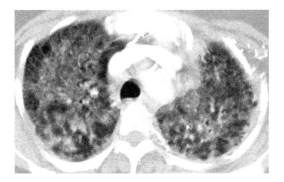

Fig. 8.55 Alveolar proteinosis in a patient with AML having myelodysplastic syndrome, neutropenic fever, and adrenal insufficiency. Axial CT of the chest shows bilateral diffuse panlobular ground-glass opacities and thickened reticular pattern giving a crazy paving appearance

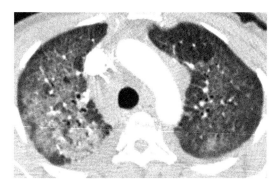

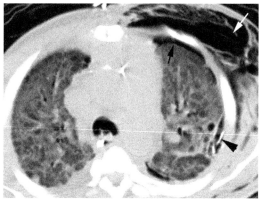

Fig. 8.56 Sarcoidosis with a crazy paving pattern. Axial CT of the chest shows with diffuse lobular ground-glass opacity with superimposed reticular markings and mediastinal lymphadenopathy

Fig. 8.57 Adult respiratory distress syndrome with crazy paving. Axial CT of the chest shows bilateral diffuse panlobular ground-glass density with crazy paving especially in the right lung. Left pneumothorax (*black arrow*) decompresses into the thoracic wall soft tissues (*white arrow*) since the lungs are rigid. Chest tube on left side (*arrowhead*) in place

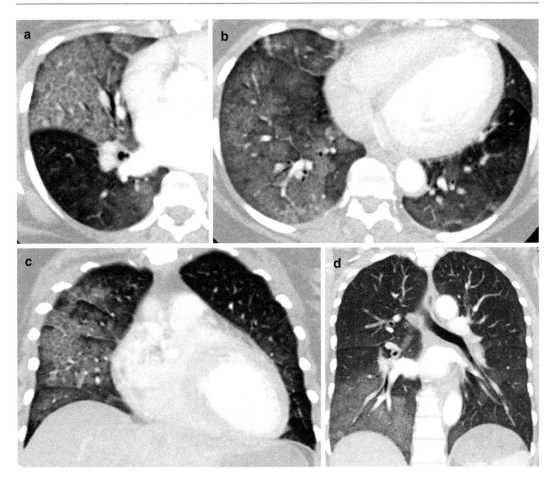

Fig. 8.58 Pulmonary contusion from motor vehicular accident with crazy paving in the right lung. Axial CT (**a**, **b**) and coronal reformatted images (**c**, **d**) show diffuse lobular ground-glass attenuation more at the right side with thick reticular pattern

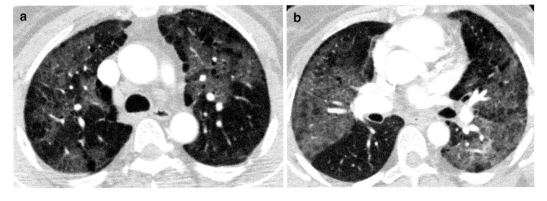

Fig. 8.59 Cryptogenic organizing pneumonia with crazy paving. (**a**, **b**) Axial CT of the chest shows with diffuse lobular ground-glass density and prominent reticular markings

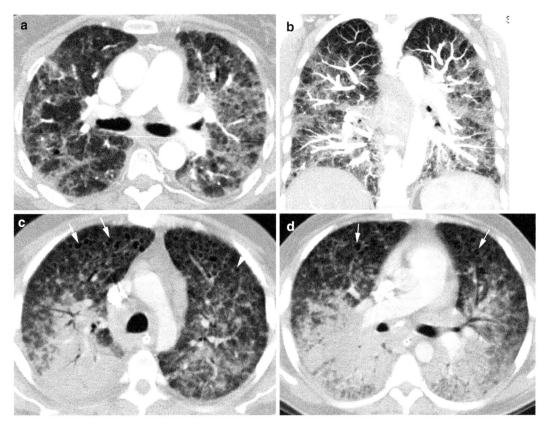

Fig. 8.60 Pneumocystis infection in two patients. Patient 1: (**a**, **b**) Axial and coronal reformatted CTs show bilateral lobular ground-glass densities with crazy paving pattern. Patient 2: (**c**, **d**) ARDS with PJP infection. Axial CT shows multiple small cyst (*arrows*), diffuse ground-glass lobular densities with crazy paving pattern, and areas of bilateral confluent lobular consolidations

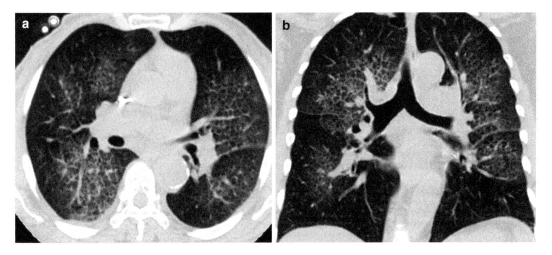

Fig. 8.61 Alveolar hemorrhage with crazy paving. Patient was ANCA positive. Lobular ground-glass density in both lungs, prominent septa bilaterally with upper lobe predominance

Mosaic Attenuation

Imaging Features
1. Patchy areas of black and white lungs
2. Infiltrative process adjacent the normal lung
3. Normal lung is denser than adjacent lung with air trapping
4. Hyperperfused lung adjacent to the oligemic lung

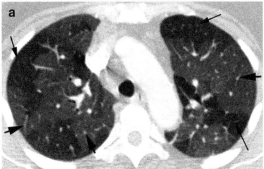
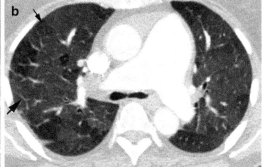

Fig. 8.62 Idiopathic pulmonary hypertension with mosaic perfusion. Axial CT in the upper and mid-lung (**a**, **b**) shows lobular low-attenuation areas of poor perfusion with decreased vascular size (*thin arrows*), and the white lung of normal perfusion has larger vessels (*thick short arrows*). (**b**) Main pulmonary artery is dilated

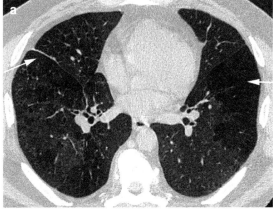
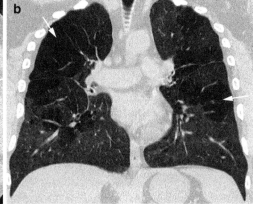

Fig. 8.63 Mosaic perfusion in bronchiolitis obliterans. Patient was exposed to toxic fumes and dust, then developed obstructive sleep apnea. (**a**, **b**) Axial and coronal reformatted CTs show large areas of low density of both lungs with decreased vascularity from bronchiolitis obliterans with air trapping (*arrows*)

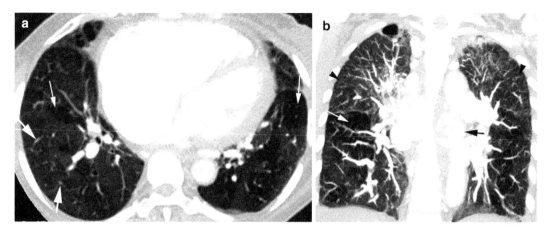

Fig. 8.64 Sarcoidosis with mosaic perfusion. History of sarcoidosis and exposure to biofuel and birds. (**a**) Axial and (**b**) coronal reformatted images show mosaic perfusion more at lung bases with lobular low-density areas with decreased vascularity (*thin white arrow*). Ground-glass density of the normal lung showing larger vessels (*thick arrow*). Small perilymphatic nodules are seen in the upper lungs (*arrowheads*) and calcified hilar lymph nodes (*black arrow*) from sarcoidosis

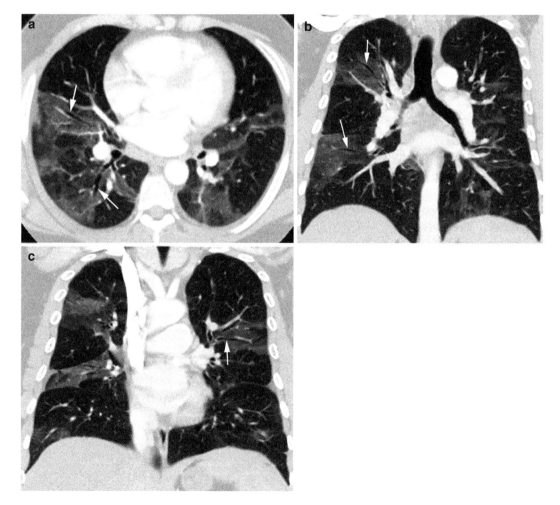

Fig. 8.65 Asthma with mosaic attenuation. History of asthma exacerbation with cocaine and heroin use. (**a–c**) Axial and coronal reformatted CTs show diffuse wedge-shaped areas of ground-glass densities of perfused lung around bronchi (*arrows*) with prominent vessels. The low-attenuated air trapped lungs show smaller vessels

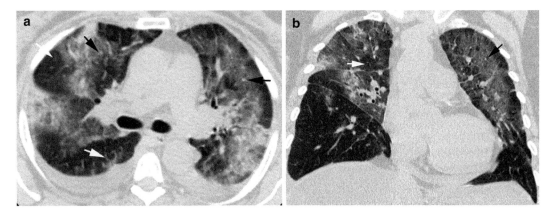

Fig. 8.66 Pneumonia with mosaic pattern. Legionella pneumonia. (**a**, **b**) Axial and coronal reformatted CTs show ground-glass infiltration interspersed with normal lungs. The vessels in the infiltrate (*black arrow*) are the same as the normal lung (*white arrow*)

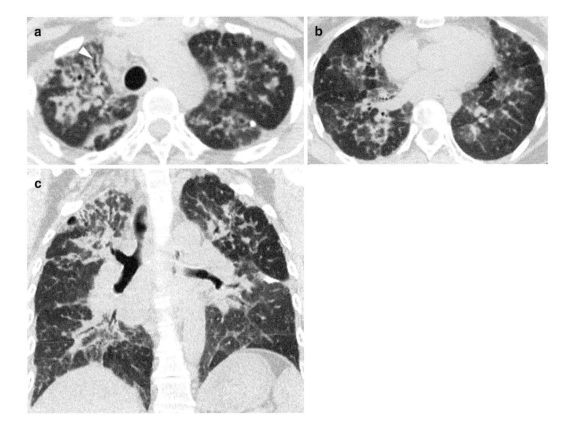

Fig. 8.67 Chronic hypersensitivity pneumonitis. (**a–c**) Axial and coronal reformatted CTs show mosaic attenuation pattern with ground-glass lobules and traction bronchiectasis (*arrowhead*) with upper lobe preponderance

Interlobular Septal Thickening

Diagnosis
Smooth Interlobular Septal Thickening

Imaging Features
1. Connective tissue polyhedral septa thickened.
2. Well seen in the apical, anterior, and lateral aspect of the upper lobes, anterior and lateral aspect of the middle lobe and lingual, anterior and diaphragmatic surfaces of the lower lobes.

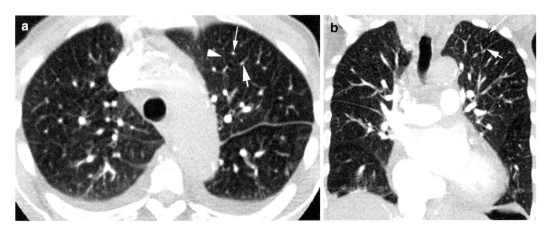

Fig. 8.68 Smooth septal thickening in CHF. A patient with atrial flutter and ejection fraction of 20 % and biatrial enlargement. (**a**) Axial CT shows diffuse interlobular septal thickening (*arrowhead*) in the upper lungs with prominent centrilobular artery (*thin long arrow*) and septal pulmonary vein (*short arrow*). (**b**) Coronal reformatted image shows the septal thickening more in the upper lungs with thick septa with vein (*short arrow*) and central pulmonary artery (*long arrow*)

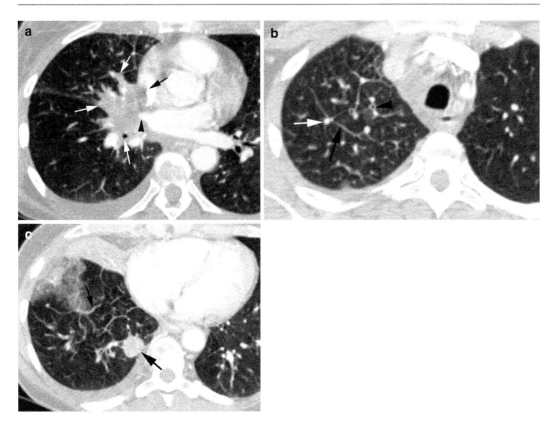

Fig. 8.69 Vascular congestion by hilar mass. (**a**) Axial CT of the chest shows right hilar mass narrowing the distal superior vena cava (*black arrow*), encasing the right superior pulmonary vein (*arrowhead*) and right lower lobe bronchus and spreading along bronchovascular distribution (*white arrows*), and impeding venous return. (**b**, **c**) Axial CT shows engorgement of the pulmonary veins in the secondary lobule (*white arrow*) and with smooth interlobular septal thickening (*thin black arrow*). The artery and bronchus are in the center of the lobule (*arrowhead*). Metastasis of the right lower lobe (*thick black arrow*)

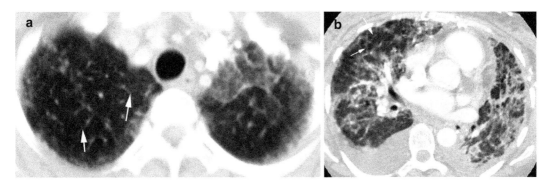

Fig. 8.70 Alveolar proteinosis in AML patient. (**a**) Axial CT shows smooth septal thickening (*arrows*) of the right upper lobe and ground-glass density with crazy paving in the left upper lobe. (**b**) One year later the lungs show increased pulmonary densities with mosaic pattern and smooth septal thickening (*arrows*) and small right pleural effusion

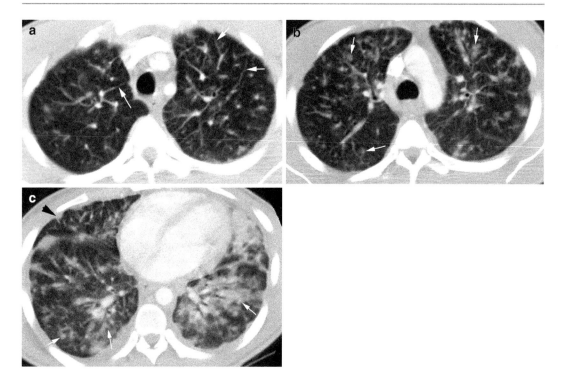

Fig. 8.71 AIDS-related Kaposi's sarcoma. (**a**) Axial CT shows smooth septal thickening best seen in the lung apices (*white arrows*). (**b**, **c**) Axial CT shows centrilobular nodules in peribronchovascular distribution (*arrows*), a few pleural-based nodules (*arrowhead*), and small right pleural effusion (**c**)

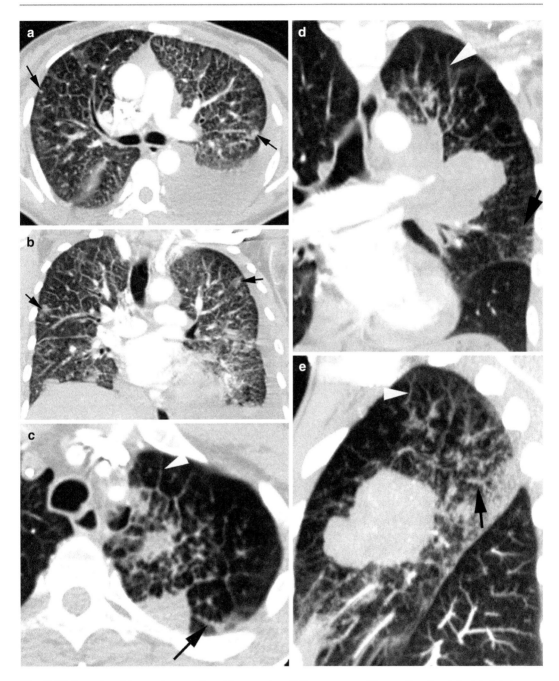

Fig. 8.72 Lymphangitic carcinomatosis with smooth interlobular septal thickening. Patient 1: metastasis from rectal adenocarcinoma. (**a**, **b**) Axial and coronal CTs show diffuse smooth interlobular septal thickening in both lungs with multiple nodular metastasis (*arrows*). Patient 2: Lung cancer with smooth and nodular interlobular septal thickening. (**c–e**) Axial, coronal, and sagittal reformatted images show smooth septal thickening in the lung apex (*arrowhead*) and nodular septal thickening (*arrow*) in posterior part of the apicoposterior segment of LUL

Diagnosis
Nodular Interlobular Septal Thickening

Imaging Features
1. Beaded appearance of the interlobular septa
2. Perilymphatic pattern associated with interstitial thickening or nodules involving

(a) Subpleural region
(b) Peribronchovascular interstitium in peri-hilar region
(c) Centrilobular peribronchovascular interstitium

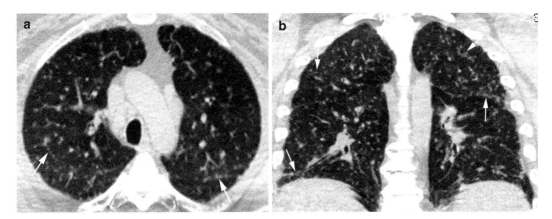

Fig. 8.73 Sarcoidosis. (**a, b**) Axial and coronal reformatted CTs showing nodularity of the septa (*arrows*), nodularity of the pleural surface, and diffuse centrilobular nodules

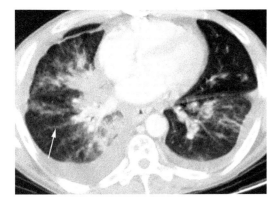

Fig. 8.74 Kaposi's sarcoma. Axial CT shows nodular septal thickening (*arrow*) and bilateral pleural effusion. Large soft tissue mass extending from the infrahilar region along the bronchovascular distribution

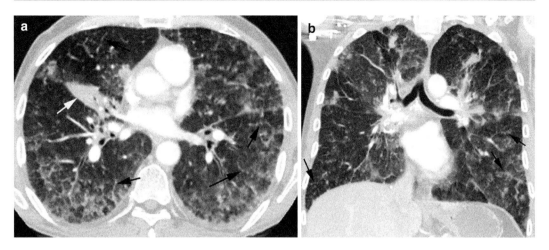

Fig. 8.75 Nodular septal thickening in acute myeloid leukemia. (**a**, **b**) Axial and coronal reformatted CTs show diffuse nodular septal thickening (*black arrows*), focal area of mass-like consolidation (*white arrow*), and diffuse patchy ground-glass densities

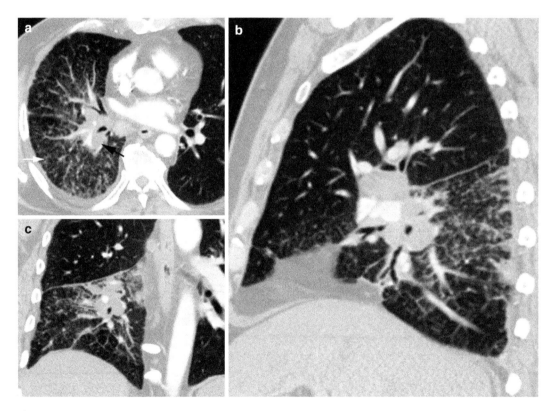

Fig. 8.76 Cryptoccocal pneumonia in HIV-positive patient. (**a–c**) Axial, sagittal, and coronal reformatted images show interstitial infiltrate in the right lower lobe with nodular septal thickening (*white arrow*) and right hilar adenopathy (*black arrow*)

Diagnosis
Irregular Septal Thickening

Imaging Features
1. Fibrosis and honeycombing
2. Distortion of lung parenchyma

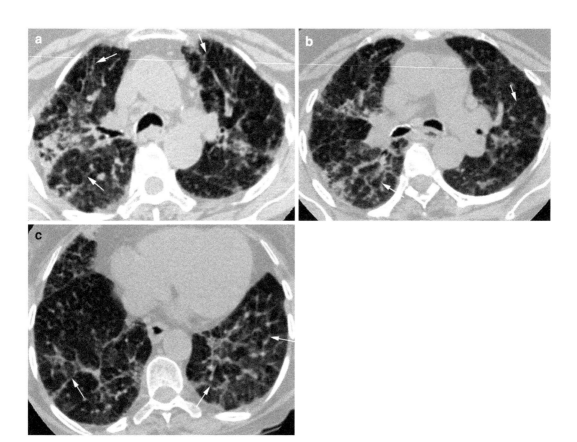

Fig. 8.77 Irregular septal thickening from 35 years of biomass fuel exposure (wood). (**a–c**) Axial CT shows irregular septal thickening (*arrows*) more in the upper lungs with ground-glass lobular densities and mosaic attenuation

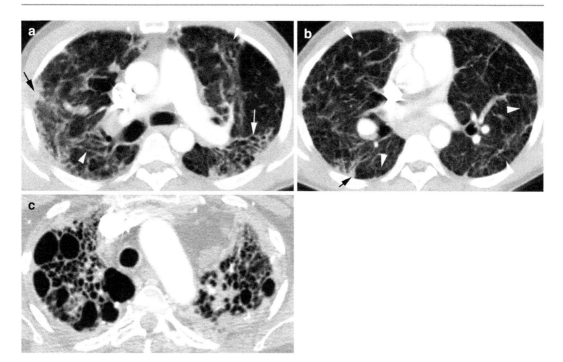

Fig. 8.78 End-stage sarcoidosis. Patient 1: (**a**, **b**) Axial CT show bronchiectasis left upper lobe (*arrow*), irregular septal thickening (*arrow heads*) and fibrotic pleural thickening (*black arrow*). Patient 2: (**c**) Axial CT shows honeycombing and cavitation and irregular septal thickening

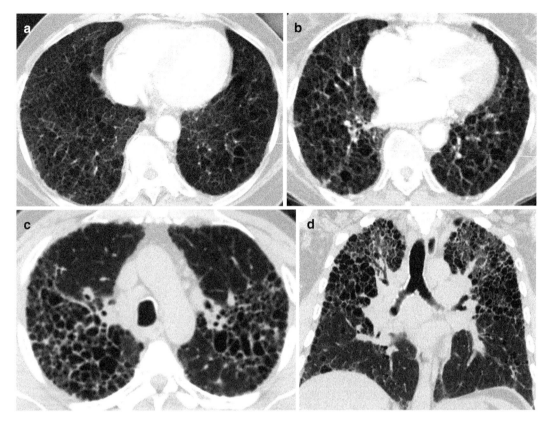

Fig. 8.79 Honeycombing in three patients. (**a**) Fibrotic NSIP in a patient with SLE. (**b**) IPF. (**a, b**) Axial CT of the chest shows clustered cystic spaces of the lung surrounded by thickened irregular septa more in lung bases. (**c, d**) In axial and coronal reformatted CTs in HP, the honeycombing has upper lobe predominance

Tuberculosis

Imaging Features

Primary TB

1. In adults dense homogeneous consolidation in any lobe; predominance in lower and middle lobe suggestive of TB.
2. Under 2 years, lobar segmental atelectasis often in the anterior segment of the upper lobe and medial segment of the middle lobe.
3. Lymphadenopathy is the hallmark, common in right paratracheal hilar stations, can be bilateral.
4. Nodes larger than 2 cm with low attenuation is suggestive of active disease.
5. LAD can be the sole feature in infants.
6. Miliary disease shows as diffuse small 2–3 mm nodules, slight lower lobe predominance, random distribution, can coalesce to form focal or diffuse consolidation in any form of disease.
7. Pleural effusion usually unilateral.

Postprimary TB

1. Predilection for apical and posterior segments of the upper lobes.
2. Patchy poorly defined consolidation.
3. Cavitation is the hallmark and are multiple within the consolidation with thick irregular wall in untreated cases.
4. Tree-in-bud appearance in endobronchial spread.
5. Tuberculomas are round oval sharply marginated lesions, single or multiple.
6. Cavitation may be complicated with mycetomas producing air crescent sign.
7. Calcified mediastinal lymph nodes may erode into the bronchus causing broncholithiasis.

TB in acquired immunodeficiency syndrome

1. Depends on level of immune suppression
2. Higher prevalence of mediastinal and/or hilar lymphadenopathy
3. Lower prevalence of cavitation

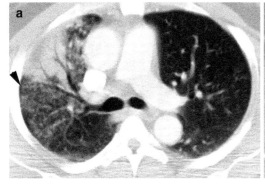
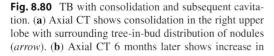
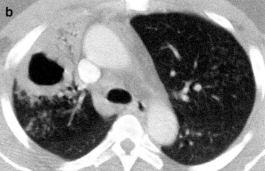

Fig. 8.80 TB with consolidation and subsequent cavitation. (**a**) Axial CT shows consolidation in the right upper lobe with surrounding tree-in-bud distribution of nodules (*arrow*). (**b**) Axial CT 6 months later shows increase in consolidation in RUL with cavitation. Nodules in RUL surrounding the cavitation have decreased but increased in the left upper lung

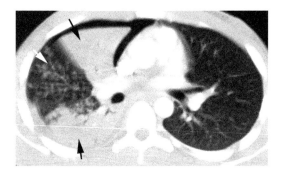

Fig. 8.81 TB consolidation. Axial CT shows two areas of consolidation (*black arrow*), endobronchial dissemination with tree-in-bud distribution (*white arrow*) and small spontaneous pneumothorax

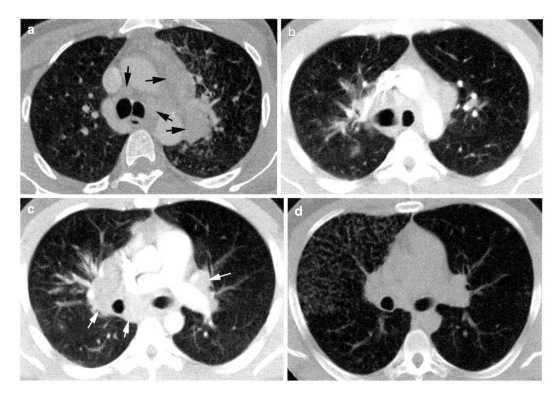

Fig. 8.82 TB lymphadenopathy. Two patients with TB having hilar and mediastinal LAD and centrilobular nodules. Patient 1 is HIV positive: (**a**) Axial CT shows mediastinal LAD (*arrows*) and lung nodules mostly left perihilar. Patient 2: (**b, c**) bilateral hilar LAD (*arrows*), very little lung nodules but peribronchial thickening in right perihilar region. (**d**) Six months later the hilar LAD has improved but the bronchocentric nodules have increased in RUL

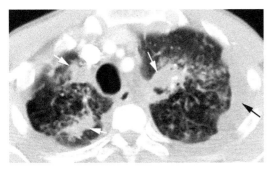

Fig. 8.83 Tuberculomas. Three solid nodules with sharp margins in both upper lungs (*white arrows*) with multiple surrounding centrilobular nodules and left pleural effusion (*black arrow*)

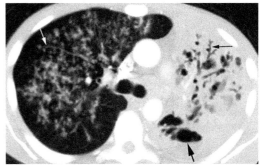

Fig. 8.84 TB, acute and chronic. Axial CT shows TB with tree-in-bud appearance of the (*white arrow*) right lung. Chronic TB in left upper lobe with chronic fibrosis causing loss of volume, traction bronchiectasis (*thin black arrow*), and cavitation (*thick black arrow*)

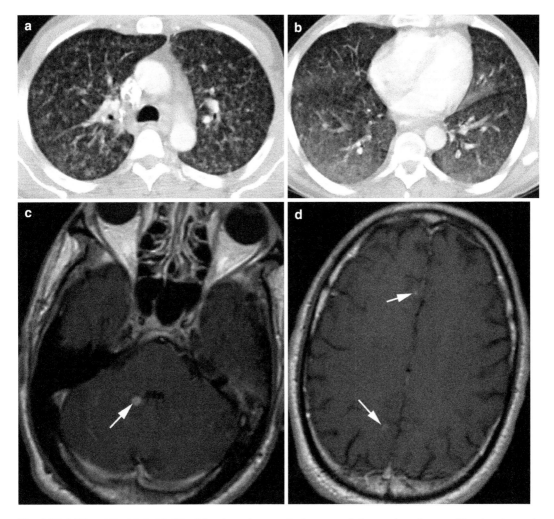

Fig. 8.85 Miliary TB. (**a**) Axial CT of the chest shows diffuse punctuate nodules in bilateral lungs.(**b**) Axial CT with the same patient shows coalescence of the nodules in the lung bases, giving ground-glass density. (**c**, **d**) MRI of brain post-gad shows tuberculomas with enhancing nodules (*arrows*). The nodule near the fourth ventricle (*arrow* in **c**) shows small central cavitation

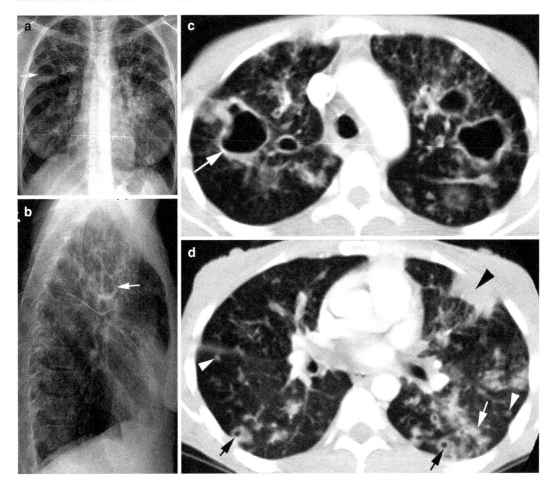

Fig. 8.86 Acute or chronic TB. (**a**, **b**) PA and lateral chest x-ray shows bilateral diffuse reticular nodular infiltrations and cavities more in the upper lungs with air-fluid level in an RUL cavity (*arrow*). (**c**) Axial CT shows multiple thick-walled cavities in the upper lungs with air-fluid level in an RUL cavity (*arrow*). (**d**) Axial CT shows focal consolidation in LUL (*black arrowhead*), conglomerated peribronchial nodules (*white arrow*), multiple small thick-walled cavities in posterior lungs (*black arrows*), and also scattered centrilobular nodules (*white arrowheads*)

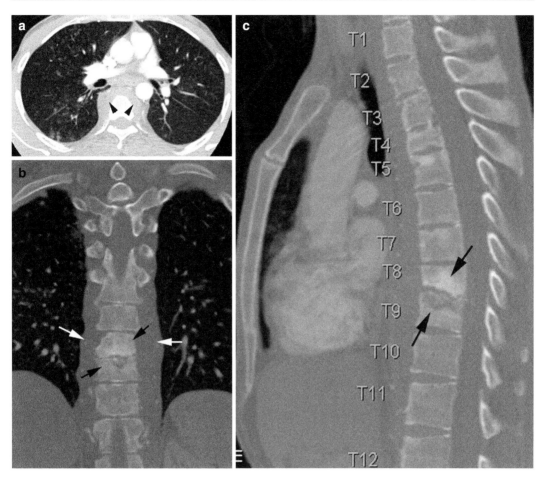

Fig. 8.87 Miliary TB with tuberculous spondylitis. (**a**) Axial CT of the chest shows diffuse miliary nodules. Paravertebral tuberculous (Pott) abscess is seen around mid-thoracic vertebrae with an increase in paravertebral soft tissue thickness (*arrow heads*). (**b, c**) Coronal and sagittal reformatted CTs of thoracic vertebrae show loss disk space at T8–T9, gibbus deformity, irregular end plates (*black arrows*), decreased disk space, and sclerosis of T8 body. Increased soft tissue is again seen around T8–T9 (*white arrows*)

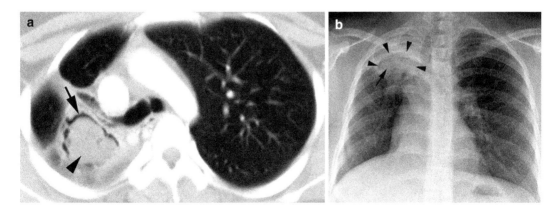

Fig. 8.88 TB mycetoma. (**a**) Axial CT of the chest shows a soft tissue mass (*arrowhead*) in a cavity surrounded by a crescent of air (*arrow*). (**b**) Chest x-ray PA view shows the mycetoma (*arrow*) in a thick-walled cavity (*arrowheads*). Both CT and chest radiograph show deviation of the superior mediastinum to the right due to fibrosis from previous TB

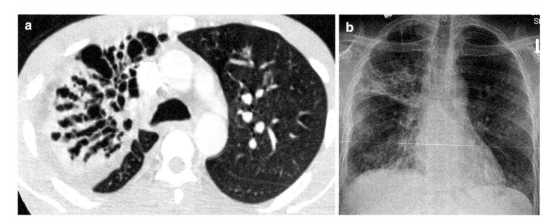

Fig. 8.89 Chronic TB with traction bronchiectasis. (**a**) Axial CT of the chest shows dilated bronchi in right upper lobe with surrounding soft tissue fibrosis causing loss of volume. (**b**) Chest radiograph PA view shows fibrotic changes in RUL posterior segment and two large bullae in the apex

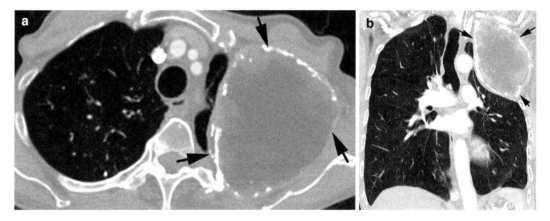

Fig. 8.90 Oleothorax. (**a**, **b**) Axial and coronal reformatted CT show deformity of left upper thoracic wall and loss of volume of left upper lobe by liquid paraffin which is surrounded by a rim of calcification (*arrows*)

Pneumocystis Infection

Imaging Features

Typical Pattern

1. Bilateral diffuse symmetric interstitial (reticular or finely granular) or ground-glass infiltrates.
2. Cystic disease is observed in one-third cases and may cause pneumothorax.
3. Distribution may vary from bilateral perihilar and lower lobe to predominantly upper lobe infiltrates.

4. Lymphadenopathy is usually not present.
5. Can progress to diffuse consolidation and adult respiratory distress syndrome.

Atypical Pattern

1. Isolated lobar disease
2. Focal parenchymal opacities or nodules
3. Cavitating nodules or masses
4. Miliary pattern
5. Endobronchial lesions
6. Pleural effusion

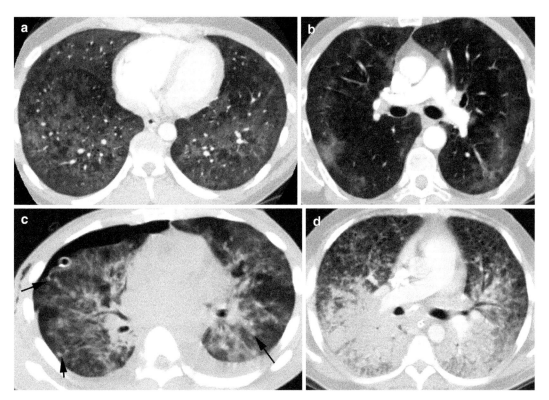

Fig. 8.91 Pneumocystis infection in different patients. Axial CT of the chest. (**a**) Diffuse ground-glass infiltration with mosaic attenuation. (**b**) Bilateral lobular ground-glass infiltration. (**c**) Diffuse ground-glass infiltration with small solid nodules (*arrows*) and spontaneous pneumothorax. (**d**) Consolidation bilateral posteriorly and small cysts anteriorly. (**e**) Ground-glass infiltration with crazy paving pattern. (**f**) Bilateral lobular ground-glass infiltration and consolidations with small bilateral pleural effusion. (**g**) Cystic pneumocystis infection with background of ground-glass density

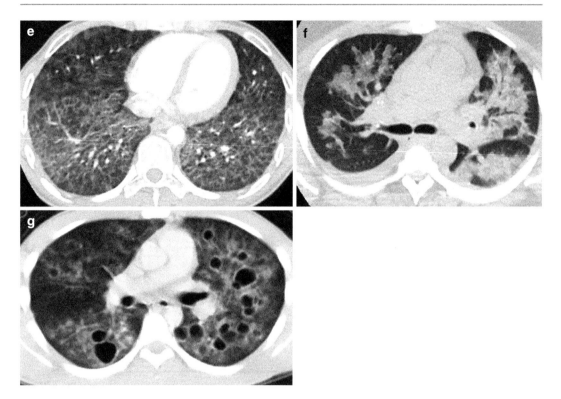

Fig. 8.91   (continued)

Hypersensitivity Pneumonitis

Imaging Features

1. Chest radiograph shows poorly defined small opacities in both lungs sometimes sparing apices and bases.
2. Ground-glass opacity with mosaic attenuation or homogeneous distribution bilaterally in middle or lung bases.

3. Chronic changes of fibrosis and traction bronchiectasis and volume loss with relative basal and extreme apical sparing.
4. Centrilobular ground-glass nodules.
5. Subpleural honeycombing mostly in mid-lung.

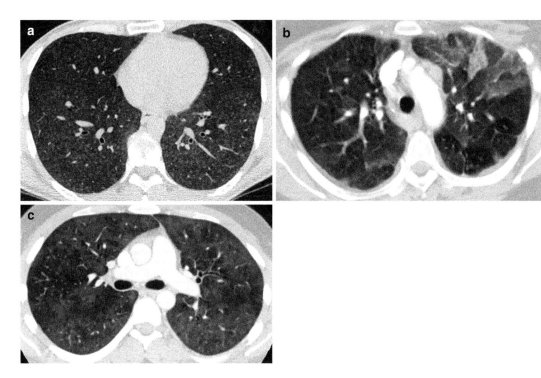

Fig. 8.92 Hypersensitivity pneumonitis. Different patients. (**a**) Axial CT of the chest shows diffuse centrilobular ground-glass nodules. (**b, c**) Diffuse bilateral lobular ground-glass densities and mosaic pattern. (**d, e**) Axial CT of chronic hypersensitive pneumonitis shows fibrotic changes with traction bronchiectasis (*arrowhead* in **d**), centrilobular nodules (*arrowhead* in **e**), lobular ground-glass opacity, and mosaic atttenuation (*arrow*) in **e**. (**f**) Chest x-ray of a patient with chronic hypersensitivity pneumonitis showing diffuse fibrotic changes with slight upper lobe predominance

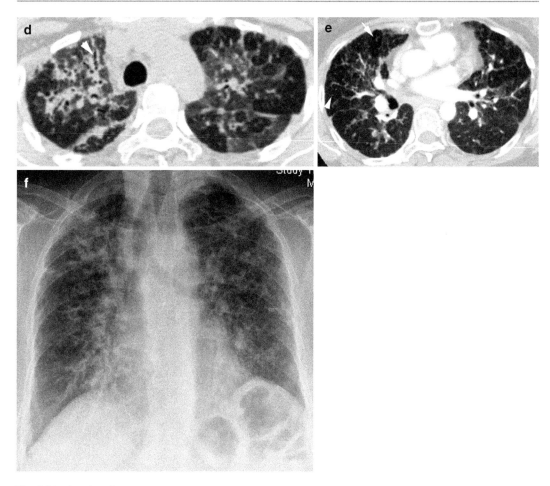

Fig. 8.92 (continued)

Sarcoidosis

Imaging Features

Common

1. Lymphadenopathy: hilar, mediastinal (right paratracheal), bilateral, symmetric and well defined.
2. Micronodules with bilateral, symmetrical distribution along lymphatics in peribronchovascular, subpleural interstitial spaces and less common in interlobular septa, in upper and middle lung.
3. Macronodules formed by coalesce of micronodules.
4. Fibrotic changes: reticular opacities, architectural distortion, traction bronchiectasis, bronchiolectasis, and volume loss.
5. Bilateral perihilar opacities.
6. Upper and mid-lung fields predominance.

Atypical

1. LAD: unilateral hilar, mediastinal only, internal mammary, paravertebral, retrocrural locations, and can have calcification
2. Air space consolidation: mass-like opacities, conglomerate masses, solitary pulmonary nodules, confluent alveolar pattern, and cavitation of nodules
3. Ground-glass opacities and mosaic attenuation
4. Linear opacities: interlobular septal thickening and intralobular linear densities
5. Fibrocystic changes: cysts, bullae blebs, emphysema, and honeycomb-like opacities with upper and mid-lung predominance
6. Miliary nodules
7. Airway involvement: mosaic attenuation, tracheobronchial abnormalities, and atelectasis
8. Pleural disease: effusion, chylothorax, hemothorax, pneumothorax, pleural thickening, and calcification
9. Mycetoma and aspergilloma

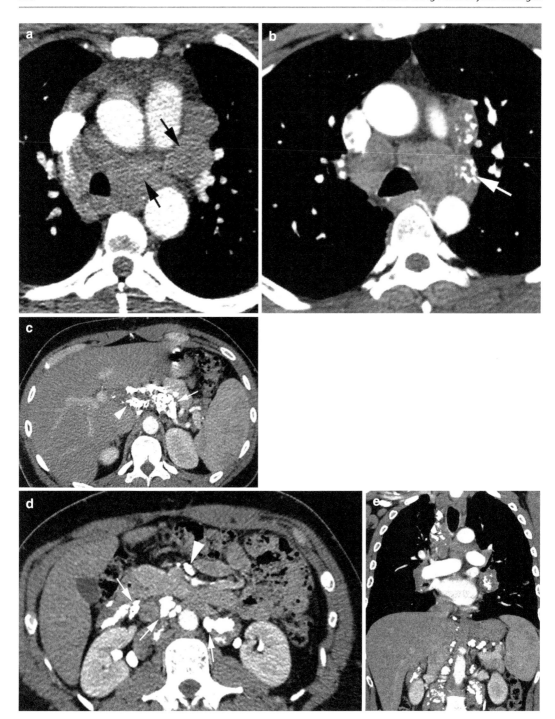

Fig. 8.93 Sarcoidosis with lymphadenopathy. (**a**, **b**) Axial CT of the chest shows (**a**) enlarged noncalcified mediastinal lymph nodes (*arrows*). (**b**) A few calcified nodes in the mediastinum (*arrow*). (**c**, **d**) Axial CT of the upper abdomen shows (**c**) calcified celiac axis (*arrow*) and periportal nodes (*arrowhead*). (**d**) Calcified nodes in retroperitoneum (*thin arrows*) and root of mesentery (*arrowhead*). (**e**) Coronal reformatted image shows the mediastinal and abdominal LAD with calcification in some nodes

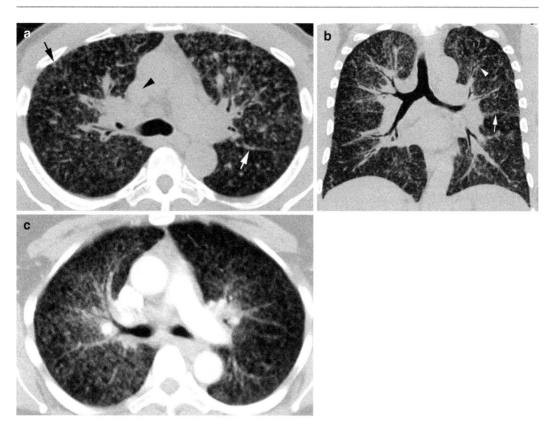

Fig. 8.94 Sarcoid micronodules. Patient 1: (**a**) Axial and (**b**) coronal reformatted images show solid micronodules in peribronchovascular (*white arrowhead*), subpleural distribution (*black arrow*) and along fissures (*thick white arrows*) with bilateral hilar adenopathy and mediastinal adenopathy (*black arrowhead*). Nodules show upper lung predominance. Patient 2: (**c**) Axial CT shows extensive micronodules in bilateral lungs

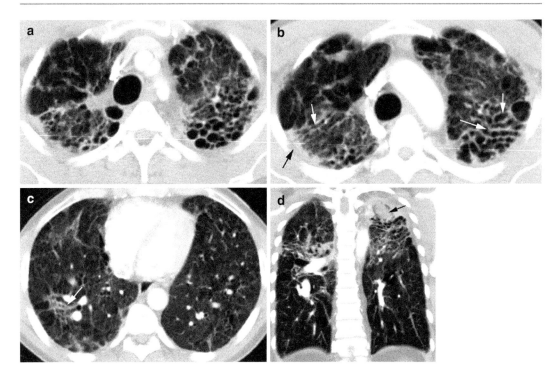

Fig. 8.95 Fibrotic stage of sarcoidosis. Axial CT (**a**) shows sarcoidosis with honeycombing of both upper lungs. (**b**) Fibrotic changes with traction bronchiectasis (*white arrow*) and pleural thickening (*black arrow*). (**c**) The mid-lung shows architectural distortion bilaterally and traction bronchiectasis (*arrow*). (**d**) Coronal reformatted CT shows fibrotic changes with upper lung predominance and mycetoma in the left apex (*arrow*)

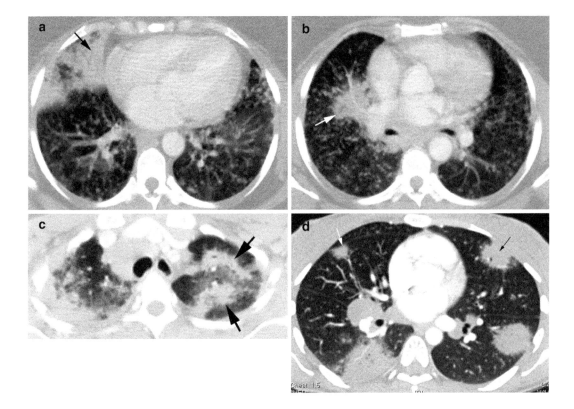

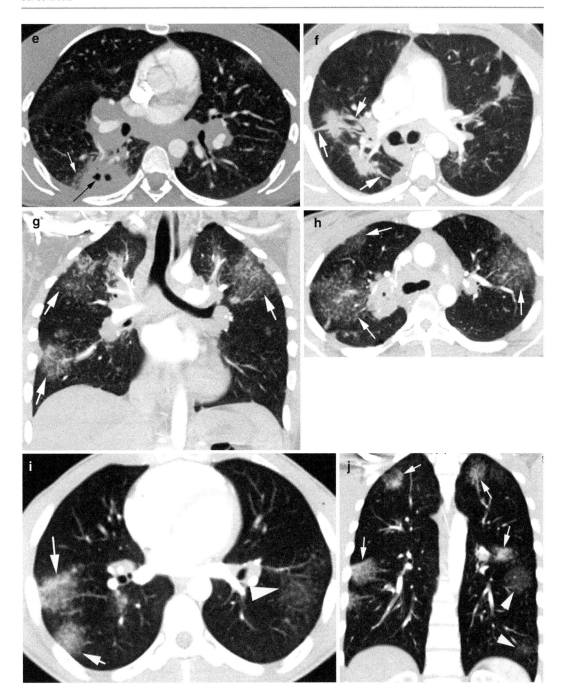

Fig. 8.96 Alveolar sarcoidosis. (**a**, **b**) Axial CT of the chest shows areas of consolidations with air bronchogram (*arrows*) and surrounding micronodules. (**c–f**) Axial CT shows large soft tissue masses (*black arrows* in **c**, *white arrow* in **d**) which are either pleural based or have pleural tags (*arrows* in **f**) with irregular margins and surrounded by micronodules (*white arrow* in **e**). Some of the nodules have central lucent cavitation (*black arrow* in **d**, **e**). (**g**, **h**). Coronal reformatted and axial CTs show conglomeration of micronodules (*arrows*) with ground-glass density (sarcoid cluster), a precursor to solid nodules. (**i**, **j**) Axial and coronal reformatted CTs show the galaxy sign with mass-forming conglomerated nodules and peripheral satellite nodules (*arrows*) and sarcoid cluster (*arrowheads*)

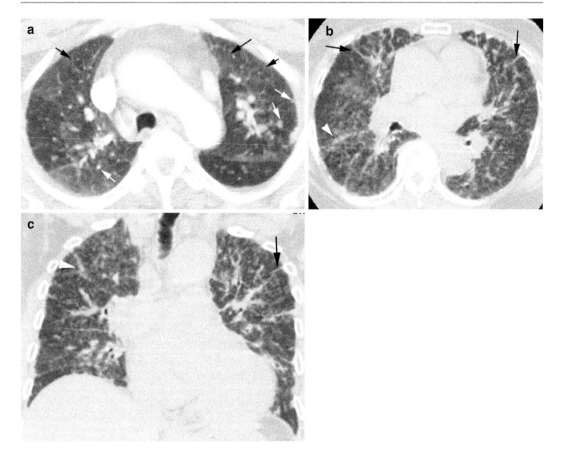

Fig. 8.97 Sarcoid with interlobular septal thickening. (**a**) Axial CT of the chest shows diffuse patchy ground-glass opacities of lung parenchyma with smooth interlobular septal thickening (*black arrows*) and centrilobular macronodules (*white arrows*). (**b**, **c**) Axial and coronal reformatted CTs show thick septal thickening (*arrows*) and nodular septal thickening (*arrowhead*)

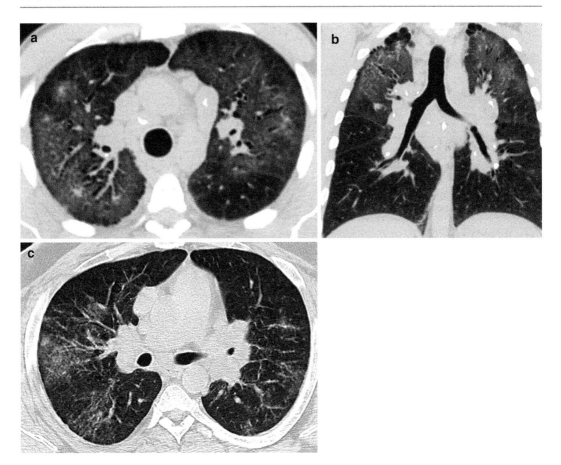

Fig. 8.98 Sarcoidosis with patchy ground-glass opacities in two patients. (**a**, **b**) Axial and coronal reformatted image shows bilateral upper lung ground-glass opacities with a few focal solid macronodules, bilateral hilar and paratracheal LAD with calcification in some nodes. (**c**) In the second patient axial CT shows bilateral patchy ground-glass densites with micronodules in peribronchovascular distribution (sarcoid cluster)

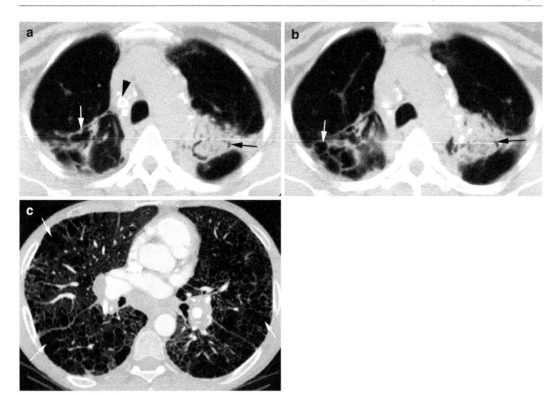

Fig. 8.99 Sarcoidosis with mycetoma, fibrocystic changes, and air trapping. (**a, b**) Axial CT shows mycetoma with air crescent sign (*thin black arrow*) in left upper lobe. Fibrocystic changes (*white arrow*) of the right upper lobe and eggshell-calcified lymph node in the mediastinum (*arrowhead*). (**c**) Different patient's axial CTs show air trapping with multiple focal areas of decrease attenuation in both mid-lungs (*arrows*) with bilateral hilar LAD

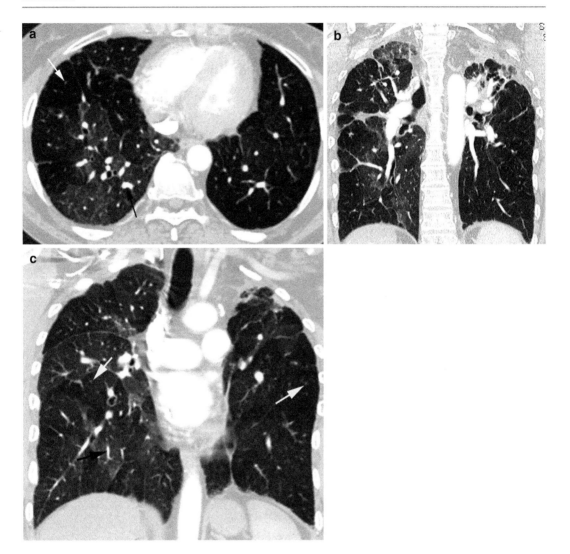

Fig. 8.100 Sarcoidosis with mosaic attenuation. History of sarcoidosis and chronic obstructive pulmonary disease. (**a**) Axial, (**b**, **c**) coronal reformatted CT in the right lung shows patchy areas of low attenuated with small vessels (*thin white arrows*) due to obstructive sarcoidosis. Adjacent ground-glass density of normal lung showing larger vessels (*black arrow*). Fibrotic changes and pleural thickening in lung apices

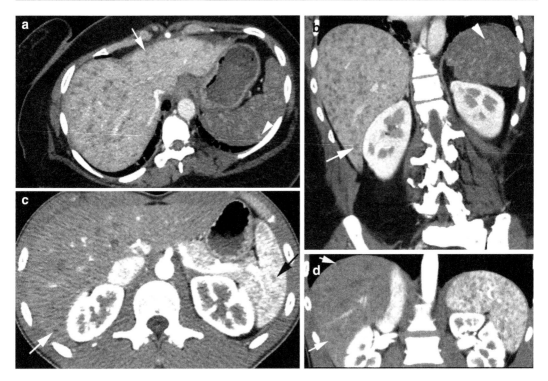

Fig. 8.101 Sarcoidosis of the liver and spleen. Patient 1: (**a**, **b**) Axial and coronal reformatted images show diffuse granulomas as low-density nodules in the liver (*arrow*) and as higher-density nodules in the spleen (*arrowhead*) since the spleen has decreased density. (**c**, **d**) Axial and coronal CTs show low-density nodules in the liver (*white arrows*) and also low-density nodules in the spleen (*black arrow*)

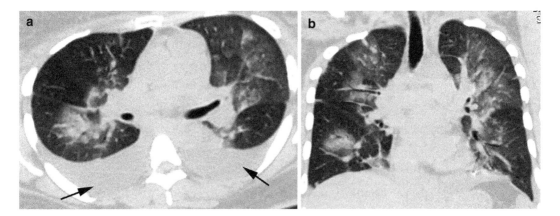

Fig. 8.102 Sarcoidosis with pleural disease. (**a**, **b**) Axial and coronal reformatted images of the chest show bilateral pleural effusion (*arrows*) and patchy ground-glass attenuation with nodules bilaterally having upper lung predominance

Silicosis

Imaging Features

1. In acute silicosis there are numerous bilateral centrilobular ground-glass nodules, patchy ground-glass opacities, and consolidation.
2. Numerous bilateral centrilobular nodules in perilymphatic distribution in paraseptal and subpleural regions.
3. Apical and posterior regions of upper lobes and apical regions of lower lobes.
4. Subpleural nodules are round or triangular shaped and may resemble pleural plaques.
5. Hilar and mediastinal lymphadenopathy may precede parenchymal lesions.
6. Calcification of lymph nodes are at the periphery with eggshell configuration.
7. Progressive massive fibrosis from expansion and conglomeration of the nodules causing soft tissue masses with irregular margins and calcification with surrounding emphysematous change.
8. Cavitation of the nodules may occur.

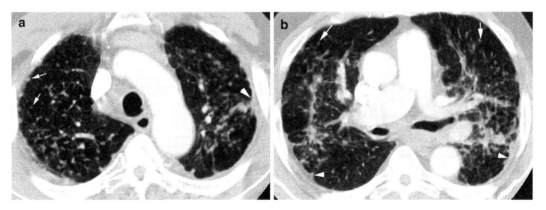

Fig. 8.103 Silicosis. (**a**, **b**) Axial CT of the chest shows multiple centrilobular nodules and subpleural nodules (*arrows*) and pleural plaques (*arrowheads*)

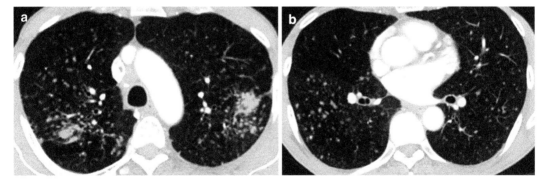

Fig. 8.104 Silicosis. Axial CT (**a**) conglomerated nodules and (**b**) diffuse centrilobular nodules less numerous in lower lung fields

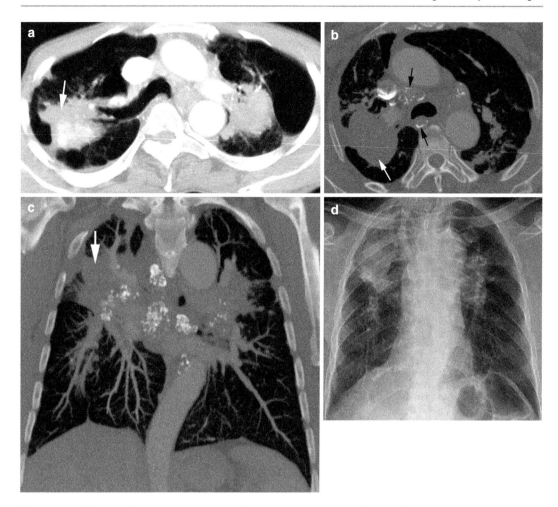

Fig. 8.105 Silicosis with progressive massive fibrosis. Axial CT (**a**, **b**) and (**c**) coronal reformatted CT show bilateral conglomerated masses with calcification (*white arrows*). (**b**, **c**) also show calcified mediastinal lymph nodes many with eggshell configuration (*black arrow*). (**d**) Chest radiograph shows large bilateral opacities in the upper lungs with upward elevation of bilateral hila

Pulmonary Aspergillosis

Imaging Features

Aspergilloma
1. Solid mass in prior cavity
2. Gravity-dependent mass with air crescent sign

Allergic bronchopulmonary aspergillosis
1. Mucoid impaction with bronchiectasis predominant in segmental and subsegmental bronchi in the upper lobes
2. Mucoid is high density or has frank calcification

Semi-invasive (chronic necrotizing) aspergillosis
1. Unilateral or bilateral segmental areas of consolidation with or without cavitation and multiple nodules
2. Aspergillous necrotizing bronchitis—endobronchial mass, obstructive pneumonitis, or collapse or hilar mass

Bronchopneumonic or airway invasive aspergillosis
1. Centrilobular nodules, tree-in-bud appearance, and peribronchial areas of consolidation

Angioinvasive aspergillosis
1. Nodules with surrounding ground-glass halo
2. Pleural-based wedge-shaped consolidation

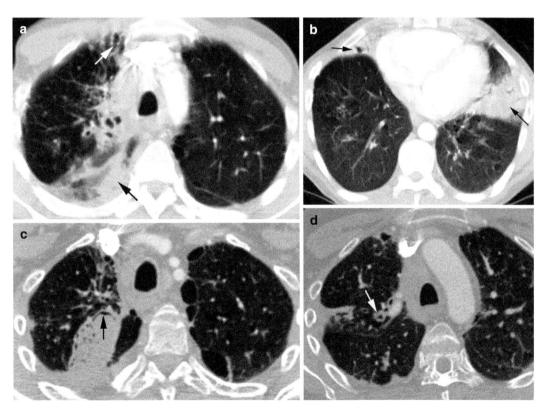

Fig. 8.106 Allergic bronchopulmonary aspergillosis in a patient with asthma. Axial CT (**a, b**) shows focal areas of atelectasis or consolidation of right upper lobe, lingular segment and middle lobe (*black arrows*). (**c**) Mycetoma of the right upper lobe with air crescent sign (*arrow*). Dilated bronchi with wall thickening (*white arrow* in **a, d**)

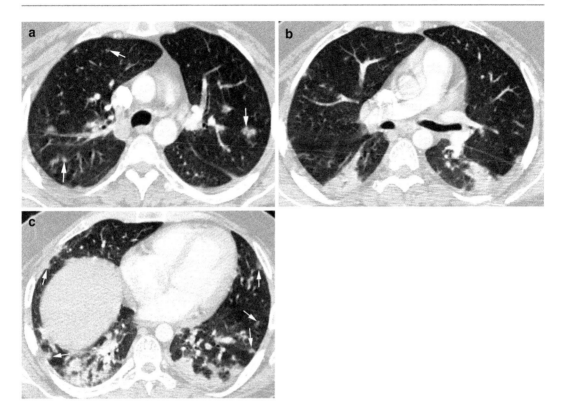

Fig. 8.107 Invasive aspergillosis in a patient with pre-B-ALL and neutropenic fever. (**a–c**) Axial CT shows multiple nodules (*arrows*) and consolidations and small pleural effusion. Some of the nodules are peripherally located and ill marginated (*arrows*)

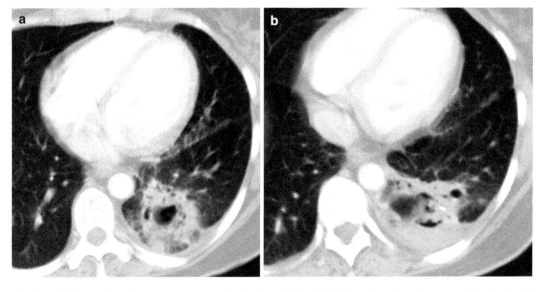

Fig. 8.108 Chronic invasive pulmonary aspergillosis in a patient with AML and neutropenic fever. (**a, b**) Axial CT shows cavitary consolidation with surrounding reticulation and pleural thickening

Interstitial Lung Disease

Diagnosis

Idiopathic Interstitial Pneumonia

Usual interstitial pneumonia and idiopathic pulmonary fibrosis: Subpleural reticular opacities, macrocystic honeycombing, traction bronchiectasis, and basal peripheral predominance

Nonspecific interstitial pneumonia

Cellular and fibrotic phases, ground-glass opacities, varying degrees of reticulation and consolidation, and microcystic honeycombing. Traction bronchiectasis in fibrotic phase, no obvious gradient, subpleural, and symmetrical

Cryptogenic organizing pneumonia

Patchy ground-glass opacities to consolidations in peribronchial or peripheral distribution with mild bronchial dilatation and basal preponderance sometimes sparing the subpleural space

Respiratory bronchiolitis–associated interstitial lung disease

Centrilobular nodules, patchy ground-glass opacities, and bronchial wall thickening with diffuse or upper lung predominance

Lymphoid interstitial pneumonia

Ground-glass opacities, perivascular cysts, septal thickening, centrilobular nodules bilaterally diffuse and symmetrical, and lower lobe predominance

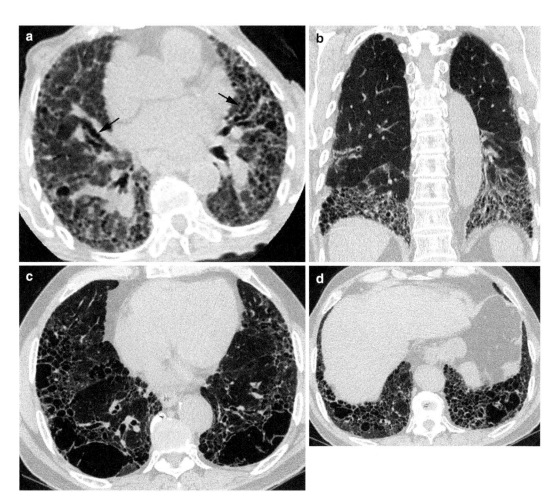

Fig. 8.109 UIP due to IPF. Two male patients with progressive shortness of breath and cough. Patient 1: (**a**, **b**) Axial and coronal reformatted CT of a 71-year-old male shows subpleural reticular opacities, honeycombing, traction bronchiectasis (*arrows*), and mild ground-glass opacity with basilar predominance. Patient 2: (**c**, **d**) Axial CT shows architectural distortion, honeycombing, and bronchiectasis. Patient has history of repeated episodes of pneumothorax

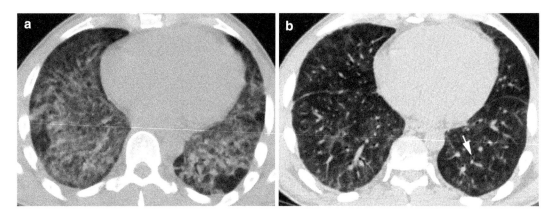

Fig. 8.110 NSIP cellular form in a 42-year-old man either methotrexate induced or from rheumatoid arthritis. Axial CT (**a**) shows diffuse ground-glass densities and reticulation in lung bases. (**b**) Improvement of ground-glass and reticular densities following treatment. Some bronchi show minimal wall thickening (*arrow*)

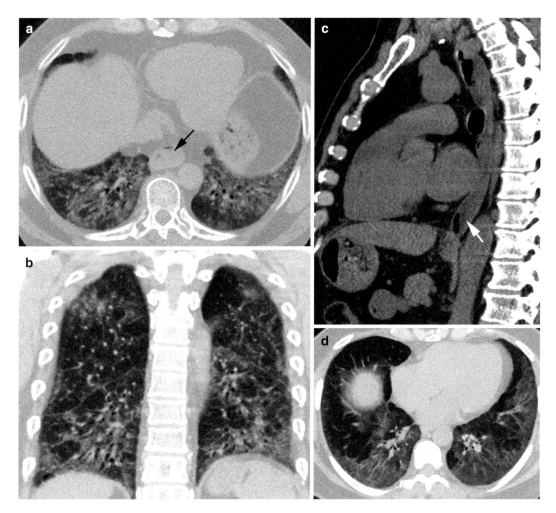

Fig. 8.111 Cellular NSIP. Ground-glass attenuation with basal predominance with fine reticulation and mild bronchiectasis. (**a–c**) A 47-year-old female with scleroderma and joint pain. Axial, coronal, and sagittal reformatted CTs also show dilated esophagus (*arrows*). (**d–f**) Axial, coronal, and sagittal reformatted CTs of a 45-year-old female with Sjogren's syndrome having dyspnea and non-pleuritic chest pain and generalized joint pain. (**g, h**) A 59-year-old female with SLE and rheumatoid arthritis having shortness of breath. Coronal reformatted and axial image also shows few scattered solid nodules (*arrows*)

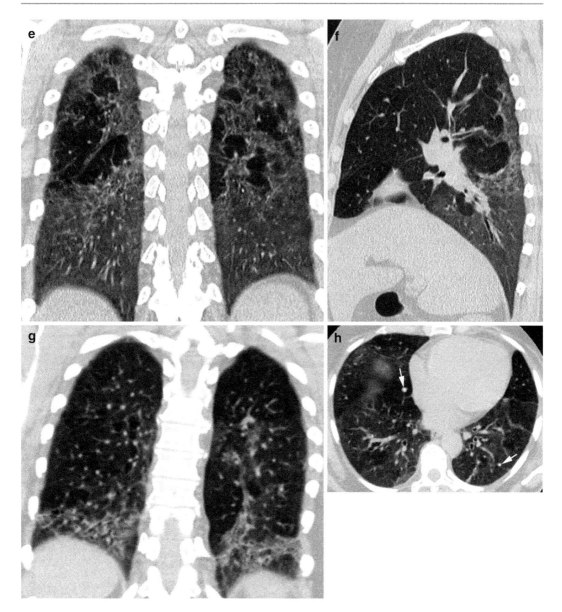

Fig. 8.111 (continued)

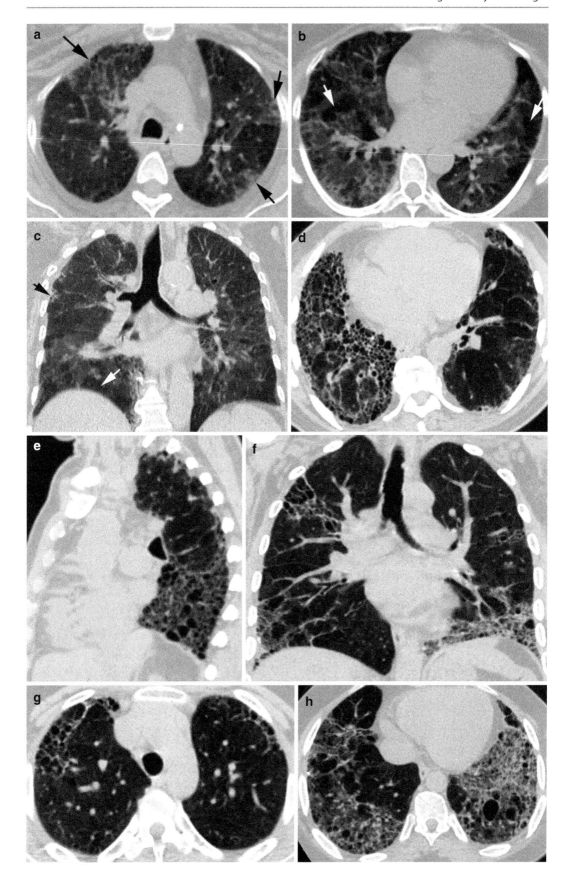

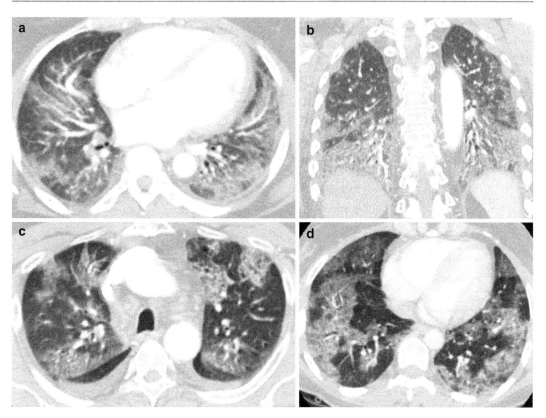

Fig. 8.113 Cryptogenic organizing pneumonia biopsy proven. (**a**, **b**) Patient with polymyositis. Axial and coronal CTs show bilateral ground-glass densities mostly peripheral and lower lobe predominance. (**c**, **d**) Axial CT of different patients shows peripheral ground-glass lobular densities. History of chronic usage of amiodarone

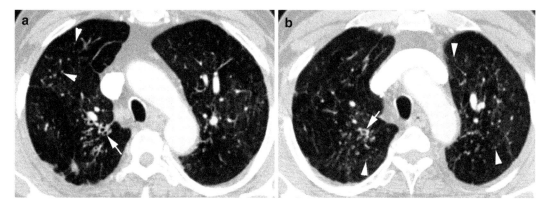

Fig. 8.114 RB-ILD in a 42-year-old male, chronic smoker. (**a**, **b**) Axial CT shows bronchial wall thickening (*arrow*) with patchy ground-glass densities and multiple centrilobular nodules (*arrowheads*)

Fig. 8.112 Fibrotic form of NSIP. Patient 1: History of RA and shortness of breath. (**a**, **b**) Axial and (**c**) coronal reformatted CTs show mild fibrotic changes with mild traction bronchiectasis in the upper lobes (*black arrows*), ground-glass densities with mosaic pattern (*white arrow*) more in the lower lobes with increased interstitial thickening of the lower lobes. Patient 2: A 72-year-old man with RA having marked shortness of breath. (**d**) Axial and (**e**) sagittal reformatted CTs show very little ground-glass density and honeycombing with basal predominance. Patient 3: History of JRA. (**f**) Coronal reformatted CT and (**g**, **h**) axial CT show fibrosis with honeycombing of both lungs with lower lobe predominance

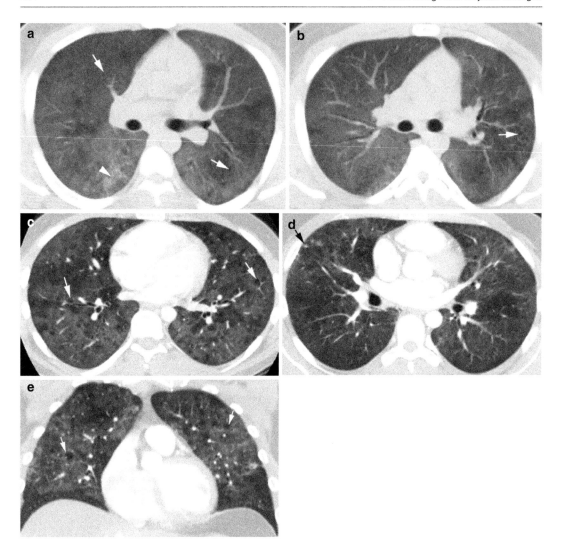

Fig. 8.115 Lymphoid interstitial pneumonia in a 22-year-old male with hyper-IgM hypogammaglobulinemia presenting with cough. (**a**, **b**) Axial CT of the chest shows bilateral diffuse ground-glass density and with perivascular cysts (*arrow*) and septal thickening (*arrowhead*). Improved with steroid therapy. Patient 2 with AIDS: (**c**) Axial CT shows diffuse ground-glass density in both lungs with multiple cysts mostly perivascular (*arrows*). (**d**, **e**) Axial and coronal reformatted CTs 10 years later show increased density of some areas of GGO and some centrilobular nodules (*black arrow*). Diffuse cysts are again seen (*white arrow*)

Pulmonary Edema

Imaging Features
1. Diffuse ground-glass attenuation—distribution depends on the etiology.
2. Interlobular septal thickening

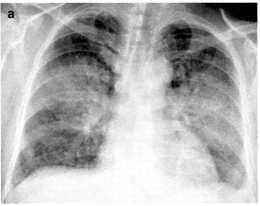 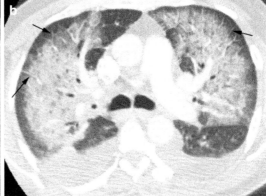

Fig. 8.116 Acute pulmonary edema. Flash pulmonary edema due to fluid overload from IV infusion. (**a**) Chest x-ray. (**b**) Axial CT of the chest. Diffuse bilateral ground-glass density with batwing distribution, sparing periphery of the lung with interlobular septal thickening (*arrows*) and bilateral pleural effusion

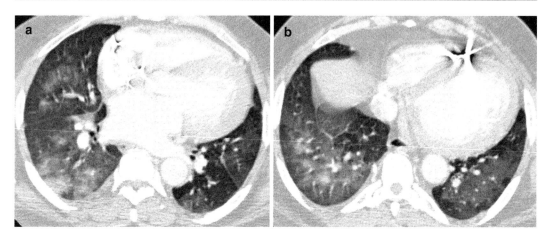

Fig. 8.117 Pulmonary edema from CHF. (**a**, **b**) Axial CT shows ground-glass densities predominant at the bases and dependent lungs. Pacemaker lead is in the right ventricle

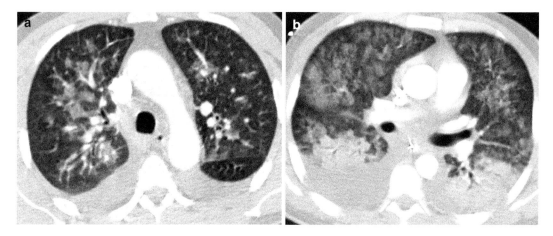

Fig. 8.118 CHF with bicuspid aortic valve and aortic stenosis. (**a**, **b**) Axial CT shows bilateral pulmonary edema with lobular ground glass densities with lower lobe predominance and bilateral pleural effusion

Adult Respiratory Distress Syndrome

Imaging Features
1. Heterogeneous areas of ground-glass opacity, usually symmetrical.

2. Consolidations usually in the vertebral-basal areas of the lungs.
3. Modest pleural effusion is common.
4. Pneumatoceles are seen later in the disease.

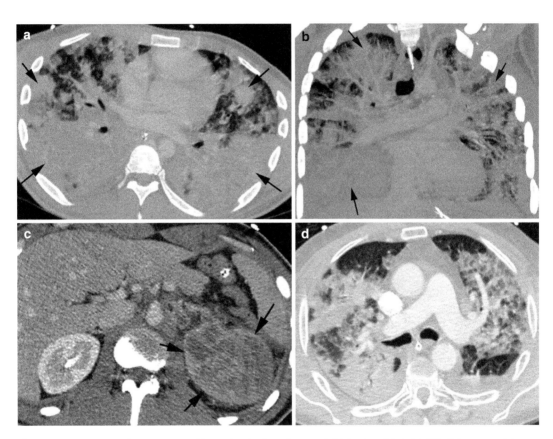

Fig. 8.119 ARDS. Patient 1 (**a–c**) with septic shock. Patient with renal cell carcinoma (rcc), lung metastasis, and pneumonia. (**a, b**) Axial and coronal reformatted CTs show diffuse patchy areas of consolidation (*black arrow*) along bronchovascular distribution and smooth interlobular septal thickening. (**c**) Axial CT of the upper abdomen shows heterogeneous enhancing RCC of the upper pole left kidney (*arrows*). Patient 2: Post-trauma. (**d**) Axial CT shows diffuse areas of solid and ground-glass densities in both lungs and small left pleural effusion

Cavitating Lesions

Diagnosis
Septic Emboli

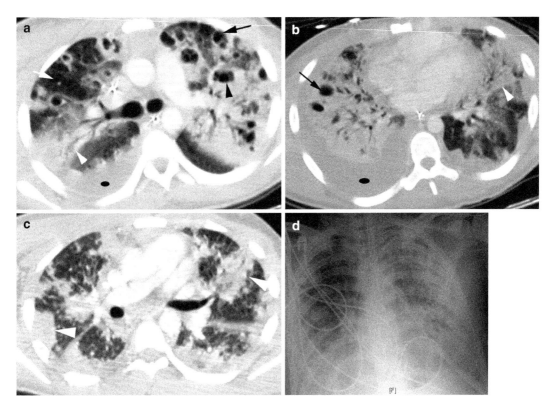

Fig. 8.120 Septic emboli with septic shock and MRSA bacteremia. (**a**, **b**) Axial CT shows multiple peripherally distributed septic emboli (*long black arrows*), some with abscess formation with air-fluid levels (*black arrowhead*), patchy areas of consolidation with air bronchogram (*white arrowhead*), interspersed normal lung (*white arrow*), and moderate right pleural effusion (ellipse). (**c**) Axial CT of the chest shows multiple subpleural consolidations (*arrowheads*). (**d**) Chest x-ray shows peripheral infiltrations due to location of septic emboli and consolidations

Diagnosis
Necrotizing Pneumonia

Imaging Findings
1. Area of consolidation
2. Cavity or cavities with no rim enhancement within the consolidation filled with fluid or with air-fluid level

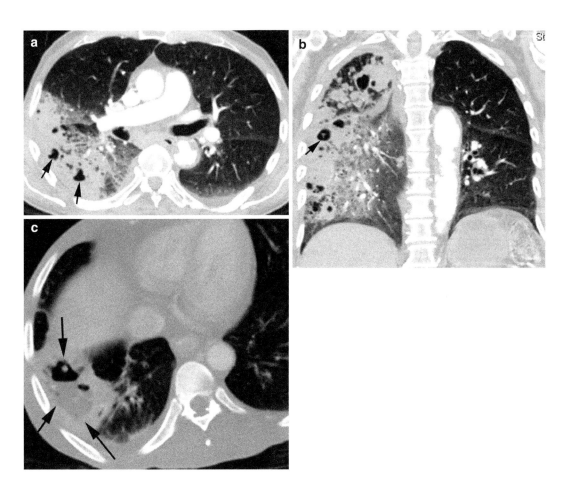

Fig. 8.121 Necrotizing pneumonia in two patients. Patient 1: (**a**, **b**) Axial and coronal reformatted CTs in a patient with prostate cancer show diffuse consolidation with surrounding ground-glass density in the right lung with multiple foci of necrosis with air and air-fluid collections (*arrows*) within the consolidated lungs with no rim enhancement. Patient 2 with diabetes, IVDU, and alcohol abuse presents with septic shock. (**c**) Axial CT shows necrotizing pneumonia of the right lung base, air-fluid collection in a consolidation (*black arrows* in **c** and *white arrows* in **d**, **f**). (**d**) Coronal reformatted CT shows the infection with gas extending inferiorly from the lung (*white arrow*) along the costal attachments of the diaphragm (*black arrow*). The adrenal gland has increased enhancement due to marked drop in blood pressure. The distal small bowel shows ischemic changes with target appearance (*arrowhead*). (**e**, **f**) Axial and sagittal reformatted CTs show the infection to invade the liver with irregularity of the right lobe near the costal margin (*black arrows* in **f** and *white arrow* in **e**). Multiple liver abscesses (*black arrows*) and small bowel ischemia (*white arrowhead*) are seen. (**g**) Axial CECT of the brain shows two abscesses in the left side with rim enhancement (*arrows*)

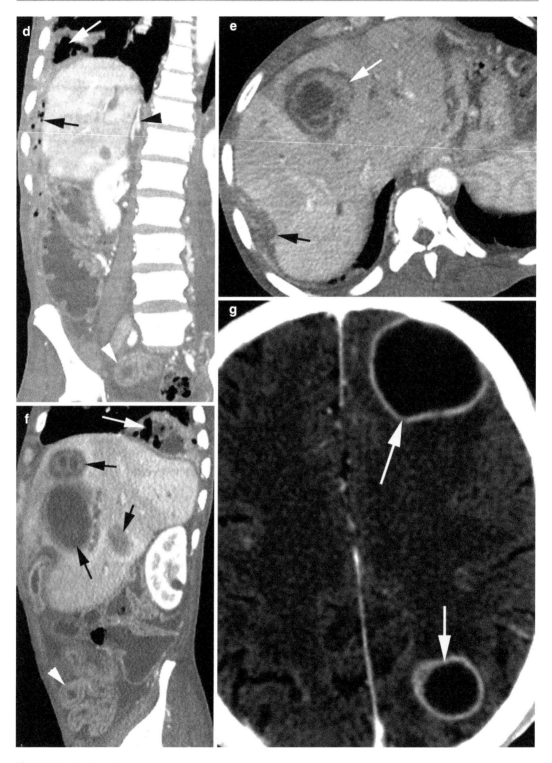

Fig. 8.121 (continued)

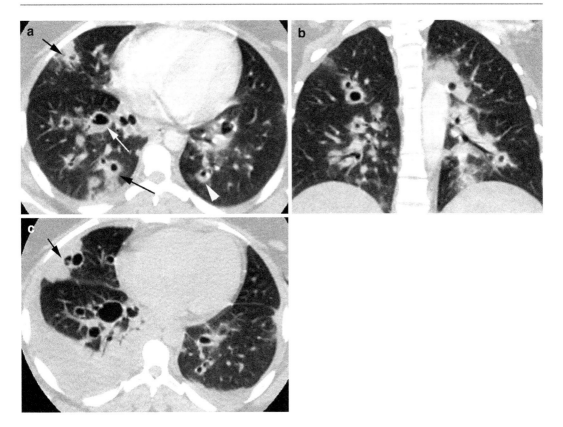

Fig. 8.122 Cavitating pneumonia due to fungal infection. Axial CT (**a**, **b**) shows multiple thick-walled cavities (*arrowhead*), some with associated consolidation (*black arrows*) and some with air-fluid levels (*white arrow*) involving the central, middle and peripheral lungs. (**c**) One month later the cavities and some consolidations (*black arrow*) have increased with bilateral pleural effusion

Diagnosis
Lung Abscess

Imaging Features
1. Thick-walled cavity with air-fluid level.
2. Inner margin is smooth.
3. Large surrounding area of parenchymal edema with ground-glass density.

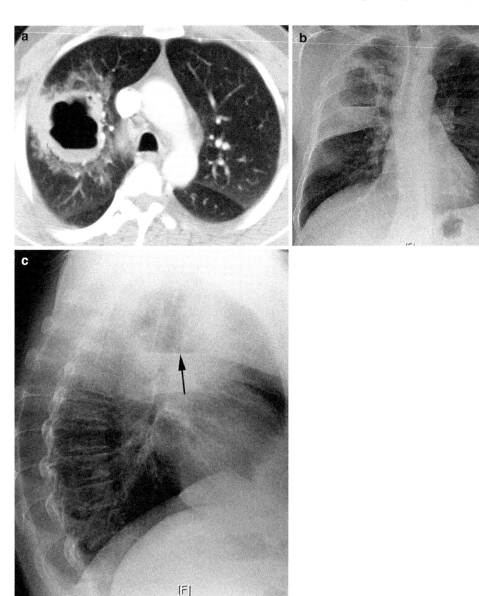

Fig. 8.123 Lung abscess. Clinical presentation of cough, chest pain, and hemoptysis. (**a**) Axial CT, (**b**, **c**) chest PA, and lateral x-rays show a thick-walled cavity with air-fluid level (*arrow*). The surrounding lung shows diffuse inflammatory changes with edema as ground-glass density

Diagnosis

Necrotic Lung Mass with Superimposed Infection

Imaging Features

1. Thick-walled mass with air-fluid level.
2. Surrounding lung parenchyma shows no significant edema.

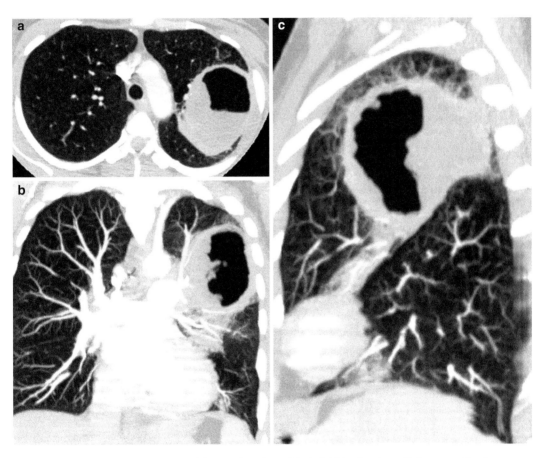

Fig. 8.124 Non-small cell lung cancer with necrosis and superimposed infection. Axial (**a**), coronal (**b**), and (**c**) sagittal reformatted CTs show large thick-walled cavity with air-fluid level and very little surrounding lung parenchymal reaction. The inner wall of the cavity is nodular and irregular

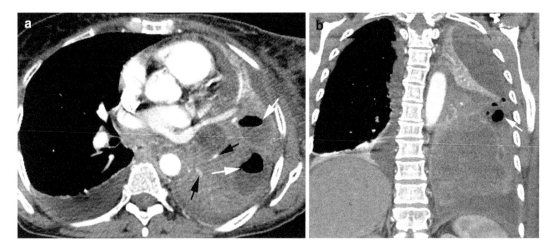

Fig. 8.125 Necrotic squamous cell carcinoma with superimposed infection. (**a**, **b**) Axial and coronal reformatted images show a large mass with prominent internal vessels (*black arrows*) and several necrotic areas, some with air-fluid collections from superimposed infection (*white arrow*)

Diagnosis

Infected Intralobar Bronchopulmonary Sequestration

Imaging Features

1. Large left lower lobe posterior segment of soft tissue mass
2. Anomalous systemic arterial supply
3. Multiple cystic spaces with gas collections and fluid levels

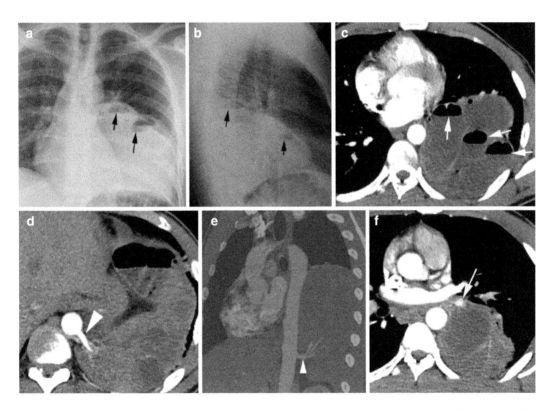

Fig. 8.126 Infected intralobar bronchopulmonary sequestration. A young patient comes in with pneumonia-like symptoms. (**a**, **b**) Chest radiograph PA and lateral views show a large soft tissue mass with air-fluid collections (*arrows*) in the paravertebral gutter of the left lower lobe posterior segment. (**c**) Axial CT of the chest shows large soft tissue mass in the left lower lobe with multiple cystic space, some having air-fluid level (*arrows*). (**d**, **e**) Axial and oblique coronal CTs show the vascular supply of the mass from the upper abdominal aorta (*arrowhead*). (**f**) Axial CT shows venous drain into the left pulmonary vein (*arrow*)

Diagnosis

Granulomatosis with Polyangiitis (Wegener's Granulomatosis)

Imaging Features

A. Nodules:
1. Single or multiple nodules from few millimeters to 10 cm in size.
2. Random distribution but can be peribronchovascular, subpleural and angiocentric, and rarely centrilobular.
3. Central cavitation common in nodules larger than 2 cm.
4. Margins may show ground-glass halo, radiating linear scarring, spiculations, and pleural tags.
B. Ground-glass opacity and consolidation
C. Pleural effusion, may have acute or chronic fibrinous pleuritis
D. Tracheal narrowing; mediastinal lymphadenopathy is uncommon

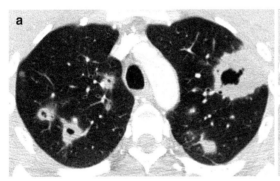
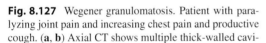
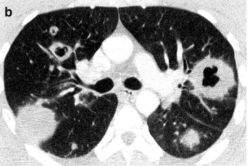

Fig. 8.127 Wegener granulomatosis. Patient with paralyzing joint pain and increasing chest pain and productive cough. (**a**, **b**) Axial CT shows multiple thick-walled cavitating nodules of varying size, ground-glass to speculated margins, and in random distribution

Diagnosis

Sarcoid Granulomatosis with Cavitation or Cyst Formation

Imaging Features

1. Multiple bilateral nodules in subpleural and peribronchovascular distribution.
2. Nodular margins are ill-defined, are irregular, and can have satellite peripheral nodules giving the galaxy sign.
3. Some nodules cavitate or heterogeneously enhance.
4. Hilar adenopathy is variable.

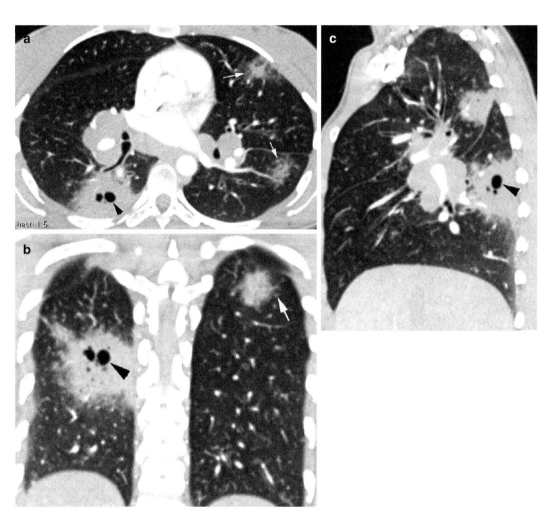

Fig. 8.128 Necrotizing sarcoid granulomatosis. (**a–c**) Axial, coronal, and sagittal CT of the chest shows a large pleural-based solid nodule in the right lower lobe with central cavities (*arrowhead*). Solid nodules are seen in the left lung with satellite nodules (*white arrows*) and with bilateral hilar adenopathy

Diagnosis
Infected Bulla

Imaging Features
1. Multiple bullae with thin walls.
2. Infected bulla has thicker wall with air-fluid level.

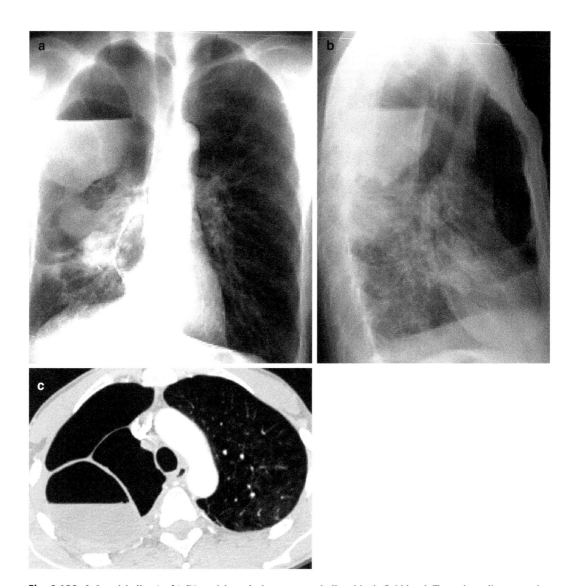

Fig. 8.129 Infected bulla. (**a**, **b**) PA and lateral chest radiograph shows thin-walled bulla with air-fluid level in the right upper lobe. (**c**) Axial CT of the chest shows the same bulla with air-fluid level. Two other adjacent noninfected bullae are seen

Pleural Disease with Acute Symptoms

R. Agarwala, *Atlas of Emergency Radiology:*
Vascular System, Chest, Abdomen and Pelvis, and Reproductive System,
DOI 10.1007/978-3-319-13042-2_9, © Springer International Publishing Switzerland 2015

Diagnosis

Tension Pneumothorax

Imaging Features

1. Plain chest radiograph shows hyperexpanded hemithorax with no lung markings and deep sulcus sign.
2. The ipsilateral lung is collapsed and the diaphragm depressed.
3. A few linear strands extend from the collapsed lung to the thoracic wall due to fibrotic adhesions.
4. The mediastinum is shifted to the contralateral side.

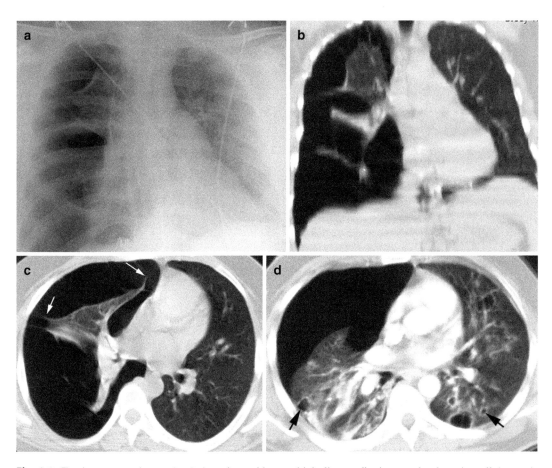

Fig. 9.1 Tension pneumothorax. (**a–c**) A patient with asthma experienced sudden shortness of breath. (**a**) Chest AP view and (**b**) coronal reformatted and (**c**) axial CT show shift of the mediastinum to the left and a deeper right costophrenic angle. The collapsed right lung shows multiple linear adhesions to the thoracic wall (*arrows*). (**d**) Axial CT of a patient with cystic pneumocystis infection shows right tension pneumothorax. Multiple cystic lesions (*arrows*) are seen bilaterally

Diagnosis

Empyema

Imaging Features

1. Large fluid and gas collection in the pleural space
2. Split pleural sign with enhancing pleura
3. Compressive collapse of the adjacent lung

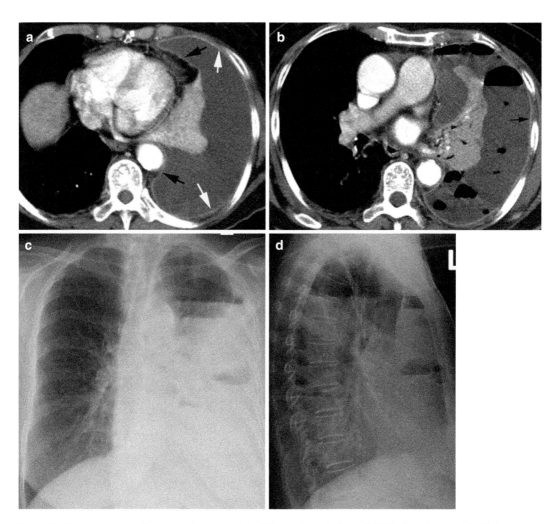

Fig. 9.2 Empyema. (**a**) Contrast-enhanced axial CT shows large pleural fluid surrounded by enhancing pleura with split pleural sign of parietal pleura (*white arrows*) and visceral pleura (*black arrows*). The left lung is collapsed. (**b**) Axial CT of the chest and (**c, d**) chest x-ray PA and lateral views 1 week later show development of gas collections in the pleural fluid with air-fluid levels. The pleura is still thick and enhancing (*arrow* in **b**)

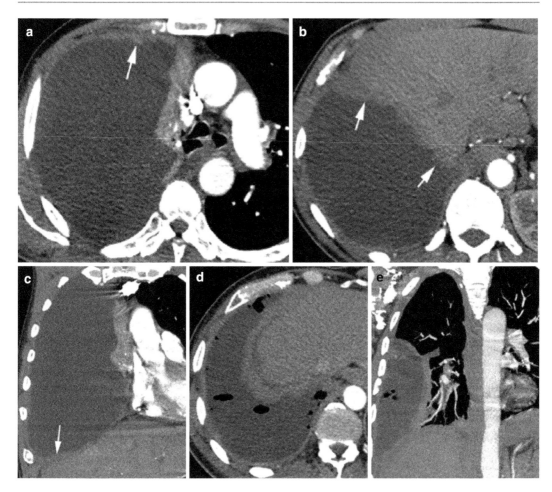

Fig. 9.3 Pleural mesothelioma with TB infection and biopsy-confirmed noncaseating granulomas. Axial (**a**, **b**) and coronal reformatted (**c**) CTs show irregular and nodular thickening of the visceral and parietal pleura (*arrows*) with enhancement similar to the intercostal muscles and liver. (**d**, **e**) Axial and coronal reformatted images show hydropneumothorax from biopsy

Diagnosis

Empyema Necessitans

Imaging Features

1. Chronic empyema which decompresses through the chest wall

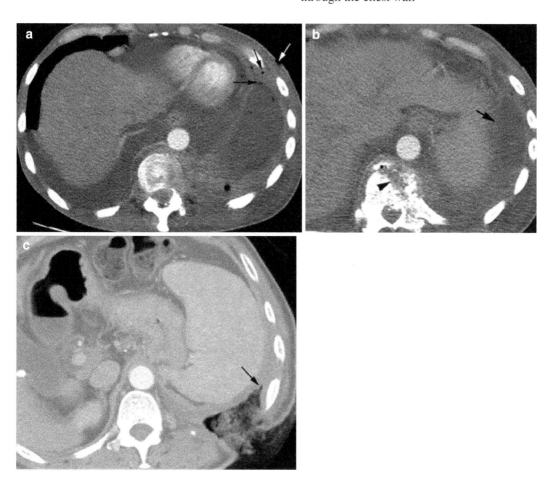

Fig. 9.4 Empyema necessitans in a patient with chronic skin boil presenting with cough, shortness of breath, and back pain. (**a**) Axial CT of the chest shows skin break (*white arrow*) and gas in the intercostal muscles (*black arrows*) tracking into the empyema with fluid and gas in the pleural space surrounded by a thick enhancing pleura. Right pleural effusion shows no enhancing pleura. (**b**) Osteomyelitis of a lower thoracic vertebra (*arrowhead*) adjacent to empyema (*arrow*) with bone destruction, small speck of gas, and thickened enhancing left paravertebral soft tissue. (**c**) The patient had decortication of the left thoracic wall with gauze packing the nonhealing skin wound showing continuity with the pleural space (*arrow*)

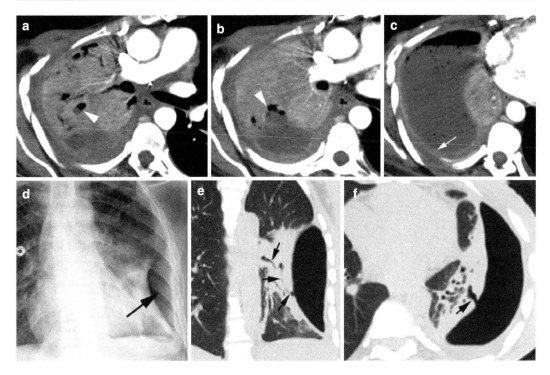

Fig. 9.5 Bronchopleural fistula. Patient 1: Metastatic breast cancer with chronic empyema. Axial contrast-enhanced CT shows (**a**) air-fluid collection in the right lower lobe bronchus (*arrowhead*) which opens up into the pleural space in the next section (*arrowhead* in **b**). (**c**) Empyema with air-fluid collection in the pleural space with a thick enhancing pleura (*arrow*). Patient 2: Trauma with persistent loculated pneumothorax. (**d**) PA chest x-ray shows loculated pneumothorax (*arrow*). (**e, f**) Coronal and sagittal reformatted images show fistulous tract (*arrows*) connecting the left lower lobe bronchus to the pneumothorax

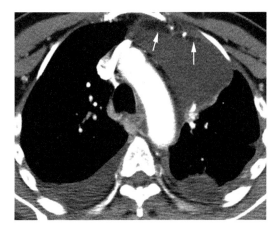

Fig. 9.6 Chylothorax. The patient developed persistent pleural collection as a complication of surgical resection of a lung nodule. Contrast-enhanced CT shows loculated fat-fluid collection (*arrows*) adjacent to the mediastinum

Diagnosis
Catamenial Hydropneumothorax

Imaging Features
1. Loculated hydropneumothorax
2. Soft tissue–enhancing nodule on the rectus abdominis muscle in the lower abdomen

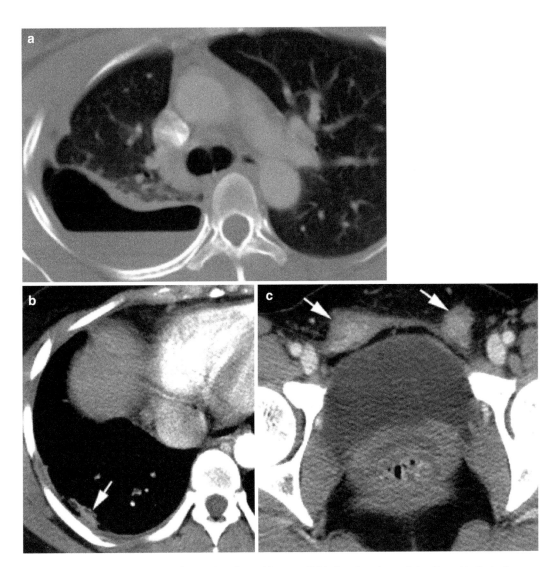

Fig. 9.7 Catamenial hydropneumothorax. A patient with known history of endometriosis complained of shortness of breath and dyspnea on exertion. (**a**) Axial CT shows loculated hydropneumothorax. (**b**) Axial CT at lower level shows pleural-based endometrioma seen as an irregular small faintly enhancing nodule adjacent to the hydropneumothorax (*arrow*). (**c**) Axial CT of the pelvis shows two enhancing nodular endometriomas in the rectus abdominis muscle, one on each side (*arrows*)

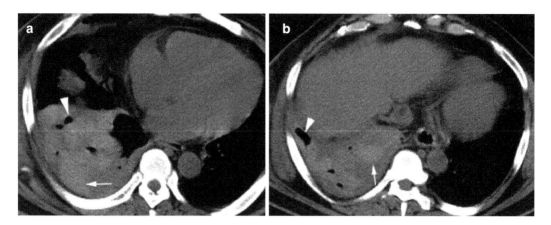

Fig. 9.8 Hemopneumothorax post-trauma. (**a**, **b**) Axial noncontrast CT shows high-density lobulated hemorrhagic fluid in the right lower pleural space (*arrow*) with pockets of air collection within it (*arrowhead*)

Fig. 9.9 Malignant mesothelioma in different patients with fatigue, increasing shortness of breath, cough, and weakness. Axial CT (**a**, **b**) shows nodular and irregular thickening of visceral and parietal pleura (*arrowhead*) with extension in the fissure (*white arrow*) and extension to the mediastinum with pericardial involvement (*black arrow*). (**c**) Nodular pleural thickening of the thoracic wall pleura (*arrow*) and mediastinal pleura (*arrowhead*). (**d**, **e**) Nodular pleural thickening is more on the left side involving diaphragmatic pleura (*arrow* in **d**), while pleural effusion more on the right side. (**e**) Axial CT of the upper abdomen showing metastasis to both the adrenal glands (*arrowheads*) and to the liver (*black arrows*). Enhancing pleural nodules are seen in the right costophrenic angle (*white arrows*)

Diagnosis

Mesothelioma

Imaging Features

1. Nodular or irregular pleural thickening with rind-like encasement of the lung
2. Variable ipsilateral hemithorax volume loss
3. Involvement of visceral and parietal pleura, interlobar fissures, and ipsilateral pleural effusion

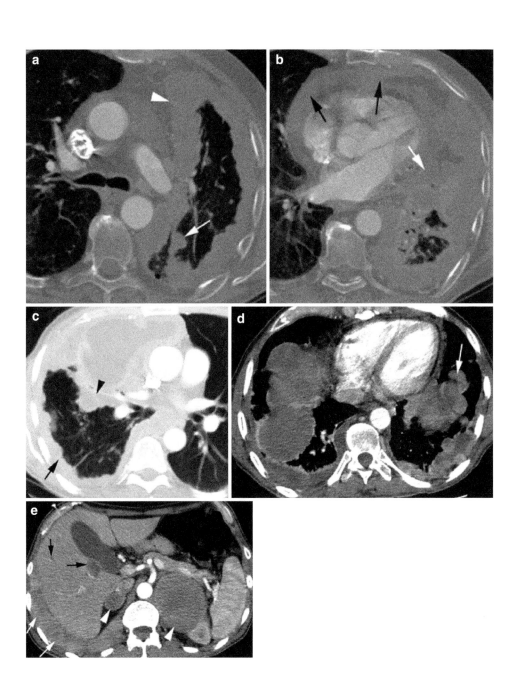

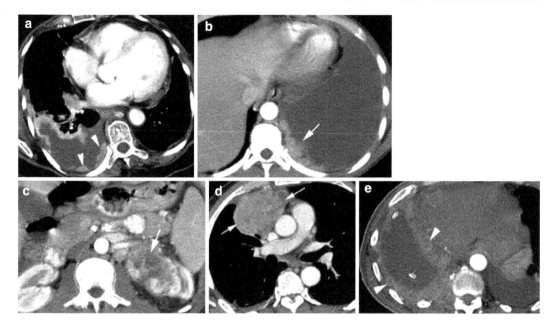

Fig. 9.10 Pleural metastasis. Axial CT (**a**) shows discrete nodular enhancing metastasis (*arrowheads*) to the parietal pleura projecting into the pleural cavity from thyroid cancer. (**b**, **c**) Ill-marginated enhancing metasta-sis (*arrow*) to the parietal pleura from renal cell carcinoma (*arrow* in **c**). (**d**, **e**) Metastasis from squamous cell carcinoma of thymus (*arrows*) to parietal and visceral pleura (*arrowheads*)

Mediastinal Disease with Acute Symptoms (Noncardiac)

10

Contents

R. Agarwala, *Atlas of Emergency Radiology:*
Vascular System, Chest, Abdomen and Pelvis, and Reproductive System,
DOI 10.1007/978-3-319-13042-2_10, © Springer International Publishing Switzerland 2015

Lymphoma

Imaging Features
1. Hilar and mediastinal lymphadenopathy
2. Multiple pulmonary nodules
3. Interstitial and alveolar infiltrates and pleural effusion

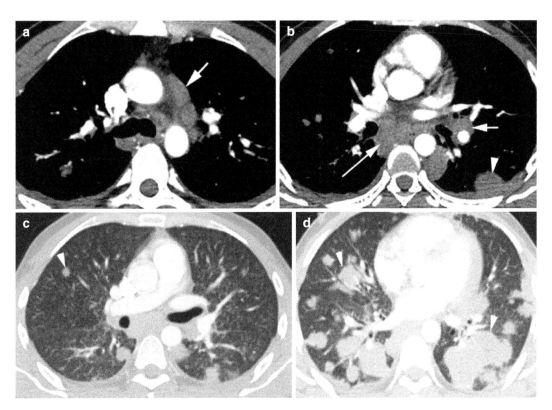

Fig. 10.1 Lymphoma with histoplasma infection in a HIV/AIDS patient. Axial CT (**a**) shows enlarged lymph nodes in the mediastinum (*arrow*), (**b**) enlarged lymph nodes in the left hilum (*short arrow*) and mediastinum (*long arrow*), and pleural-based nodule (*arrowhead*). (**c**) Diffuse centrilobular micronodules are seen bilaterally with subpleural sparing. Solid lung nodule (*arrowhead*) and pleural-based masses bilaterally. (**d**) Many of the large solid masses (*arrowhead*) in the parenchyma are seen more at the lung bases

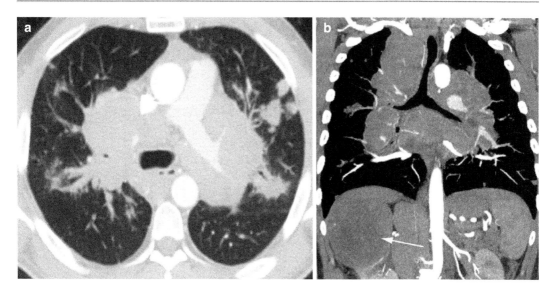

Fig. 10.2 Mediastinal and hilar LAD due to metastasis from RCC. (**a**, **b**) Axial and coronal reformatted CT show large lymph nodes in the bilateral hila and mediastinum narrowing in bilateral bronchi and with multiple solid lung nodules. A large necrotic right renal mass is seen (*arrow*)

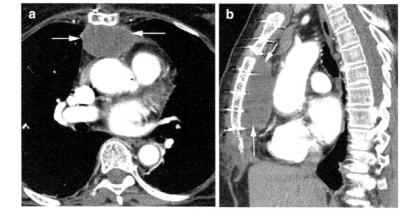

Fig. 10.3 Hematoma in the anterior mediastinum post-surgery. (**a**, **b**) Axial and sagittal reformatted images show a large well-marginated retrosternal hematoma (*arrows*) with sternotomy sutures

Thyroid Lesions

Diagnosis

Goiter

Imaging Features

1. Enlarged one or both lobes of the thyroid.
2. Nodules solid, low density, or mixed.
3. Calcifications can be coarse or microcalcification.
4. Cystic lesions.

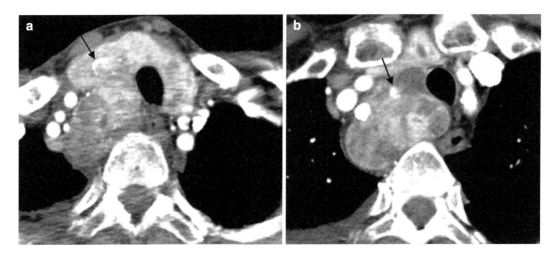

Fig. 10.4 Multinodular goiter with colloid cysts, biopsy proven. Axial CT (**a**, **b**) shows multiple low-density nodules bilaterally and retrosternal extension on the right side. Coarse calcifications is seen in the right lobe (*arrow*)

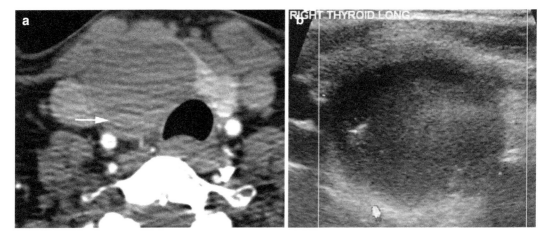

Fig. 10.5 Hemorrhage in a colloid cyst. (**a**) Axial CT shows a large cyst in the right lobe of the thyroid with dependent high-density hemorrhage (*arrow*). (**b**) Color Doppler US shows low-level echoes within the cyst in the right lobe of the thyroid with no internal vascularity and no increased vascularity of the cyst wall

Diagnosis
Thyroid Carcinoma

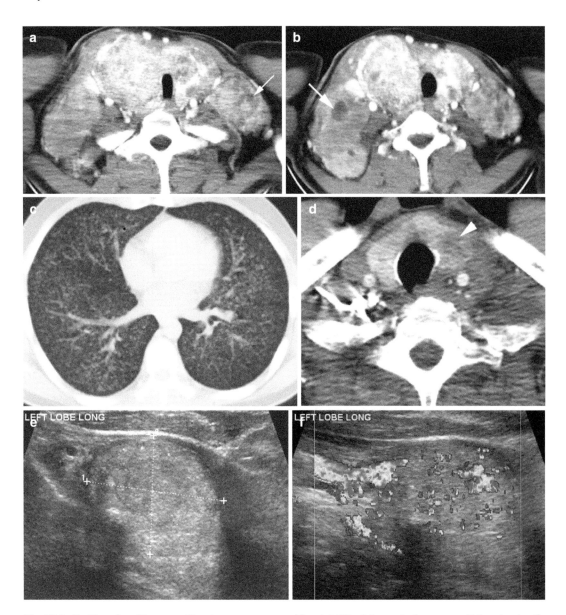

Fig. 10.6 Papillary thyroid cancer with pulmonary metastasis. Patient 1: (**a**, **b**) Axial CT neck shows both lobes of the thyroid to be enlarged, with increased vascularity and with multiple low-density foci. Low-density metastases are also seen in adjacent lymph nodes (*arrows*) bilaterally. (**c**) Axial CT of the chest shows miliary metastasis. Patient 2: (**d**) axial CT of the neck shows a small low-density ill-marginated nodule in the left thyroid lobe (*arrowhead*). (**e**, **f**) Grayscale and color Doppler ultrasound show hypervascular large heteroechoic solid mass (calipers in **e**) in the left lobe of the thyroid. (**g**, **h**) Axial and coronal reformatted CTs show macronodular metastasis to bilateral lungs

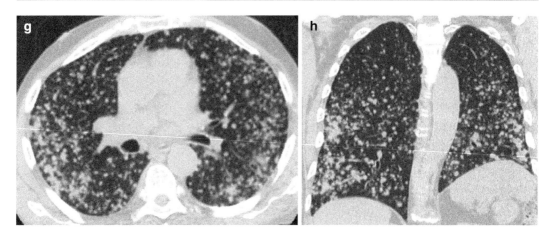

Fig. 10.6 (continued)

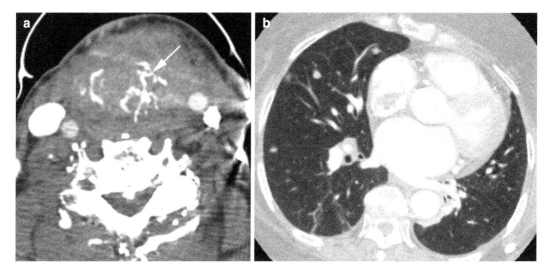

Fig. 10.7 Hurthle cell follicular thyroid carcinoma. Axial CT (**a**) of the neck shows coarse calcifications (*arrow*) in the diffusely enlarged thyroid. (**b**) Axial CT of the chest shows nodular metastases in the lungs (**b**)

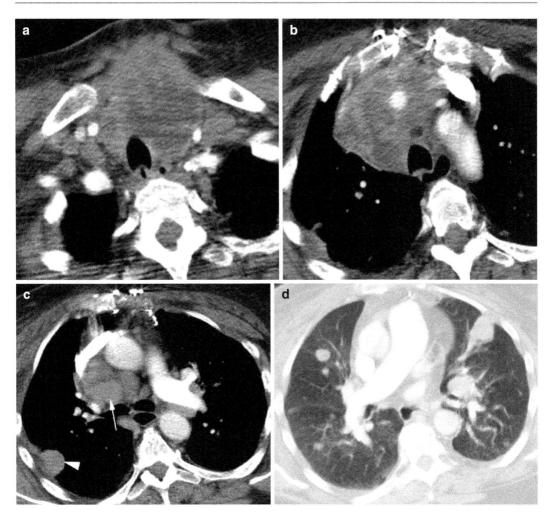

Fig. 10.8 Anaplastic thyroid carcinoma with lung metastasis. Axial CT (**a**, **b**) shows diffuse enlargement of both lobes of the thyroid with irregular low densities and with retrosternal extension of the right lobe. (**c**) Lymphadenopathy is seen at the precarinal region (*arrow*) and in the left hilum, and pleural-based metastasis is seen in the right lung (*arrowhead*). (**d**) Axial CT of the lung windowing at lower level shows multiple large solid lung metastases

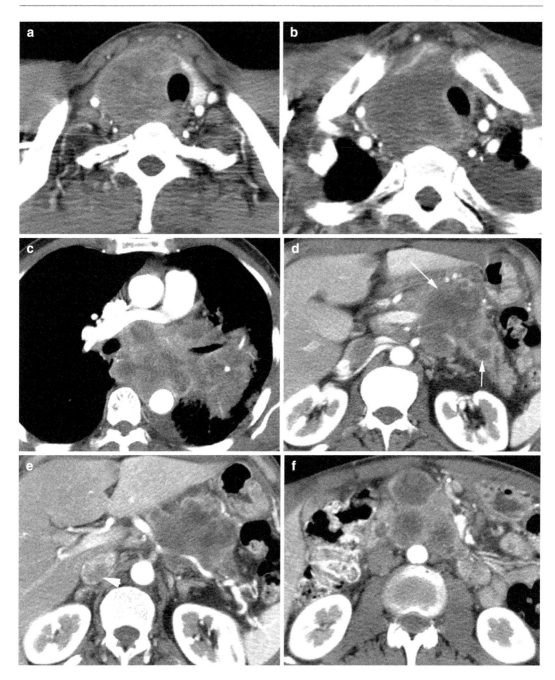

Fig. 10.9 Small cell lung cancer with metastasis to the thyroid, pancreas, adrenal gland, and mesenteric root lymph nodes. Axial CT of the chest (**a**, **b**) shows low-density metastasis to the right lobe of the thyroid. (**c**) Shows lung carcinoma in the left hilum extending into the mediastinum and shows narrowing of the left upper lobe of the bronchus. Axial CT of the abdomen (**d**–**f**) shows multiple low-density metastases to the body and tail of the pancreas (*arrows*) and right adrenal gland (*arrowhead*). (**f**) Necrotic lymph nodes at the root of mesentery

Thymic Tumors

Diagnosis
Thymic Epithelial Tumors

Imaging Features
Thymoma
1. Most are encapsulated solid lesions that can be oval, round, or lobulated.
2. Can have hemorrhage, necrosis, or cystic component.
3. Calcification may be in the capsule or throughout the mass.

4. Usually slow growing but can be aggressive and invade into the mediastinum, pleura, and pericardium.
Thymic carcinomas
1. More aggressive and invades adjacent structures
2. Calcification is more frequent and have low-density areas
3. Distant metastasis and mediastinal lymphadenopathy

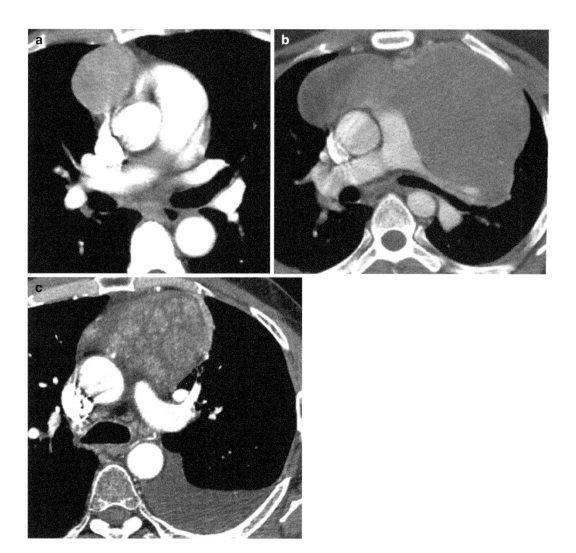

Fig. 10.10 Thymoma. (**a–c**) Axial CT of the mediastinum shows nonaggressive anterior mediastinal focal mass in three patients all with histologic diagnosis of benign thymoma. (**c**) Spindle cell benign thymoma

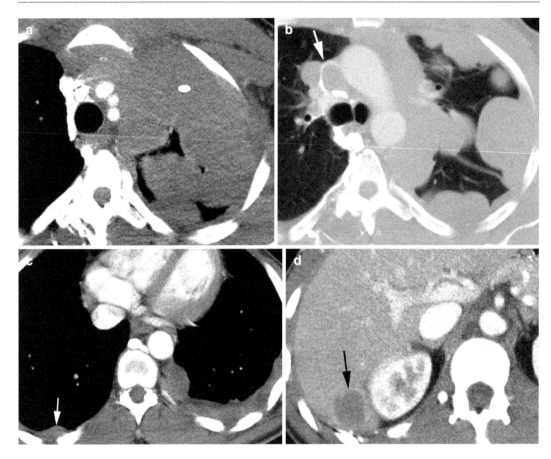

Fig. 10.11 Thymic carcinoma of three patients. Patient 1: (**a–e**) Axial and coronal reformatted CT show left anterior mediastinal mass (*ellipse* in **a**) infiltrating the pleura in the left thorax giving it a nodular appearance and with left hilar lymphadenopathy (*arrowhead* **e**). It is also compressing the superior vena cava (*white arrow* in **b**). Pleural metastasis is seen on the right side (*white arrow* in **c**) and to the liver (*black arrow* in **d**). Patient 2: (**f**) axial CT shows anterior mediastinal mass with calcification and areas of cystic degeneration. Patient 3: (**g–k**) axial and coronal reformatted CT show recurrence of thymic carcinoma with prior history of radiation therapy. Now shows curvilinear calcification of thymic mass (*arrows* in **g**, **h**) and pleural metastasis with similar calcification (*arrows* **j**, **k**). The mass shows invasion to the mediastinal pleura (*arrow* in **i**)

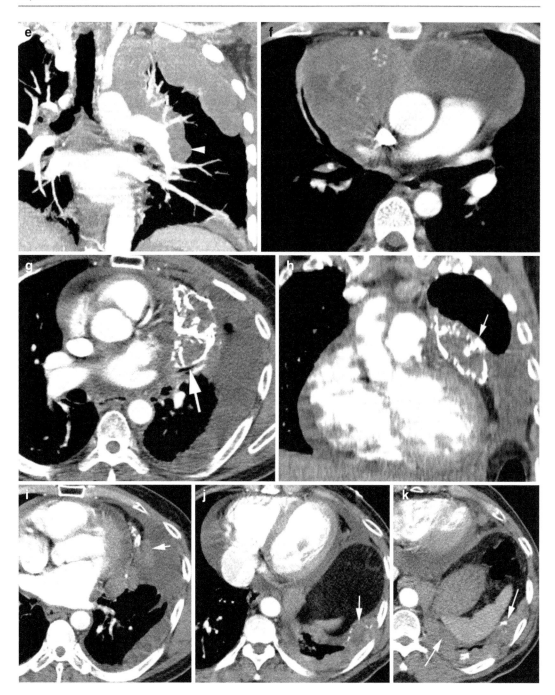

Fig. 10.11 (continued)

Diagnosis

Thymic Neuroendocrine Tumor

Imaging Features

1. Lack fibrous capsule but commonly have necrosis or hemorrhage and may have fine calcification
2. Invade to adjacent structures
3. Distant intrathoracic and extrathoracic metastasis
4. Difficult to differentiate from thymic epithelial tumors

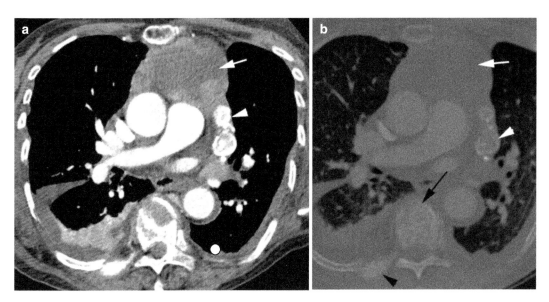

Fig. 10.12 Neuroendocrine tumor of the thymus with bony metastasis. (**a**, **b**) Axial CT shows a large anterior mediastinal mass with peripheral enhancement (*white arrows*), central necrosis, and coarse calcification (*white arrowhead*) with extension to the left hilum. Mixed metastasis is seen in the right posterior rib (*black arrowhead*) and to multiple vertebral bodies (only one shown, *black arrow*)

Diagnosis
Thymic Lymphoma

Imaging Features
1. Enlarged single or multiple masses mimic other thymic lesions
2. Difficult to distinguish from other thymic masses

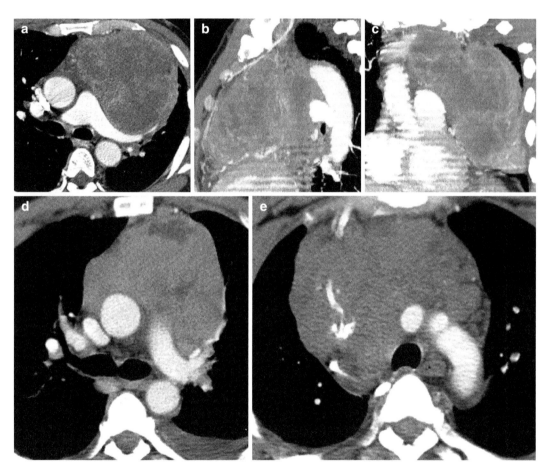

Fig. 10.13 Lymphoma in different patients. (**a–c**) B-cell lymphoma axial, sagittal, and coronal CT. (**d**) T-cell lymphoma axial CT. (**e**) Hodgkin's lymphoma axial CT

Diagnosis
Thymic Germ Cell Tumor

Imaging Features
1. Large lobulated anterior mediastinal mass.
2. Seminomas are relatively homogenous.
3. Teratomas may have one or more components of the embryonic germ cell layers.

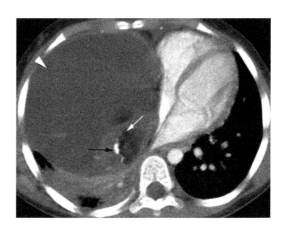

Fig. 10.14 Thymic teratoma. Axial CT shows a large anterior mediastinal mass causing leftward deviation of the mediastinum and partial collapse of the right lung. The mass shows focal area of fatty tissue (*white arrow*), calcification (*black arrow*), and fluid collection (*arrowhead*)

Nongonadal Germ Cell Tumor

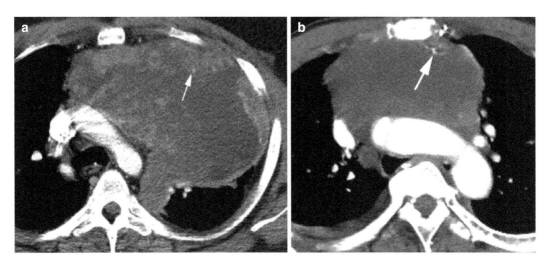

Fig. 10.15 Nongonadal seminoma in two patients. Axial CT (**a**) shows a large anterior mediastinal mass with low-density necrotic areas, enhancing solid tissue, and small specks of calcification (*arrow*). (**b**) Small calcifications (*arrow*) in the anterior mediastinal mass without significant enhancing solid tissue

Lipoma

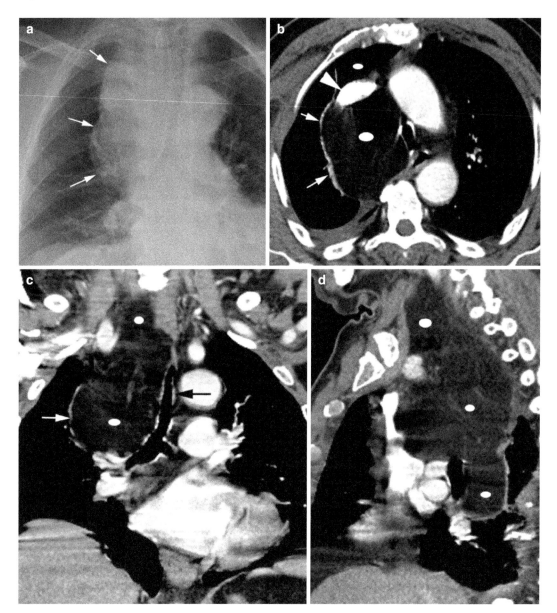

Fig. 10.16 Lipoma of the mediastinum. Chest radiograph (**a**) shows a large mass in the right paratracheal region (*arrows*) with extrinsic pressure on the trachea. (**b–d**) Axial CT and coronal and sagittal reformatted images show a large lipoma (*ellipse*) in the right side of the mediastinum extending into the neck on the medial side of the common carotid artery up to the level of the larynx. It is causing extrinsic pressure on the SVC (*arrowhead*) and is displacing the azygos vein (*thin white arrows*) and the trachea (*thick black arrow*)

Esophageal Lesions

Diagnosis
Foreign Body in the Esophagus

Imaging Features
1. Metallic coin in the esophagus posterior to the trachea as seen in lateral view

Fig. 10.17 Coin in the esophagus. (**a, b**) PA and lateral chest images show an esophageal coin with the tracheal air column anterior (*arrow*) to the coin. The rounded appearance of the coin in the lateral view is contrary to the truism

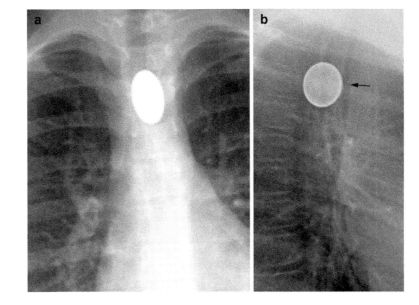

Diagnosis

Bone in the Esophagus

Imaging Features

1. Elongated calcified density in the esophagus, behind the trachea at the thoracic inlet

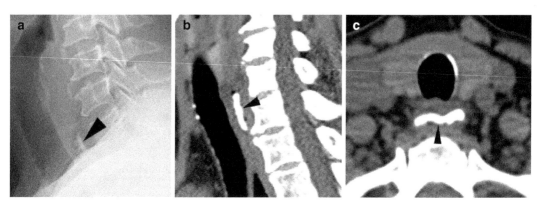

Fig. 10.18 Bone in the esophagus. (**a**) Lateral view of the neck shows a radio-opaque bone (*arrowhead*) in the esophagus at the thoracic inlet behind the trachea. (**b, c**) Sagittal reformatted and axial CTs confirm the radiographic findings (*arrow head*)

Diagnosis
Bronchoesophageal Fistula

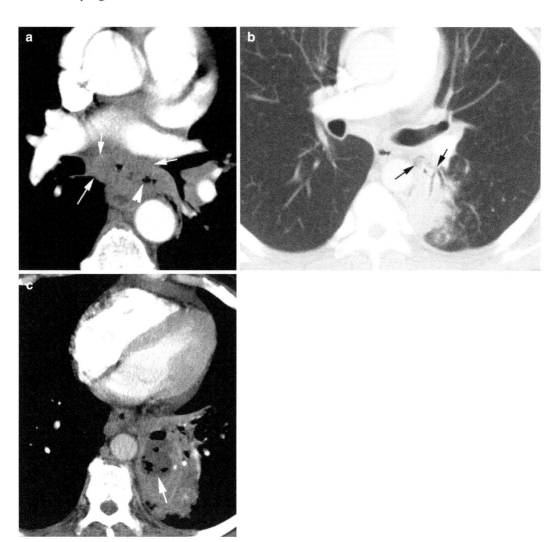

Fig. 10.19 Esophageal carcinoma with bronchoesophageal fistula and abscess formation. Axial CT (**a**) shows soft tissue mass (*white arrows*) surrounding the infra-carinal esophagus which shows perforation with gas extending outside the lumen (*arrowhead*). (**b**) Gas and fluid are seen communicating with the left lower lobe bronchus (*black arrows*). (**c**) Abscess with loculated gas and fluid collection in the consolidated lung in the left lower lobe (*thick arrow*)

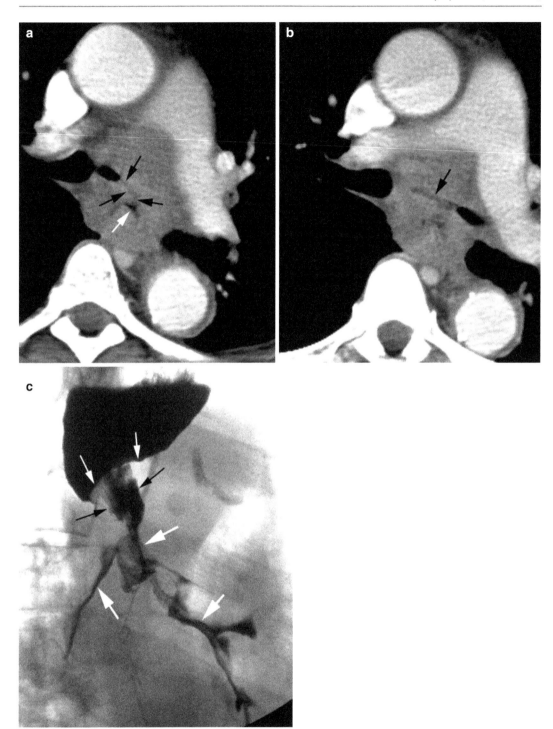

Fig. 10.20 Esophageal carcinoma at the carina encasing the left main stem bronchus with fistulous communication. (**a**) Axial CT shows a faint fistulous tract (*black arrows*) from the esophagus (*white arrow*) to the trachea. (**b**) Axial CT at a lower plane than the fistulous tract shows narrowed fluid-filled left main stem bronchus (*arrow*). (**c**) Barium swallow study contrast in the left lower lobe bronchi (*thick white arrows*) from the abrupt irregular narrowed esophagus (*black arrows*) with shelf-like transitional zone (*thin white arrows*)

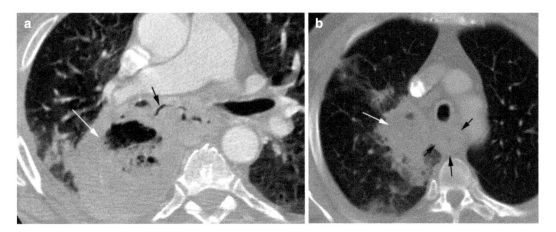

Fig. 10.21 Squamous cell carcinoma of the esophagus which has perforated into the lung parenchyma with abscess formation. Axial CT (**a**) shows perforation of the tract (*black arrow*) from the esophagus to the abscess (*white arrow* in **a** and **b**). (**b**) Mass around the esophageal lumen (*black arrows*)

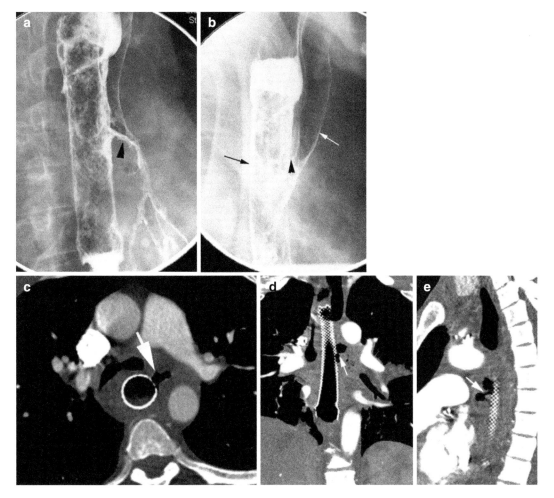

Fig. 10.22 Bronchoesophageal fistula through esophageal stent for esophageal squamous cell carcinoma. (**a**, **b**) In a barium swallow study, oblique and lateral views show barium draining into the left lower lobe bronchus (*arrowhead*). The stented esophagus (*black arrow*) is posterior to the trachea (*white arrow*). (**c**–**e**) Axial, coronal, and sagittal reformatted CT show gas leaking out of the esophageal stent (*arrows*)

Diagnosis
Esophagopleural Fistula

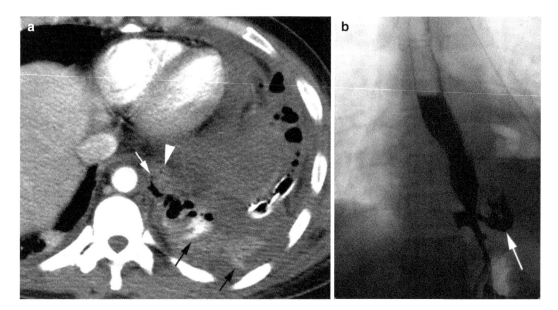

Fig. 10.23 Esophagopleural fistula and postsurgical rupture of the esophagus. (**a**) Axial CT shows perforation (*thin white arrow*) of the esophagus (*arrowhead*) with contrast and gas extravasation into the pleural space (*black arrows*). (**b**) Barium swallow study done after CT shows contrast leaking out of the distal esophagus (*arrow*)

Tracheal and Bronchial Lesions

Diagnosis
Tracheal Stenosis

Imaging Features
1. Narrowing of the trachea in CT and radiographs best seen in lateral views

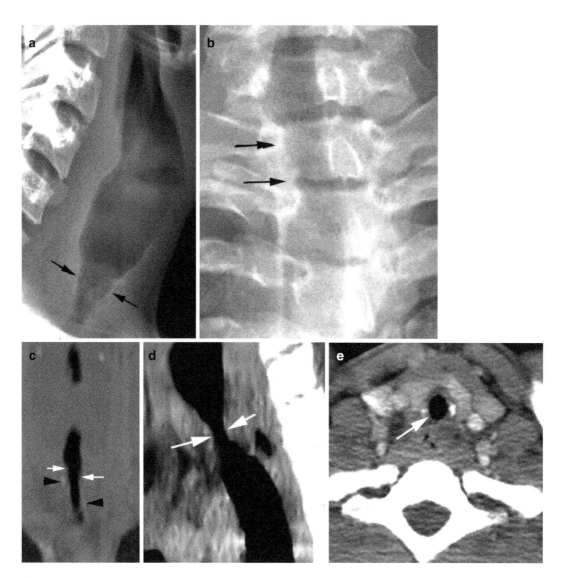

Fig. 10.24 Tracheal stenosis. A patient who has a history of asthma. (**a**, **b**) Radiographs of the neck and (**c–e**) CT of the neck in coronal, sagittal, and axial views show a focal area of narrowing of the tracheal air column (*arrows*) by smooth concentric thickening of soft tissues within the normal-appearing tracheal cartilages (*arrowhead*) at the thoracic inlet

Diagnosis
Fibrosing Mediastinitis

Imaging Features
1. Typically affects the middle mediastinum.
2. Tracheobronchial narrowing.
3. Soft tissue mass with coarse calcification.
4. Pulmonary infiltrates.
5. Diffuse form obliterates the mediastinal fat plane and encases or invades adjacent structures.

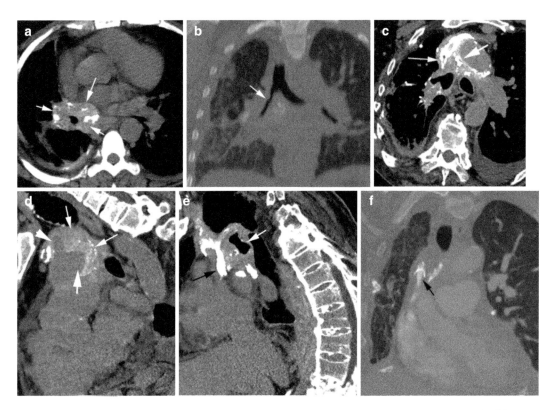

Fig. 10.25 Fibrosing mediastinitis in two patients. Patient 1: (**a**, **b**) Axial and coronal reformatted noncontrast CT show high-density soft tissues with calcification surrounding the right lower lobe bronchus causing irregular narrowing (*arrow*). The right lung shows diffuse infiltrates and fibrosis with loss of volume. Patient 2: (**c**, **d**) Axial and sagittal reformatted CT show diffuse high-density soft tissues with calcification in the superior mediastinum (*thin arrows*) and the right hilum encasing the proximal arch of the aorta (*thick white arrow*), the origin of the brachiocephalic artery (*arrowhead*). (**e**, **f**) Sagittal and coronal reformatted CTs show the fibrosing tissue with calcification constricting the proximal SVC and innominate vein (*black arrow*) and right main stem bronchus (*white arrow*). Thoracic vertebrae show ankylosing spondylitis and the right lung shows fibrosis with loss of volume

Fig. 10.26 Tracheobronchomegaly (Mounier-Kuhn syndrome). CT axial (**a**, **b**), coronal, (**c**) and sagittal (**d**) reformatted images show marked dilatation of the trachea and bilateral main stem bronchi with bronchiectasis more at the bases. Saclike outpouchings are seen in the trachea (*arrows*) (**e**) Axial CT lower lungs show bilateral cystic bronchiectasis

Diagnosis
Tracheobronchomegaly

Imaging Features
1. Dilatation of the trachea and central bronchi
2. Saclike outpouching between tracheal cartilages
3. Bronchiectasis

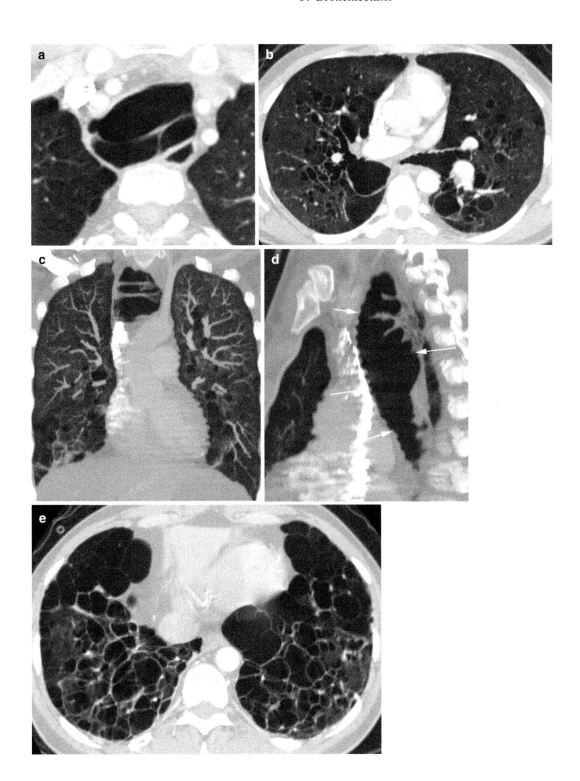

Diagnosis
Bronchogenic Cyst

Imaging Features
1. Mostly well-circumscribed mass with variable attenuation
2. Mostly cystic but can be solid
3. Can have milk of calcium

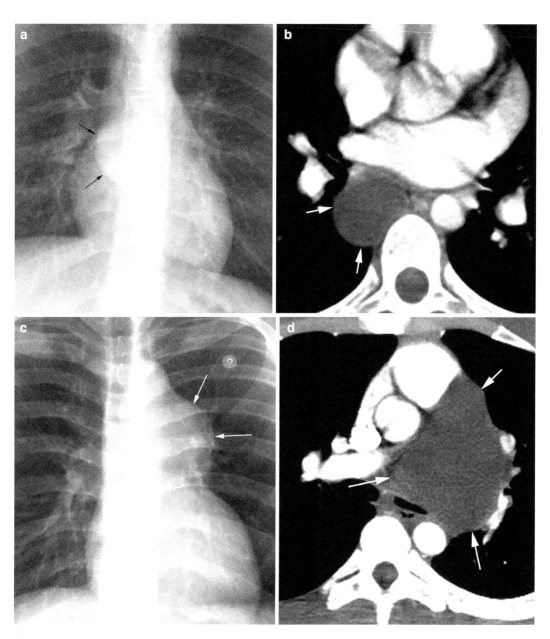

Fig. 10.27 Bronchogenic cyst in two patients as incidental finding. Patient 1: (**a**) PA of the chest and (**b**) axial CT show a low-density cyst at the carina (*arrows*). Patient 2: (**c**) PA of the chest and (**d–f**) axial, coronal, and sagittal reformatted CTs show a cyst in the AP window (*arrows*) causing extrinsic compression on the left main stem bronchus

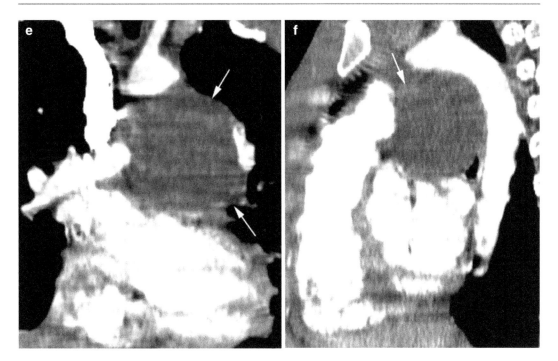

Fig. 10.27 (continued)

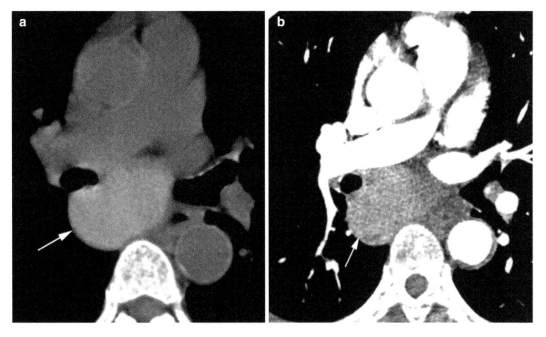

Fig. 10.28 Bronchogenic cyst with increased density. Incidental finding on a 75-year-old female with ischemic chest pain. (**a**) Axial CT of the chest shows high density in a cyst at the carina (*arrow*) and is probably from milk of calcium. (**b**) No enhancement is seen in postcontrast image (*arrow*)

Diagnosis
Bronchial Carcinoid

Imaging Findings
1. Smooth well-defined mass in central bronchus.
2. Can have irregular or ill-defined margins and can be aggressive and invade the mediastinum.
3. Hilar or perihilar mass ranging from 2 to 5 mm.
4. Usually have eccentric calcification but can have diffuse calcification resembling broncholithiasis.
5. Cavitation is rare.
6. Can have associated hilar and mediastinal lymphadenopathy.
7. May or may not enhance with contrast.

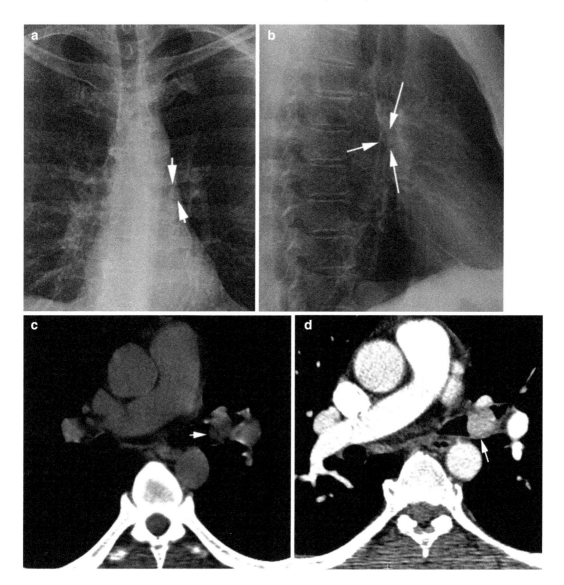

Fig. 10.29 Bronchial carcinoid. (**a**, **b**) PA and lateral chest x-ray show a well-marginated mass in the left main stem bronchus (*arrows*). (**c**, **d**) Axial precontrast and postcontrast CTs of the chest show a soft tissue nodule in the left main stem bronchus with diffuse uniform enhancement (*arrow*)

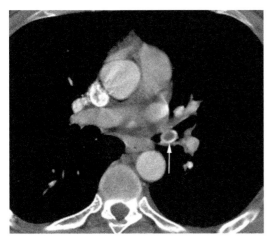

Fig. 10.30 Endobronchial carcinoid. Axial post-enhancement CT shows a focal endobronchial mass with peripheral enhancement (*arrow*)

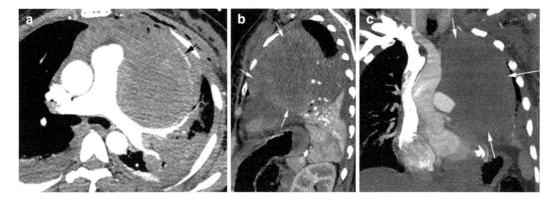

Fig. 10.31 A carcinoid anterior mediastinum. (**a–c**) Axial, sagittal, and coronal reformatted CT show a large mildly heterogeneous mass (*white arrows*) in the anterior mediastinum on the left side displacing vessels (*black arrow*) and mass effect on the mediastinum showing poor enhancement

Diagnosis

Broncholithiasis

Imaging Features

1. Calcification within a bronchus usually in the lower lobe.
2. The affected bronchus can be fluid filled from chronic hemoptysis.
3. Centrilobular nodules surrounding the bronchus from endobronchial spread of fluid.
4. Multiple calcified lymph nodes in the hila.

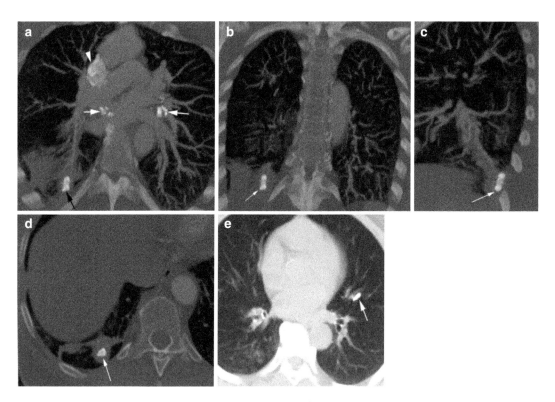

Fig. 10.32 Bilateral broncholithiasis. (**a–d**) Partial axial, coronal, and sagittal reformatted and true axial CTs of the chest show calcified bilateral hilar (*white arrows*) and azygos (*arrowhead*) lymph nodes. A large calcified lymph node is seen in the distal right lower lobe bronchus (*black arrow* in **a**, *white arrow* in **b–d**) (**e**) Broncholith is also seen within the lingular bronchus (*white arrow*)

Diagnosis

Tooth in the Bronchus

Imaging Features

1. Tooth with metallic crown in the RLL bronchus
2. Surrounding lung infiltration from aspiration

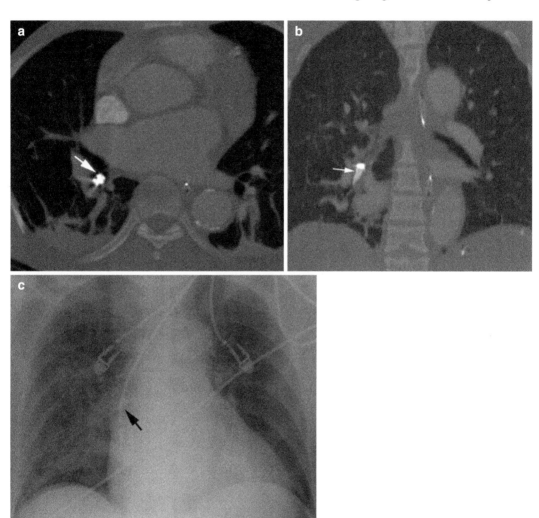

Fig. 10.33 Tooth in the right lower lobe bronchus. (**a, b**) Axial and coronal reformatted images show tooth in the RLL bronchus (*arrow*). Streak artifacts are from metallic crown. Bilateral lower lobe infiltrations are from aspiration. (**c**) PA chest radiograph shows tooth in the right hilum (*arrow*) with surrounding infiltration from aspiration

Diagnosis
Endobronchial Mucus

Imaging Features
1. Frothy soft tissue filling airways
2. The RLL bronchus commonly affected

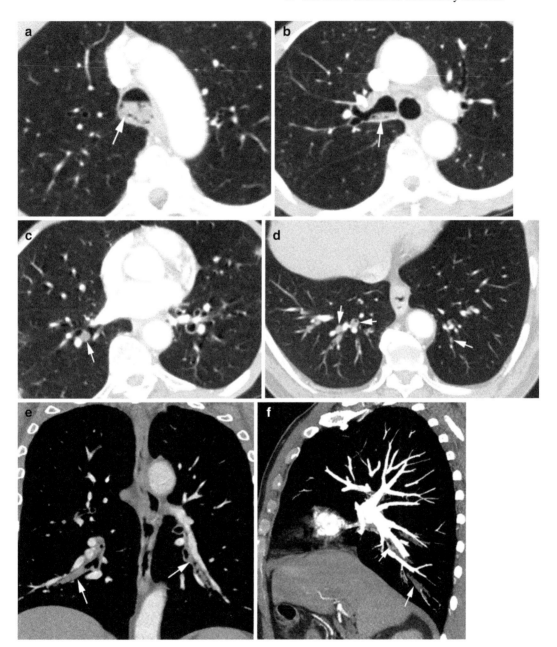

Fig. 10.34 Mucus in the tracheobronchial tree in two patients. Patient 1: (**a**, **b**) Axial CT shows frothy mucus with air-fluid level in the distal trachea and right main stem bronchus (*arrows*). (**c**, **d**) Axial CT of the lower lobes shows fluid-filled bronchi (*arrows*) between pulmonary artery anteriorly and the pulmonary vein posteriorly. Patient 2: (**e**, **f**) Coronal and sagittal reformatted images show fluid-filled bronchi between the pulmonary artery anteriorly and the vein posteriorly in both lower lobes (*arrows*)

Bibliography

1. Abbott GF, Rosado-de-Christenson ML, Franks TJ, et al. From the archives of the AFIP: pulmonary Langerhans cell histiocytosis. Radiographics. 2004;24:821–41.
2. Abbott GF, Rosado-de-Christenson ML, Frazier AA, et al. Lymphangioleiomyomatosis: radiologic-pathologic correlation. Radiographics. 2005;25:803–28.
3. Attili AK, Kazerooni EA. Lymphangioleiomyomatosis. Radiology. 2007;244:303–8.
4. Attili AK, Kazerooni EA, Gross BH, et al. Smoking-related interstitial lung disease: radiologic-clinical-pathologic correlation. Radiographics. 2008;28:1383–98.
5. Austin JHM, Garg K, Aberle D, et al. Radiologic implications of 2011 classification of the adenocarcinoma of the lungs. Radiology. 2013;266:62–71.
6. Aviram G, Fishman JE, Boiselle PM. Thoracic manifestation of AIDS. Appl Radiol. 2003;32:11–21.
7. Benveniste MFK, Rosado-de-Christenson ML, Sabloff BS, et al. Role of imaging in the diagnosis, staging and treatment of thymoma. Radiographics. 2011;31:1847–61.
8. Burrill J, Williams CJ, Bain G, et al. Tuberculosis: a radiologic review. Radiographics. 2007;27:1255–73.
9. Capobianco J, Grimberg A, Thompson BM, et al. Thoracic manifestations of collagen vascular diseases. Radiographics. 2012;32:33–50.
10. Chong S, Lee KS, Chung MJ, et al. Pneumoconiosis: comparison of imaging and pathologic findings. Radiogaraphics. 2006;26:59–77.
11. Criado E, Sanchez M, Ramirez J, et al. Pulmonary sarcoidosis: typical and atypical manifestations at high-resolution CT with pathologic correlation. Radiographics. 2010;30:1567–86.
12. Desai SR, Wells AU, Suntharalingam G, et al. Acute respiratory syndrome caused by pulmonary and extra-pulmonary injury: a comparative CT study. Radiology. 2001;208:689–93.
13. Desai SR, Wells AU, Suntharalingam G, et al. Acute respiratory distress syndrome caused by pulmonary and extrapulmonary injury: a comparative CT study. Radiology. 2001;218:689–93.
14. Eisenhuber E. The tree-in bud sign. Radiology. 2002;222:771–2.
15. Franquet T, Muller NL, Ginenez A, et al. Spectrum of pulmonary aspergillosis: histologic, clinical and radiologic finding. Radiographics. 2001;21:825–37.
16. Franquet T, Muller NL, Gimenez A, et al. Spectrum of pulmonary aspergillosis: histologic, clinical and radiologic findings. Radiographics. 2001;21:825–37.
17. Frazier AA, Rosado de Christenson ML, Stocker JT, et al. Intralobar sequestration: radiologic-pathologic correlation. Radiographics. 1997;17:725–45.
18. Frazier AA, Rosado-de-Christenson MI, Galvin JR, et al. Pulmonary angiitis and granulomatosis: radiologic-pathologic correlation. Radiographics. 1998;18:687–710.
19. Glueucker T, Capasso P, Schnyder P, et al. Clinical and radiologic features of pulmonary edema. Radiographics. 1999;19:1507–31.
20. Goodman LR, Fumagalli R, Tagliabue P, et al. Adult respiratory distress syndrome due to pulmonary and extrapulmonary causes: CT, clinical, and functional correlations. Radiology. 1999;213:545–52.
21. Goodman LR, Fumagalli R, Tagliabue P, et al. Adult respiratory distress syndrome due to pulmonary and extrapulmonary causes: CT, clinical and functional correlations. Radiology. 1999;213:545–52.
22. Greiwe AC, Miller K, Farver C, et al. Pulmonary Langerhans cell histiocytosis. Radiographics. 2012;32:987–90.
23. Hansell DM. Thin-section CT of the lung: the Hinterland of normal. Radiology. 2010;256(3):695–711.
24. Hansell DM, Bankier AA, MacMahon H, et al. Fleischner society: glossary of terms for thoracic imaging. Radiology. 2008;246:697–722.
25. Harisinghani MG, McLoud TC, Shepard JO, et al. Tuberculosis from head to toe. Radiographics. 2000;20:449–70.
26. Hartman TE, Tazelaar HD, Swensen SJ, et al. Cigarette smoking: CT and pathologic findings of associated pulmonary diseases. Radiographics. 1997;17:377–90.
27. Hirschmann JV, Pipavath SNJ, Godwin JD. Hypersensitivity pneumonitis: a historical, clinical, and radiologic review. Radiographics. 2009;29:1921–38.
28. Howling SJ, Hansell DM, Wells AU, et al. Follicular bronchiolitis: thin-section CT and histologic findings. Radiology. 1999;212:637–42.
29. Jeung MY, Gasser B, Gangi A, et al. Bronchial carcinoid tumors of the thorax: spectrum of radiologic findings. Radiographics. 2002;22:351–65.
30. Johkoh T, Muller NL, Colby TV, et al. Nonspecific interstitial pneumonia: correlation between thin-section CT findings and pathologic subgroups in 55 patients. Radiology. 2002;225:199–204.
31. Johnson GL, Fishman EK, Hruban RH. CT evaluation of thymoma: spectrum of disease. Appl Radiol. 1997;26:13–20.
32. Kenney HH, Agrons GA, Shin JS. Invasive pulmonary aspergillosis: radiologic and pathologic findings. Radiographics. 2002;22:1507–10.
33. Kligerman ST, Groshong S, Brown KK, et al. Nonspecific interstitial pneumonia: radiologic, clinical and pathologic considerations. Radiographics. 2009;29:73–87.
34. Koyama T, Ueda H, Togashi K, et al. Radiologic manifestations of sarcoidosis in various organs. Radiographics. 2004;24:87–104.
35. Kraus GJ. Split pleural sign. Radiology. 2007;243:297–8.
36. Kuhlaman JE, Singha MK. Complex disease of the pleural space: radiographic and CT evaluation. Radiographics. 1997;17:63–79.
37. Kuhlman JE. Pneumocystic infections: the radiologist's perspective. Radiology. 1996;198:623–35.
38. Lalani TA, Kanne JP, Hatfield GA, et al. Imaging findings in systemic lupus erythematosus. Radiographics. 2001;24:1069–86.
39. Leung AN. Pulmonary tuberculosis: the essentials. Radiology. 1999;210:307–22.
40. Levine MS. Achalasia and diffuse esophageal spasm: spectrum of findings and complementary roles of barium studies and manometry. Appl Radiol. 2006;35:19–26.
41. Lynch DA, Travis WD, Muller NL, et al. Idiopathic interstitial pneumonias: CT features. Radiology. 2005;236:10–21.

42. Mahfouz M. Necrotizing pneumonia: sequential finding on chest radiography. Egypt J Bronchol. 2009;3: 86–9.

43. Martinez F, Chung JH, Digumarthy SR, et al. Common and uncommon manifestations of Wegener granulomatosis of chest CT: radiologic-pathologic correlation. Radiographics. 2012;32:51–69.

44. McAdams HP, Rosado-de-Christenson ML, Templeton PA, et al. Thoracic mycoses from opportunistic fungi: radiologic-pathologic correlation. Radiographics. 1995; 15:271–86.

45. Miller BH, Rosado-de-Christenson MI, McAdams HP, et al. Thoracic sarcoidosis: radiologic-pathologic correlation. Radiographics. 1995;15:421–37.

46. Miller BH, Rosado-de-Christenson ML, Mason AC, et al. Malignant pleural mesothelioma: radiologic-pathologic correlation. Radiographics. 1996;16: 613–44.

47. Moon WJ, Jung SL, Lee JH, et al. Benign and malignant thyroid nodules: US differentiation—multicenter retrospective study. Radiology. 2008;247:762–70.

48. Mueller-Mang C, Grosse C, Schmid K, et al. What every radiologist should Know about idiopathic interstitial pneumonias. Radiographics. 2007;27:595–615.

49. Nasseri F, Eftekhari F. Clinical and radiologic review of the normal and abnormal thymus: pearls and pitfalls. Radiographics. 2010;30:413–28.

50. Nishino M, Ashiku SK, Kocher ON, et al. The thymus: a comprehensive review. Radiographics. 2006;26: 335–48.

51. Ridge CA, Bankier AA, Eisenber RL. Mosaic attenuation. Am J Roentgenol. 2011;197:W970–7.

52. Sahin H, Brown KK, Curran-Everett D, et al. Chronic hypersensitivity pneumonitis: CT features—comparison with pathologic evidence of fibrosis and survival. Radiology. 2007;244:591–8.

53. Shida H, Chiyotani K, Honma K, et al. Radiologic and pathologic characteristics of mixed dust pneumoconiosis. Radiographics. 1996;16:483–98.

54. Shin MS, Jackson RM, Ho KJ. Tracheobronchomegaly (Mounier-Kuhn syndrome): CT diagnosis. Am J Roentgenol. 1988;150:777–9.

55. Silva CIS, Muller NL, Lynch DA, et al. Chronic hypersensitivity pneumonitis: differentiation from idiopathic pulmonary fibrosis and nonspecific interstitial pneumonia by using thin-section CT. Radiology. 2008;246:288–97.

56. Sumikawa H, Johkoh T, Ichikado K, et al. Usual interstitial pneumonia and chronic idiopathic interstitial pneumonia: analysis of CT appearance in 92 patients. Radiology. 2006;241:258–66.

57. Ujita M, Renzoni EA, Veeraraghavan S, et al. Organizing pneumonia: perilobular pattern at thin-section CT. Radiology. 2004;232:757–61.

58. Vandermeer FQ, Wong-You-Cheong J. Thyroid nodules: when to biopsy. Appl Radiol. 2007;36:8–18.

59. Wand ZF, Reddy GP, Gotway MB, et al. Malignant pleural mesothelioma: evaluation with CT, MR imaging, and PET. Radiographics. 2004;24:105–19.

60. Wang ZJ, Reddy GP, Gotway MB, et al. Malignant pleural mesothelioma: evaluation with CT, MR imaging and PET. Radiographics. 2004;24:105–19.

61. Watadani T, Sakai F, Johkoh T, et al. Interobserver variability in the CT assessment of honeycombing in the lungs. Radiology. 2013;266:936–44.

62. Webb WR. Thin-section CT of the secondary pulmonary lobule: anatomy and the image—the 2004 Fleischner lecture. Radiology. 2006;239:322–38.

Part III

Abdomen and Pelvis

Trauma

Contents

R. Agarwala, *Atlas of Emergency Radiology:*
Vascular System, Chest, Abdomen and Pelvis, and Reproductive System,
DOI 10.1007/978-3-319-13042-2_11, © Springer International Publishing Switzerland 2015

Liver

Diagnosis
Penetrating Grade III Liver Laceration

Imaging Features
1. Hematoma: subcapsular >50 % surface area and rupture with active bleeding
2. Hematoma: intraparenchymal >10 cm
3. Laceration: capsular tear, >3 cm in depth

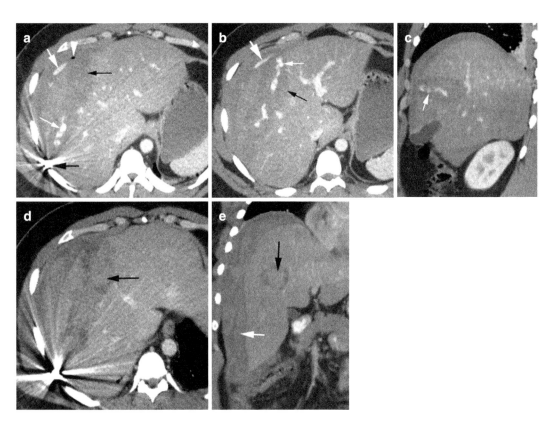

Fig. 11.1 Penetrating liver laceration grade III by gunshot injury. Contrast-enhanced CT (**a**, **b**) axial and (**c**) coronal reformatted images show linear low-density laceration of the liver (*thin black arrow*) with high-density contrast mixed with active hemorrhage (*thin white arrow*) within it which is also extending into the subphrenic space (*thick white arrow*), a bullet adjacent to the rib (*thick black arrow*) and with small focus of gas (*arrowhead*). (**d**, **e**) Axial and coronal reformatted CTs 1 week later show high-density hematoma in the laceration (*black arrow*) and perihepatic space (*white arrow*) but no active hemorrhage

Diagnosis
Laceration of the Liver, Tear of the Diaphragm,
and Pulmonary Contusion

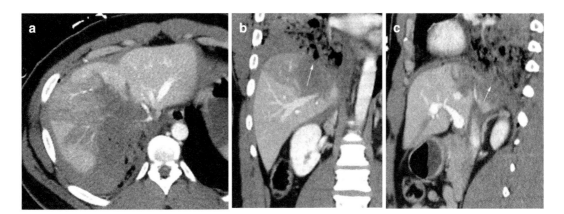

Fig. 11.2 Liver laceration, lung contusion, and tear of the diaphragm from penetrating trauma. (**a**) Axial CT and (**b**) coronal and (**c**) sagittal reformatted images show low-density laceration of the dome of the right lobe of the liver continuous with the adjacent pulmonary contusion. The diaphragm is discontinuous posteriorly (*arrow*)

Diagnosis

Subcapsular Hemorrhage

Imaging Features

1. High-density hemorrhagic fluid extending from the liver parenchyma into the subcapsular space
2. Fluid contouring the liver and deforming the liver surface

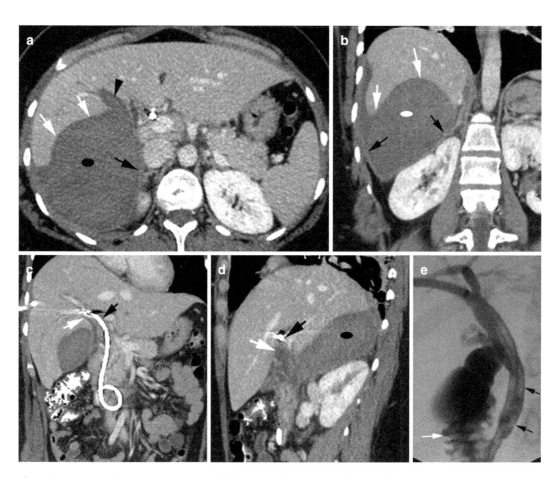

Fig. 11.3 Subcapsular hemorrhage from PTC drain placement. History of laparoscopic cholecystectomy and impacted stone in CBD followed by PTC drain placement. (**a, b**) Axial CT and coronal reformatted images show a thin linear capsule (*black arrows*) surrounding the hemorrhagic fluid (*ellipse* also in **d**) that is compressing and deforming the liver surface (*white arrows*) and is extending from the liver parenchyma (*arrowhead*). (**c, d**) Coronal and sagittal reformatted images show hemorrhage tract (*white arrow*) extending from near the biliary drain (*black arrow*). (**e**) T-tube cholangiogram shows multiple stones in the common bile duct as filling defects (*black arrows*) with contrast flowing into the duodenum (*white arrow*)

Diagnosis

Biloma

Imaging Features

1. Laceration of the liver parenchyma
2. Large well-marginated fluid collection at the site of the previous laceration

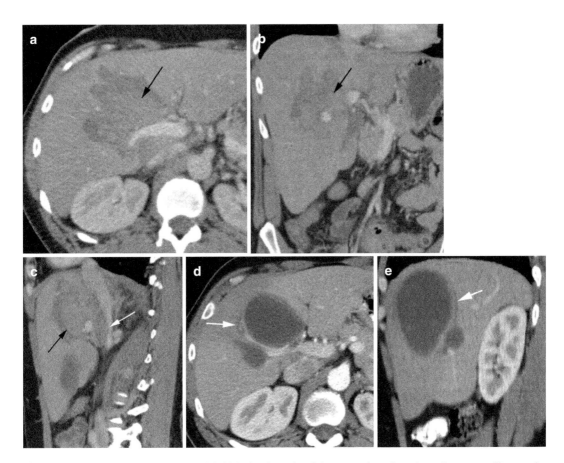

Fig. 11.4 Liver laceration grade IV with high-density hematoma from blunt trauma and well-marginated biloma replacing the hematoma a month later, which was drained. Axial CT and coronal and sagittal reformatted images (**a–c**) show laceration with hematoma (*black arrow*) involving porta hepatis and causing mass effect on the IVC (*white arrow* in **c**). (**d, e**) Axial and sagittal reformatted images 1 month later show two loculated low-density fluid collections continuous with the biliary duct (*white arrow*) which were drained

Diagnosis
Injury to the Biliary Tract

Imaging Findings
1. Air in the biliary tree
2. Biliary fluid and gas contained within the liver capsule
3. Laceration of the liver from penetrating trauma
4. Spillage of contrast from the bile ducts by ERCP study

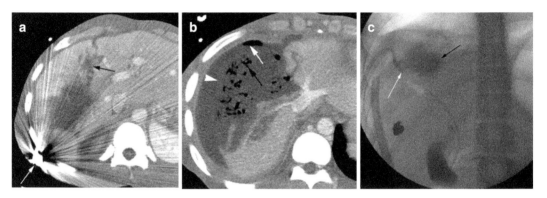

Fig. 11.5 Laceration of the liver and injury to the biliary ducts. Axial CT (**a**) shows laceration of the right lobe of the liver (*black arrow*) by a bullet (*white arrow*). (**b**) At a higher level than (**a**), gas is seen in the biliary tree (*black arrow*), and large biloma is seen with layered gas (*white arrow*) distending the liver capsule and outside the liver parenchyma (*arrowhead*). (**c**) ERCP examination shows leakage of contrast (*black arrow*) with drainage catheter (*white arrow*)

Diagnosis

Subcapsular Hepatic Active Bleeding by Angiogram

Imaging Features

1. Loculated parenchymal and subcapsular hematoma
2. No active hemorrhage in postcontrast study
3. Active hemorrhage by angiogram

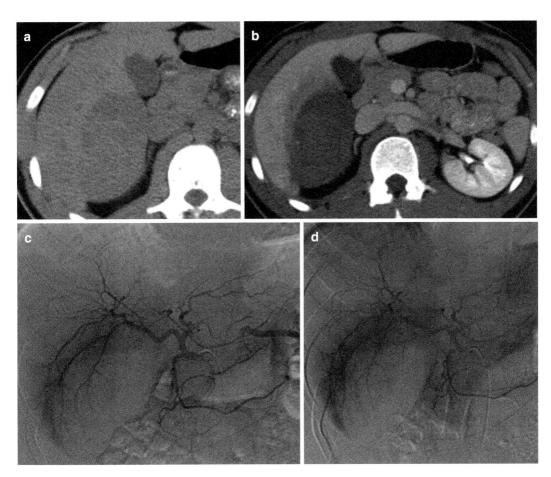

Fig. 11.6 Hematoma involving the liver parenchyma and subcapsular region with active bleeding by angiogram, with history of blunt trauma. Axial CT (**a**) precontrast shows high-density hematoma involving segment VI and protruding inferiorly with subcapsular extension. (**b**) Postcontrast study does not show active hemorrhage within the hematoma. (**c**) Angiogram of the hepatic artery shows faint blush of extravasation in the early part of the study. (**d**) Delayed phase of the study shows increased extravasation of contrast

Spleen

Diagnosis

Splenic Laceration

Imaging Features

1. Laceration of the spleen with or without active intraparenchymal bleed from disruption of trabecular vessels
2. Capsular tear with active intraperitoneal bleed
3. Parenchymal and subcapsular hematoma

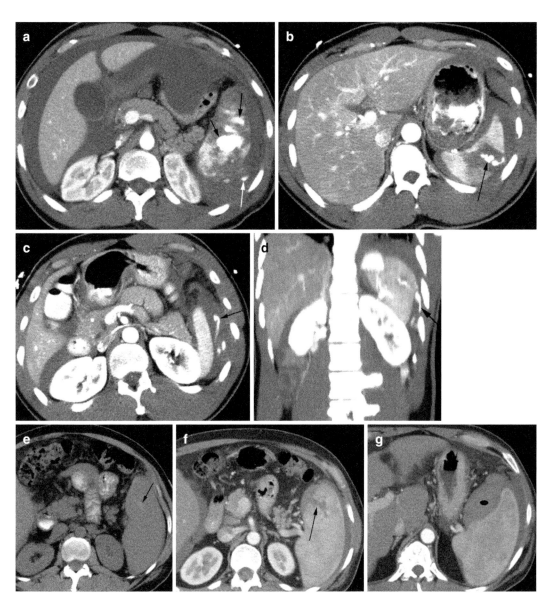

Fig. 11.7 Splenic laceration in different patients. Patient 1: (**a**) axial contrast-enhanced CT following blunt trauma shows grade III laceration with injury to the trabecular vessels and intraparenchymal pooling of contrast (*black arrows*). Cortical tear is also seen with active bleeding into the peritoneal cavity (*white arrow*). Patient 2: (**b, c**) axial and (**d**) coronal reformatted CTs following penetrating wound show active bleeding from the spleen into the peritoneal cavity (*arrows*). Patient 3: (**e**) axial noncontrast image shows linear high-density hematoma within laceration (*arrow*). (**f, g**) CECT shows linear tear of the spleen (*arrow*) and large subcapsular hemorrhage (*ellipse*)

Pancreas

Diagnosis
Pancreatic Tear

Imaging Features

1. Linear lucent line through the neck with complete separation of the neck and body
2. Laceration of the pancreas with several incomplete lines through the pancreas
3. Surrounding hemorrhage and/or pancreatic fluid

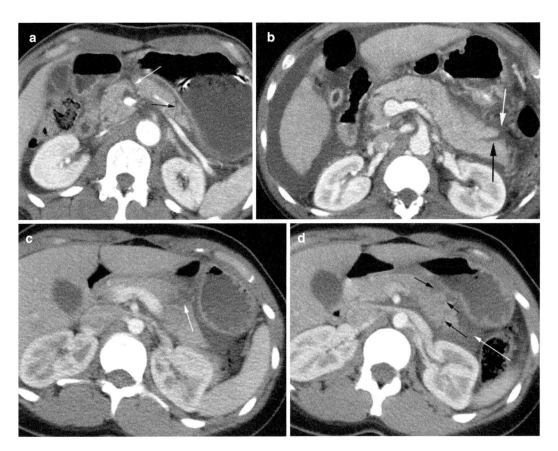

Fig. 11.8 Tear and laceration of the pancreas in three patients with trauma. Patient 1: (**a**) axial CT shows complete tear of the neck (*white arrow*) and at the tail (*black arrow*). The surrounding low-density fluid is leaking pancreatic fluid from the tear of the pancreatic duct. Patient 2: (**b**) axial CT following a stab wound shows incomplete tear at the tail of the pancreas (*black arrow*) with surrounding small high-density hematoma (*white arrow*). Patient 3: (**c**, **d**) axial CT shows multiple incomplete tears of the tail of the pancreas (*black arrows*) with surrounding high-density hematoma (*white arrow*)

Kidneys

Diagnosis
Renal Laceration and Hematoma

Imaging Features
1. Sharp tear through the renal parenchyma
2. Hemorrhagic fluid within the tract of the tear and the subcapsular space

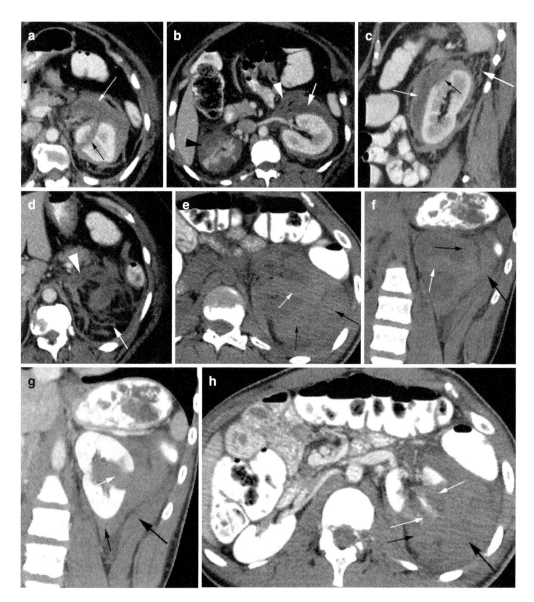

Fig. 11.9 Laceration of the kidney from stab injury in two patients. Patient 1: (**a–d**) axial CT shows grade III laceration with sharp contour of the tear (*black arrow* **a** and **c**) and hemorrhagic fluid in the subcapsular space (*thin white arrow*). Hemorrhagic fluid is also thickening the perirenal septa (*thick white arrow* **c, d**) and anterior renal fascia (*white arrowhead* **b, d**). The right kidney shows infarction with decreased cortical perfusion (*black arrowhead*) (history of drug abuse). Patient 2: (**e–h**) precontrast axial (**e**) and coronal reformatted images (**f**) show high-density acute hemorrhage in the renal parenchymal tear (*thin white arrow*), in the subcapsular space (*thin black arrow*) and perirenal space (*thick black arrow*). Postcontrast coronal reformatted (**g**) and axial (**h**) CT images show the same findings. Axial image shows multiple linear tears through midpole of the kidney involving the cortex and medulla

Diagnosis

Grade IV Laceration of the Kidney

Imaging Features

1. Parenchymal laceration through the cortex, medulla, and collecting system
2. Main renal artery or vein injury with contained hemorrhage

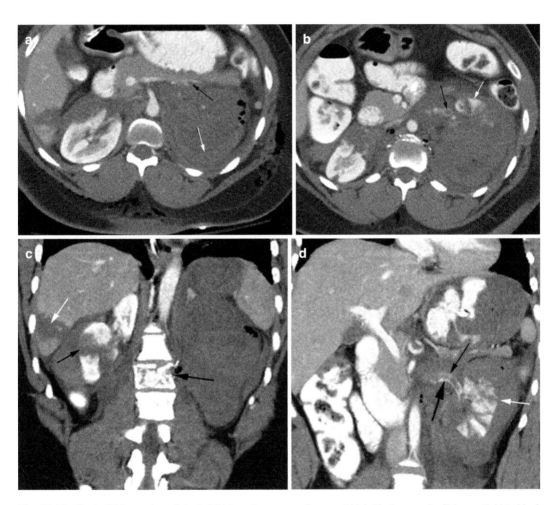

Fig. 11.10 Grade IV laceration of the left kidney from gunshot injury with most of the left kidney devascularized. (**a**, **b**) Axial CT and (**c**, **d**) coronal reformatted images show small area of enhancement in upper pole and midpole of the left kidney (*white arrow* **b**, **d**). Thrombus is seen in the left renal vein (*thin black arrow* **a**, **b**). The left renal artery (*thick black arrow* in **d**) is small (*thin black arrow* showing vein). Hematoma is seen in the subcapsular region (*white arrow* in **a**). (**c**) Fracture is seen midpole of the right kidney (*thin black arrow*), adjacent liver (*white arrow*), and lumber vertebra (*thick black arrow*)

Diagnosis

Renal Laceration with Active Bleeding and
Colon Perforation

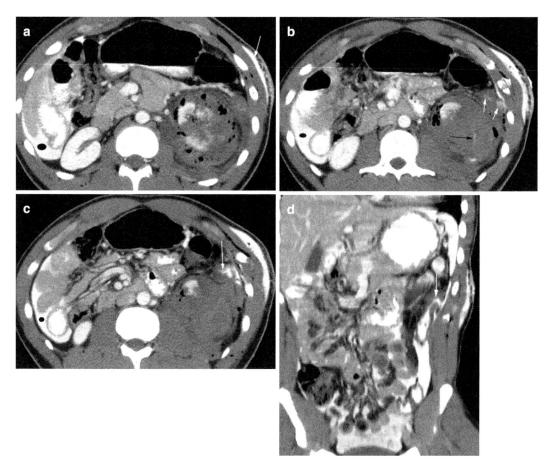

Fig. 11.11 Gunshot injury with left renal laceration and tear of the left colon. (**a**) Axial contrast-enhanced CT shows extensive laceration of the lower half of the left kidney with hematoma in the renal parenchyma and the subcapsular space with extensive pneumatosis. Spillage of enteric contrast is also seen in subcutaneous tissues (*white arrow*). (**b**) Axial CT higher than (**a**) shows linear extravasation of enteric contrast into the hematoma in the anterior pararenal space (*white arrows*) from the left colon. Active extravasation of IV contrast is seen in the lower renal pole (*black arrow*). (**c**, **d**) Axial and coronal reformatted images show tear of the left colon (*white arrow*) with enteric contrast spilling into the anterior pararenal hematoma and peritoneal cavity (*ellipse*) mostly in the right side of the abdomen

Ureter

Diagnosis
Perforation of the Ureter

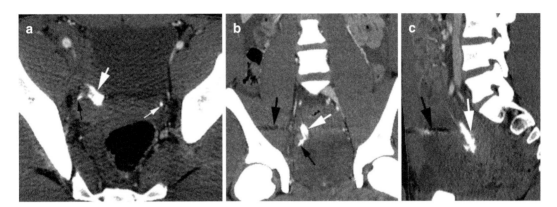

Fig. 11.12 Perforation of the ureter by gunshot injury. CECT (**a–c**) axial, coronal, and sagittal reformatted images show extravasation of contrast (*thick white arrow*) from the distal right ureter (*thin black arrow*). The left ureter (*thin white arrow* in **a**) is normal. Beam hardening artifacts are seen from the bullet (*thick black arrow* **b**, **c**)

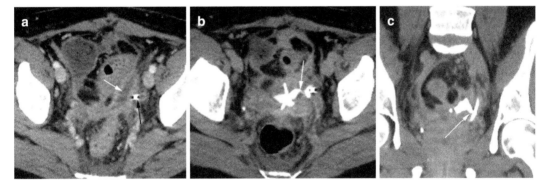

Fig. 11.13 Injury of the ureter with urinoma during hysterectomy. CECT axial (**a**) in the arterial phase shows fluid collection (*white arrow*) medial to the stent in the left ureter (*black arrow*). (**b**) Delayed-phase axial and (**c**) coronal reformatted images show extravasation of contrast (*arrow*) from the stented ureter collecting into the fluid collection (urinoma) seen in (**a**)

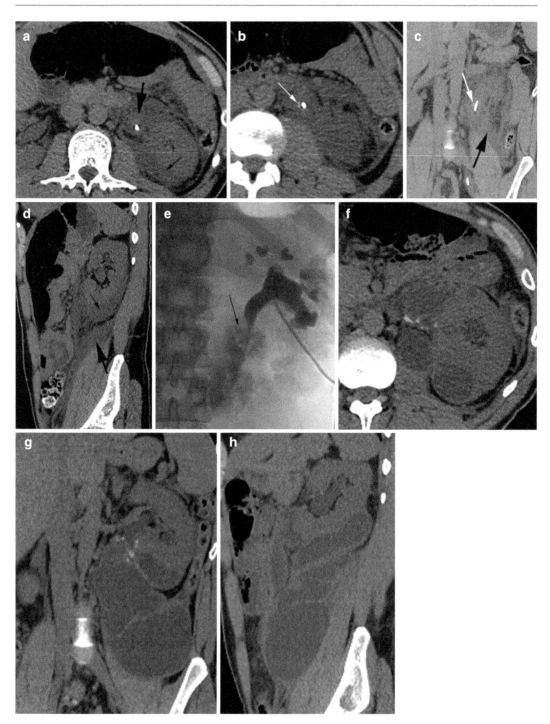

Fig. 11.14 Urinoma post-ureteroscopy. Noncontrast axial CT (**a**, **b**) and coronal (**c**) and sagittal (**d**) reformatted images show large low-density diffuse fluid in the subcapsular space (*thin black arrow*) and perirenal space (*thick black arrow*). A stone is seen adjacent to the stent (*white arrow*). (**e**) Nephrostogram shows leakage of contrast from the proximal right ureter (*arrow*). (**e–g**) Noncontrast CT done 1 month later: (**e**) axial, (**f**) coronal, and (**g**, **h**) sagittal reformatted images show multiple loculations of the urinoma

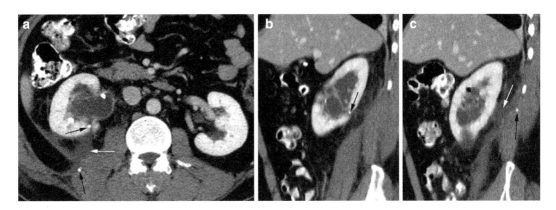

Fig. 11.15 Urinoma as a result of percutaneous nephrostomy. CECT axial (**a**) and sagittal reformatted images (**b**, **c**) show one stone in the nephrostomy tract in the renal cortex and one in the quadratus lumborum muscle (*black arrows*) with urinoma (*white arrows*) along the tract

Bladder

Diagnosis
Bladder Rupture

Imaging Features
1. Tear of the bladder wall
2. Hematoma of the bladder wall
3. Spilled contrast into the peritoneal and extra-peritoneal spaces

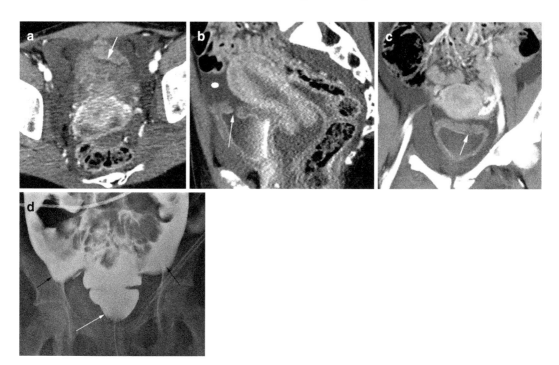

Fig. 11.16 Intraperitoneal bladder rupture. History of motor vehicular accident. CECT axial (**a**), sagittal (**b**), and coronal (**c**) reformatted images show tear of the dome of the bladder (*arrows*) with urine in the peritoneal cavity (*ellipse*). (**d**) Retrograde cystogram shows contrast spilling into the peritoneal cavity (*black arrows*) from the bladder with catheter (*white arrow*)

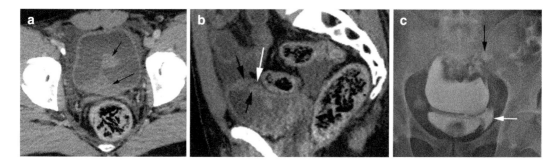

Fig. 11.17 Intra- and extraperitoneal bladder rupture form MVC. CECT (**a**) axial and (**b**) sagittal reformatted images show thrombus in the bladder wall around the tear (*black arrows*) with linear tear seen in sagittal view (*white arrow*). Cystogram (**c**) shows extravasated contrast into the peritoneal cavity surrounding the sigmoid colon (*black arrow*) and retroperitoneum (*white arrow*)

Urethra

Diagnosis
Ruptured Urethra

Imaging Features
1. Contrast within the corpora cavernosum and corpus spongiosum
2. Extravasated contrast in the perineum which is continuous with subcutaneous tissues of the anterior abdominal wall

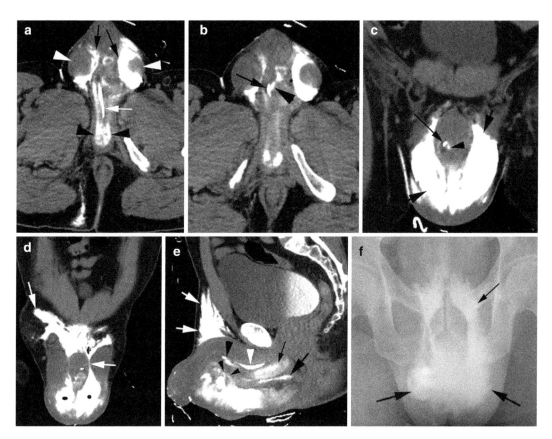

Fig. 11.18 Injury to the penile urethra from GSW. (**a**) CECT axial (**a**) image shows extravasated contrast in the corpus spongiosum (*black arrowheads*) on either side of the contrast-filled urethra (*white arrow*) and contrast in the tunica vaginalis space (*thick black arrows*) bilaterally surrounding the testes (*arrowheads*). (**b**) Axial CT and (**c**) coronal reformatted images show site of urethral rupture (*long arrow*) with extravasation of contrast (*arrowhead*) (*thick black arrowhead* also in **e**) and pooling of contrast outside the deep fascia (*short thick arrow*). (**d**) Coronal reformatted image shows that contrast in subcutaneous soft tissues at the ventral aspect of the penis (*ellipse*) is tracking to the lower abdominal wall subcutaneous tissues ventral to the rectus abdominis muscles bilaterally (*arrow*). (**e**) Sagittal reformatted image shows injury of the corpus spongiosum ventral to the urethra (*white arrow head*) containing high-density contrast (*thin black arrow*). Contrast is also seen outside the corpus spongiosum but within the deep fascia (*thick black arrow*). Tear of fascia in the mid-penis ventrally (*small black arrowheads*) with contrast pooling in the subcutaneous space. Contrast tracking to the lower anterior abdominal wall (*thin white arrows*). (**f**) Retrograde urethrogram shows similar findings with contrast in the undersurface of the penis (*thick black arrows*) and anterior abdominal wall (*thin black arrow*)

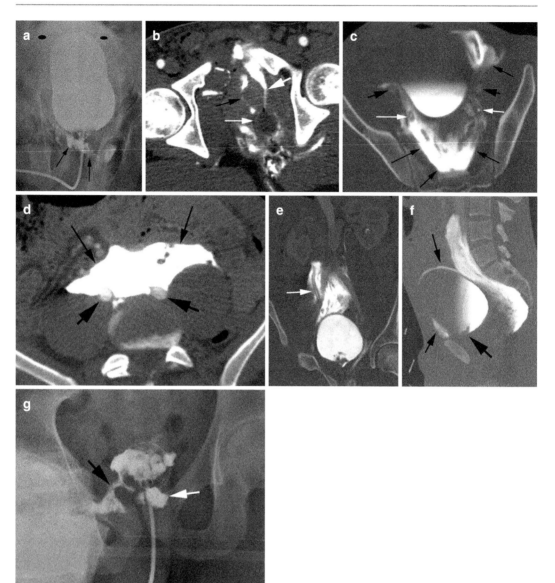

Fig. 11.19 Ruptured prostatic urethra and bladder base from gunshot injury. Cystogram (**a**) shows extravasation of contrast from the prostatic urethra (*thin black arrows*). High-density contrast around the dome of the bladder is contrast in the retroperitoneum (*ellipse*) from previous CT study. Axial CT (**b**) done before the cystogram shows a Foley catheter inferior to the prostatic urethra (*thin white arrow*) with small irregular contrast within the prostatic urethra (*black arrow*). Extravasated contrast from the tip of the catheter is curving around the prostate (*thick white arrow*) toward the symphysis pubis. Axial CT (**c**, **d**) and (**e**) coronal reformatted images show that extravasated contrast in the perineum from the catheter is tracking around the bladder (*thin black arrows*) to the retroperitoneal space posteriorly curving over the psoas muscles, surrounding the common iliac arteries (*thick black arrows*) and the ureters (*white arrow*). (**f**) Sagittal reformatted image shows contrast extending anteriorly in the space of Retzius (*thin short arrow*) and curving posteriorly over the dome of the bladder (*long arrow*). The bladder base is irregular (*thick black arrow*). Cystogram done a few days later (**g**) shows contrast leaking from the bladder base on the right side (*black arrow*) and from the prostatic urethra (*white arrow*)

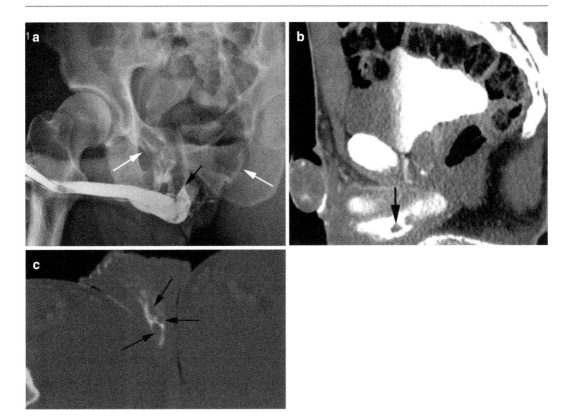

Fig. 11.20 Rupture of the posterior urethra from straddle injury. (**a**) Urethrogram shows obstruction of the posterior urethra (*black arrow*). Flexible cystoscopy showed ventral disruption of the urethra distal to the external sphincter. Vascular intravasation of contrast is seen (*white arrows*). CT sagittal reformatted image (**b**) and axial image (**c**) show multiple thrombi causing filling defect within the urethra (*arrows*)

Bowel

Diagnosis
Bowel and Mesenteric Trauma.

Imaging Features
1. Bowel wall defect
2. Extraluminal air in the peritoneal or retroperitoneal spaces or intramural
3. Extraluminal enteric contrast
4. Extravasation of contrast from vessels
5. Focal bowel wall thickening
6. Mesenteric fat stranding with focal fluid and hematoma
7. Intraperitoneal and retroperitoneal fluid

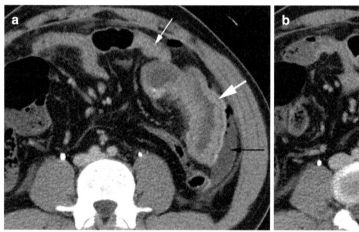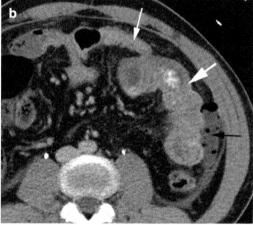

Fig. 11.21 Small bowel tear from seat belt injury. Axial CT (**a**, **b**) shows a loop of dilated small bowel with thick walls (*thick white arrow*). Focal extraluminal gas mixed with fluid is seen adjacent to it (*black arrow*). The rest of the small bowels show normal architecture (*thin white arrow*)

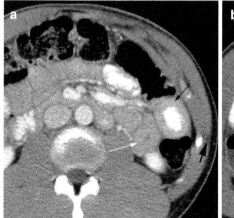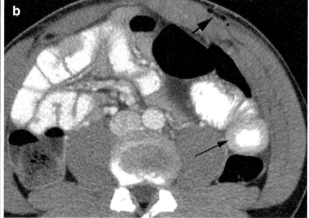

Fig. 11.22 Small bowel wall hematoma from penetrating trauma. Axial CT (**a**, **b**) shows mural hematoma in a loop of small bowel (*black arrow*). The thick wall has higher density than the other collapsed loops (*white arrow*). Stab wound defects are seen in the adjacent abdominal wall (*thick black arrow*)

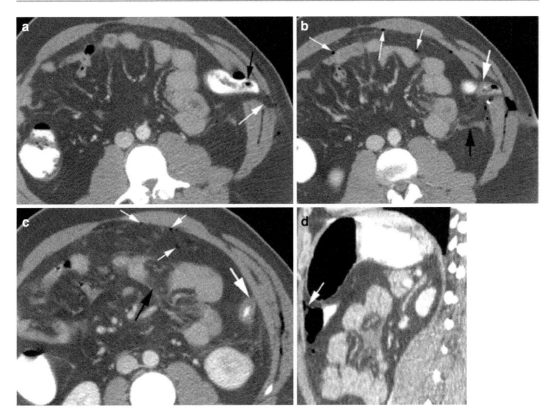

Fig. 11.23 Large and small bowel injury from gunshot injury. Axial CT (**a**) shows protrusion of the mid-descending colon (*black arrow*) through strap muscle defect (*white arrow*). (**b, c**) Axial CT proximal to (**a**) shows wall thickening (*thick white arrow*) of the nondilated colon which was ischemic at surgery and was resected. Hemorrhagic fluid is seen adjacent to the injured colon and in the small bowel mesentery (*black arrow*). Small specks of pneumoperitoneum (*thin short white arrows*) are seen. (**d**) Sagittal reformatted image shows small bowel perforation with gas leakage (*arrow*)

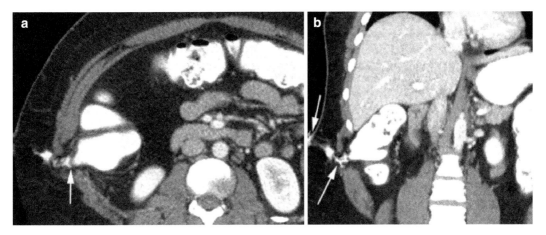

Fig. 11.24 Perforation of the right colon with leakage of contrast. History of stab wound to the right flank. CT axial (**a**) and coronal reformatted images (**b**) show leakage of contrast from the ascending colon through the defect in the strap muscles extending to the skin (*arrows*)

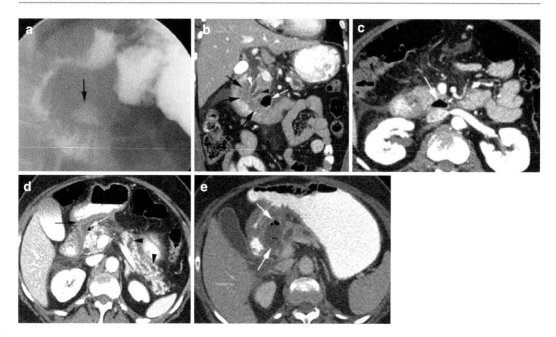

Fig. 11.25 Duodenal perforation post-ERCP. History of distal CBD and proximal PD stricture with sphincterotomy. (**a**) Barium swallow study shows perforation of the third portion of the duodenum with extravasation of contrast (*arrow*). CT coronal reformatted (**b**) and axial (**c**) images show air leaking from the third part of the duodenal sweep (*white arrow*), stricture of the CBD (*white arrowhead*) and PD (*black arrowhead*), and edema of the duodenal sweep medial wall (*black arrows*). Axial CT (**d**) shows gas and fluid in the duodenal groove (*white arrow*) and edema of the adjacent stomach and duodenum (*black arrow*) and a dilated pancreatic duct (*arrowheads*). (**e**) Axial CT a week later shows abscess in the duodenal groove (*arrows*)

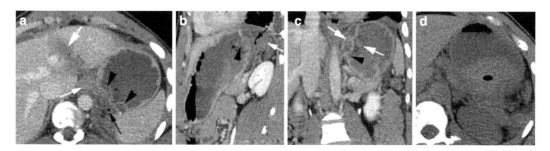

Fig. 11.26 Laceration of the stomach and liver from gunshot injury. CT axial (**a**), sagittal (**b**), and coronal (**c**) reformatted images show wall irregularity of the fundus of the stomach posteriorly (*arrowheads*) with surrounding hematoma (*thin white arrows*), extraluminal gas (*black arrow*), and laceration of the left lobe of the liver (*thick white arrow*). (**d**) Unenhanced CT shows large intraluminal high-density hemorrhage (*ellipse*) within the stomach

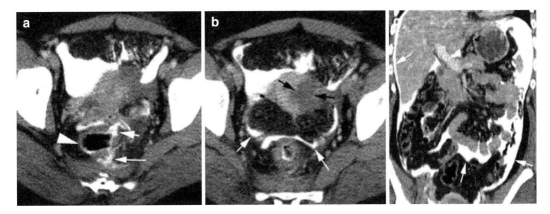

Fig. 11.27 Tear of the rectosigmoid colon and uterus from GSW (surgically repaired) with extravasation of enteric contrast into the peritoneal cavity and retroperitoneum. CT axial (**a**, **b**) shows extravasation of enteric contrast from the rectosigmoid colon (*arrowhead*) into the peritoneal cavity anteriorly (*short white arrow*) and posteriorly to the retroperitoneal space (*long white arrow*). Low density in the left side of the body and fundus of the uterus (*black arrows*) is uterine tear and hematoma. (**c**) Coronal reformatted image shows intraperitoneal extravasated contrast surrounding the bowel loops and liver (*arrows*)

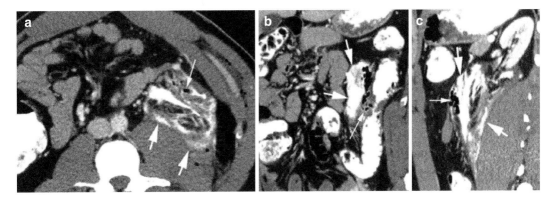

Fig. 11.28 Tear of the descending colon with retroperitoneal extravasation of enteric contrast from GSW. CT axial (**a**), coronal (**b**), and sagittal (**c**) reformatted images show perforation of the descending colon with contrast (*thick arrows*) and air leaking out (*thin arrow*) into the surrounding retroperitoneum anterior to the psoas muscle

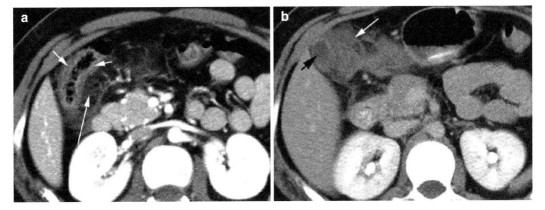

Fig. 11.29 Hematoma of the wall of the hepatic flexure with surrounding hemorrhage and edema from blunt trauma. Axial CT (**a**) shows high-density wall thickening of hepatic flexure (*short white arrows*) and edema of the mesentery medial to it (*long white arrow*). (**b**) Axial CT at higher plane shows diffuse high-density hematoma (*white arrow*) in the adipose tissue medial to the gallbladder (*black arrow*)

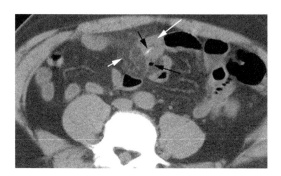

Fig. 11.30 Foreign body perforation of the small bowel.
Axial CT shows linear opaque foreign body (*short black
arrow*) penetrating the thick small bowel wall (*long white
arrow*) with surrounding mesenteric edema (*short white
arrow*) and small focus of perforated extraluminal air
(*long black arrow*)

Diaphragm

Diagnosis
Traumatic Diaphragm Tear

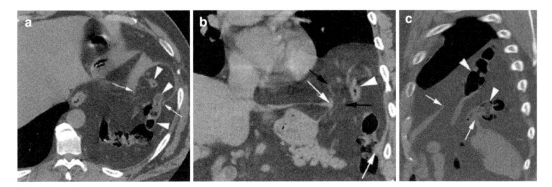

Fig. 11.31 Diaphragmatic tear. History of old trauma. CT axial (**a**), coronal (**b**), and (**c**) sagittal reformatted images show tear of the left hemidiaphragm with herniation of the splenic flexure (*arrowheads*) along with the mesentery (*thin black arrows*) into the thorax through the torn ends of the diaphragm (*thin white arrow*)

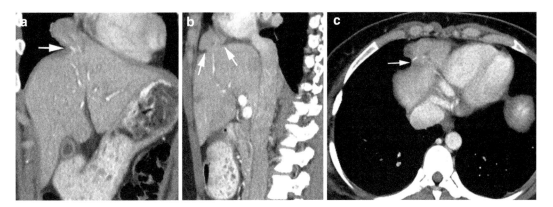

Fig. 11.32 Herniation of the liver through diaphragm defect. CT coronal (**a**) and sagittal (**b**) reformatted images show focal protrusion of the dome of the liver through a defect in the diaphragm (*arrows*). (**c**) Axial CT shows a lobulated liver adjacent to the right heart border with a narrow neck (*arrow*). The vascularity of the herniated liver is continuous with the rest of the liver

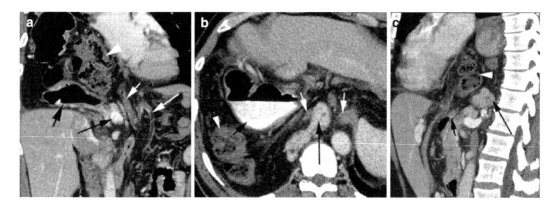

Fig. 11.33 Herniation through the esophageal hiatus. CT (**a**) coronal reformatted image shows herniation of a loop of the jejunum (*short white arrow*), mesentery (*long white arrow*), and pancreas (*long black arrow*) at the hiatal defect. The stomach (*short black arrow*) and colon (*arrowhead*) are in the thorax. Axial image (**b**) shows separation of both leaves of the diaphragm (*white arrows*). The pancreas (*long black arrows*), stomach (*short black arrow*), and colon (*arrowhead*) are in the thorax. (**c**) Sagittal reformatted image shows the colon (*arrowhead*) and pancreas (*long black arrow*) in the thorax and the duodenum (*short black arrow*) at the hiatus

Diseases of the Liver

Contents

R. Agarwala, *Atlas of Emergency Radiology:*
Vascular System, Chest, Abdomen and Pelvis, and Reproductive System,
DOI 10.1007/978-3-319-13042-2_12, © Springer International Publishing Switzerland 2015

Biliary System

Biliary Stones

Diagnosis
Gallstones

Imaging Features
Sonogram:
1. Echogenic foci with acoustic posterior shadow in dependent portion of GB.
2. Cholesterol stones are echogenic with comet tail artifacts and may float.

CT:
1. Calcified stones have high density.
2. Noncalcified stones have low density and may not be visible.
3. Cholesterol stones usually have lower attenuation than bile.
4. Mercedes-Benz sign of nitrogen gas in the center of cholesterol crystal.

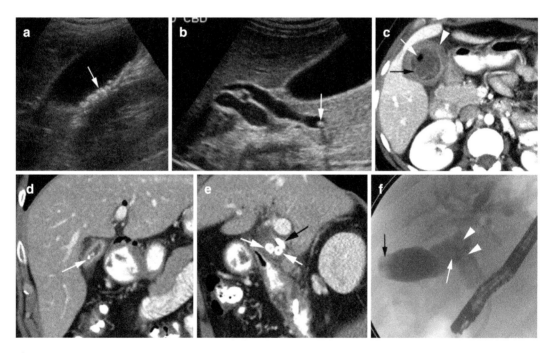

Fig. 12.1 Gallstones. Ultrasound of the gallbladder (**a**) shows multiple highly reflective echogenic foci within the GB with posterior acoustic shadowing (*arrow*). (**b**) Echogenic stone with echo shadow at the distal end of the dilated common bile duct (*arrow*). (**c**) Axial CT shows low-density stones with rim calcifications (*black arrow*), small gas collection in one stone (*white arrow*), and acute cholecystitis with GB wall thickening (*arrowhead*). (**d**) Coronal reformatted CT image shows multiple high-attenuated calcified stones in contracted GB (*arrow*). (**e**) CT Sagittal reformatted image shows stones in cystic duct (*white arrows*) and stent in common hepatic duct (*black arrow*). (**f**) ERCP study shows stones in the gallbladder (*black arrow*), cystic duct (*white arrow*), and CBD (*arrowheads*)

Diagnosis

Mirizzi Syndrome

Imaging Features

1. Gallstone impacted in the distal cystic duct or Hartmann's pouch of the gallbladder causing extrinsic compression on the common hepatic duct

2. Dilatation of common hepatic and intrahepatic biliary ducts and normal caliber of the common bile duct

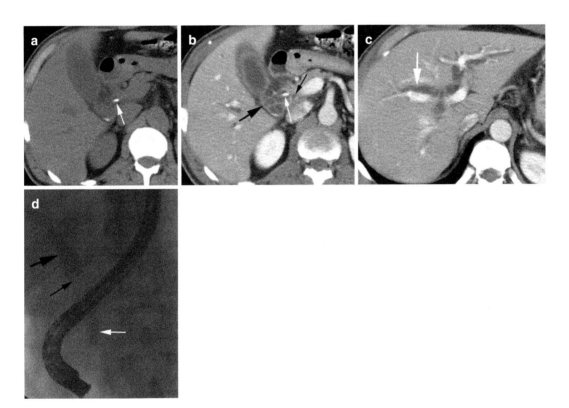

Fig. 12.2 Mirizzi syndrome. (**a**) Axial CT precontrast study shows gallstone in the distal cystic duct at the junction with the common hepatic duct (*white arrow*). (**b**, **c**) Axial CECT shows dilatation of the cystic duct (*thick black arrow*) and intrahepatic bile ducts (*thick white arrow*) with stone at the distal cystic duct (*thin white arrow*). Common bile duct at head of the pancreas is not dilated (*thin black arrow*). (**d**) ERCP examination shows stone at the junction of the cystic duct and common hepatic duct (*thin black arrow*) with dilatation of ducts proximal to the stone (*thick black arrow*) and CBD not dilated (*white arrow*)

Diagnosis
Cholesterol Sludge

Imaging Features
1. Floating stones
2. Comet tail artifacts

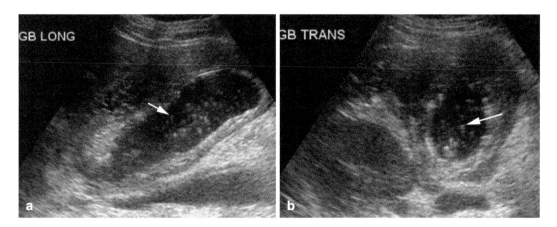

Fig. 12.3 Cholesterol sludge. Ultrasound of the gallbladder (**a**, **b**) shows multiple echogenic floating crystals with comet tail artifacts (*arrow*)

Diagnosis
Cholesterolosis of the Gallbladder

Imaging Features

1. Multiple nonmobile echogenic foci within the gallbladder wall with ring-down artifacts and no shadowing
2. May be a patchy localized form or diffuse form

Hyperplastic Cholecystosis

Diagnosis
Cholesterolosis of the Gallbladder

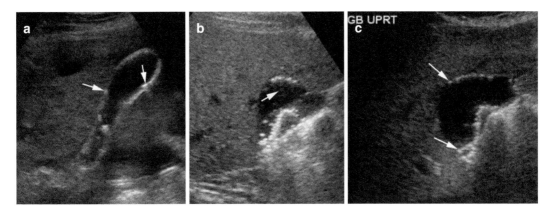

Fig. 12.4 Cholesterolosis of the gallbladder. Ultrasound of the gallbladder in patient 1 (**a**) shows multiple echogenic foci in the gallbladder wall with ring-down artifacts (*arrows*). Patient 2: (**b, c**) Supine and upright position of the patient shows multiple nonmobile echogenic foci in the dependent and nondependent gallbladder wall with distal comet tail artifacts (*arrow*)

Diagnosis

Adenomyomatosis

Imaging Features

1. Types—diffuse, segmental, or focal
2. Brightly echogenic nonmobile nonshadowing polypoid masses in the gallbladder wall with distal comet-tail artifact

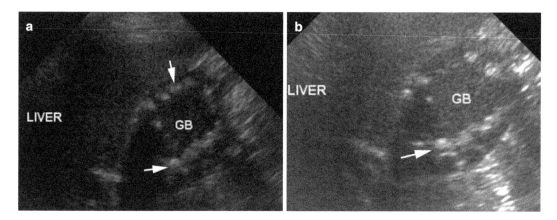

Fig. 12.5 Adenomyomatosis. (**a, b**) Sonogram of the gallbladder (marked as *GB*) shows diffuse nodular echogenic polypoid masses in the gallbladder wall (*arrows*) with comet-tail artifacts

Biliary Gas

Diagnosis
Emphysematous Cholecystitis

Imaging Features
Sonogram:
1. High echogenicity of the gallbladder wall with posterior dirty shadowing
2. Can involve dependent and nondependent wall depending upon extent of involvement
3. Does not move with change of position

CT:
1. Curvilinear gas in the wall of the gallbladder.

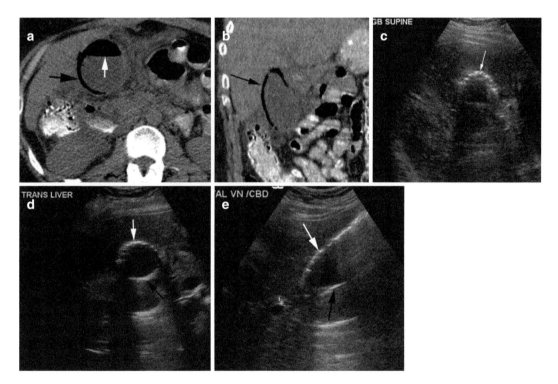

Fig. 12.6 Emphysematous cholecystitis. (**a**, **b**) Axial and coronal reformatted CT shows curvilinear gas in the wall of the gallbladder (*black arrow*). Intraluminal air has air-fluid level (*white arrow*). Ultrasound of the same gallbladder (**c–e**) show bright echogenicity of the gallbladder wall with reverberation artifacts involving both anterior (*white arrow*) and posterior walls (*black arrow*)

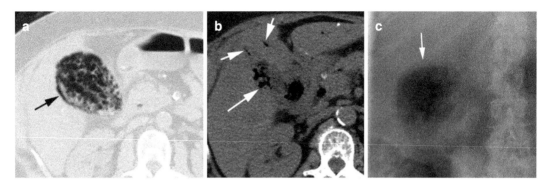

Fig. 12.7 Emphysematous cholecystitis. Axial CT (**a**, **b**) shows extensive sloughing of the gallbladder mucosa with gas collection in the wall of the gallbladder (*arrow* in **a** and *long arrow* in **b**) and air in the bile ducts (*short arrows*). (**c**) Flat plate of the abdomen shows irregular gas collection in the gallbladder (*arrow*)

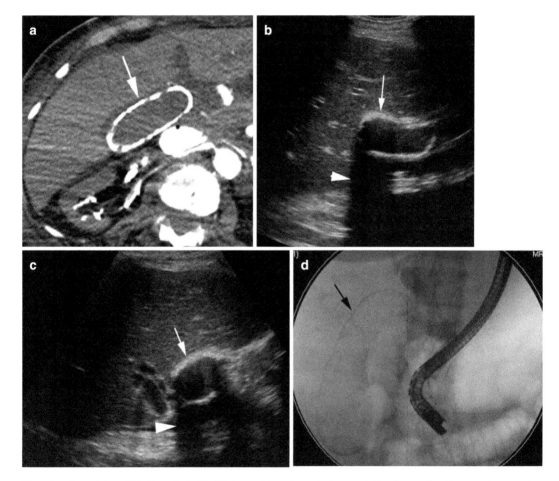

Fig. 12.8 Porcelain gallbladder. (**a**) Axial CT shows diffusely thickened and calcified gallbladder wall (*arrow*). (**b**, **c**) Ultrasound in longitudinal and transverse views of the gallbladder shows diffusely thickened echogenic wall (*arrow*) from calcification and with posterior negative shadowing (*arrowhead*). (**d**) ERCP study shows the gallbladder with calcified wall (*arrow*)

Diagnosis
Wall Echo Shadow (WES) Sign

Imaging Features

1. Two parallel curvilinear echogenic lines separated by a thin hypoechoic space
2. Acoustic shadowing distal to the echogenic line in the far field

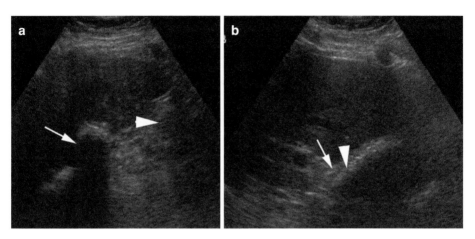

Fig. 12.9 Wall echo shadow (WES) sign. Ultrasound shows (**a**) the gallbladder filled with stones with a negative posterior shadow (*thin arrow*). A focal echogenic area with dirty shadow is seen from bowel loops filled with gas (*arrowhead*). (**b**) The outer thinner component (*thin arrow*) is the wall, and echogenic thicker layers (*arrowhead*) are the stones with thin layer of hypoechoic bile between the two layers

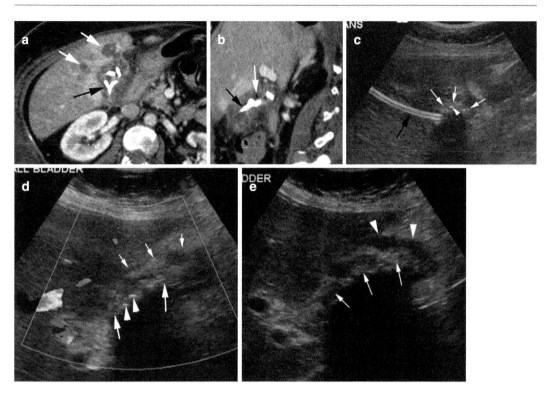

Fig. 12.10 WES sign from cholecystostomy catheter. A patient with acalculous cholecystitis and abscess. (**a**) Axial CT shows a catheter coiled within the gallbladder (*black arrow*). The gallbladder bed shows increased enhancement with small abscesses (*white arrows*). (**b**) Sagittal reformatted image shows small gas bubbles (*white arrow*) adjacent to the catheter (*black arrow*). (**c**) Grayscale ultrasound shows linear catheter (*black arrow*) in the liver parenchyma. Coiled catheter within the gallbladder has ill-defined curvilinear intermediate echogenicity (*white arrows*) with a few echogenic gases

(*arrowhead*). (**d**) Color Doppler shows increased vascularity around the gallbladder fossa region surrounding the WES sign caused by thick wall (*small white arrows*), echogenic coiled catheter (*thick white arrows*), and few gas bubbles (*arrowheads*) forming the second parallel line with posterior shadowing. Small amount of bile is forming the irregular sonolucency between the two echogenic lines. (**e**) Grayscale US shows the gallbladder wall (*arrowheads*) surrounding the coiled catheter posterior to it (*thin arrow*) with distal negative shadowing and small sonolucent bile between the two lines

Diagnosis
Pneumobilia

Imaging Features

1. Bright echoes in the gallbladder with reverberation artifacts
2. Echoes change in position and rise to nondependent wall in upright position

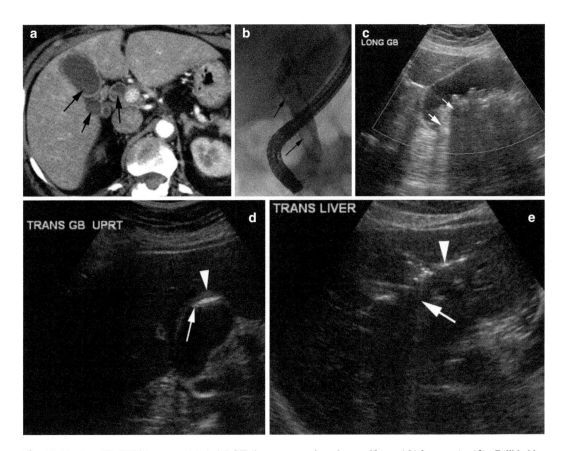

Fig. 12.11 Post-ERCP biliary gas. (**a**) Axial CT shows layered sludge in the gallbladder and bile ducts (*arrows*). (**b**) ERCP shows a stone-filled common bile duct (*arrows*). (**c**) Post-ERCP supine gallbladder ultrasound shows multiple-layered stones and gas in the gallbladder. Stones have negative shadows (*thin arrow*) while the gas has reverberation artifacts (*thick arrow*). (**d**) Gallbladder ultrasound in upright position shows gas (*arrow*) rising to the fundus hugging the gallbladder wall (*arrowhead*). (**e**) Gas in intrahepatic bile ducts with bright echoes (*arrowhead*) and reverberation artifacts (*arrow*)

Diagnosis

Gallstone Ileus

Imaging Features

1. Chronic cholecystitis
2. Fistula with duodenum is common
3. Rigler's triad: Impacted stone in the small bowel, SBO and pneumobilia

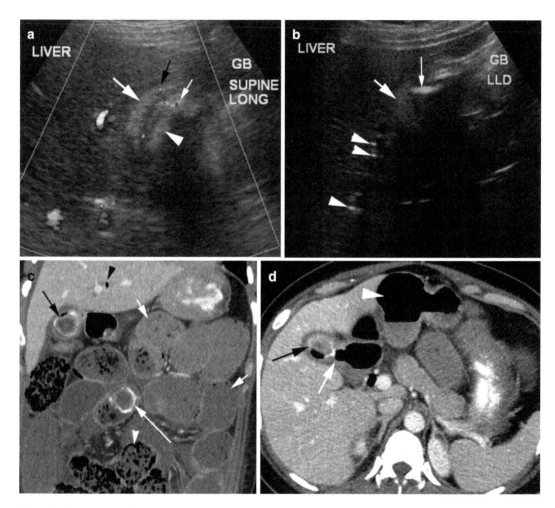

Fig. 12.12 Gallstone ileus. Middle-aged female with chronic right upper quadrant pain now with colicky abdominal pain. US study done first shows WES sign. (**a**) Color Doppler study shows thick-walled gallbladder (*thick white arrow*) with increased vascularity in the wall (*black arrow*). Large stone within lumen with echo shadow (*arrowhead*). Twinkling artifacts from small gas foci adjacent to stone (*thin arrow*). (**b**) Grayscale decubitus view shows air collection (*thin arrow*) in the fundus of the thick-walled gallbladder (*thick arrow*) and echogenic gas in biliary tracts (*arrowheads*). (**c**) Coronal reformatted CT shows large stone in mid-small bowel (*long arrow*) causing obstruction with bowel dilatation (*short arrows*) with small bowel feces sign (*white arrowhead*). Stone with gas is seen in the gallbladder (*black arrow*) and gas biliary duct (*black arrowhead*). (**d**) Axial CT shows fistula (*white arrow*) of duodenum with gallbladder filled with stone and gas (*black arrow*) and dilated stomach (*arrowhead*)

Cholangitis

Imaging Features
1. Irregular narrowing and dilated intrahepatic biliary ducts with wall thickening and surrounding edema
2. Gas, stones, debris, and/or pus in intrahepatic biliary ducts
3. Liver abscesses with dilated ducts

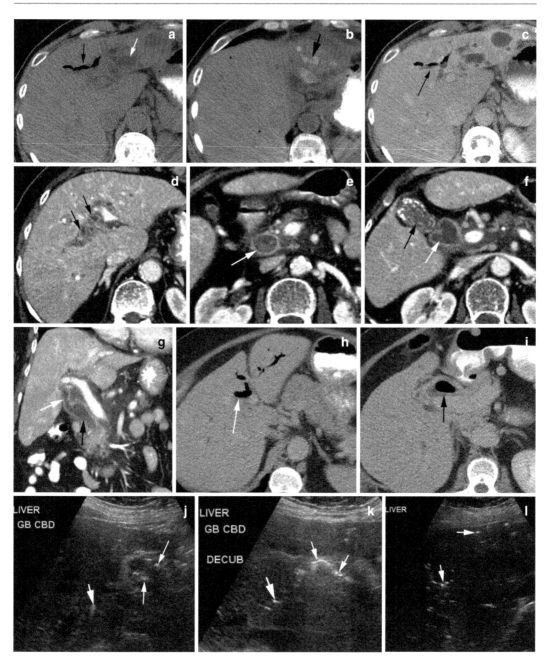

Fig. 12.13 Ascending cholangitis in three patients. Patient 1 (**a**–**c**). Noncontrast axial CT (**a**, **b**) shows pneumobilia (*thin black arrow*), dilated ducts (*white arrow*), and stones in some dilated ducts (*thick black arrow*). (**c**) CECT shows layered dependent debris in gas-filled ducts (*arrow*). Patient 2 (**d**–**g**). Axial CECT shows (**d**) thick-walled dilated ducts at porta hepatis with surrounding edema (*arrows*). (**e**) Dilated CBD filled with stones and sludge (*arrow*). (**f**) Contracted gallbladder with stones from chronic cholecystitis (*black arrow*) and dilated hepatic and common hepatic ducts (*white arrow*). (**g**) Coronal reformatted image shows dilated common hepatic (*white arrow*) and CBD (*black arrow*). Patient 3 (**h**–**l**). Axial CT (**h**) shows pneumobilia of the left lobe (*arrow*). (**i**) Gas in the gallbladder lumen (*arrow*). Ultrasound (**j**) shows gas within the gallbladder (*thin white arrows*) as hyperechoic foci with dirty shadowing. (**k**) GB gas moves and gathers in the nondependent portion in decubitus position (*thin white arrows*). Bright echoes with dirty shadowing within the liver are from pneumobilia (*thick white arrows* in **j**–**l**)

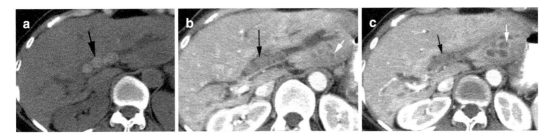

Fig. 12.14 Recurrent pyogenic cholangitis with pigment stones. (**a**) Noncontrast axial CT better shows stones in dilated intrahepatic bile ducts (*black arrow*). (**b, c**) Postcontrast axial CT at different levels shows multiple small clustered abscesses in the left lobe (*white arrows*) adjacent to the dilated ducts with stones (*black arrow*)

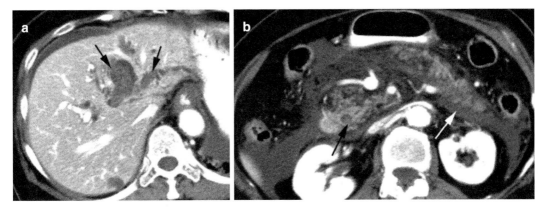

Fig. 12.15 Recurrent oriental cholangitis with gallstone pancreatitis. Postcontrast axial CT (**a**) shows dilated intrahepatic biliary ducts with pigment stones (*arrows*). (**b**) Stone in CBD (*black arrow*), IEP with mild heteroge- neous pancreatic enhancement, and diffuse acute peripan- creatic fluid collection in the anterior pararenal space (*white arrow*)

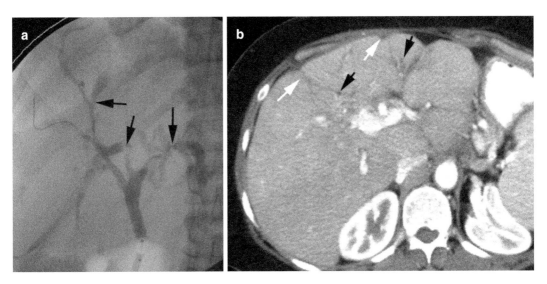

Fig. 12.16 Primary sclerosing cholangitis. ERCP exami- nation (**a**) shows multifocal strictures (*black arrow*) and focal ectasia of intrahepatic biliary ducts adjacent to stric- tures. (**b**) Axial CECT shows scarring of the liver (*white arrows*) with mild intrahepatic biliary dilatation in the affected lobe (*black arrows*)

Biliary Papillomatosis

Imaging Feature
1. Dilated intra- and extrahepatic bile ducts
2. CT—multiple nodules within the ducts which can enhance or not enhance

3. ERCP—single or multiple nodular intraductal filling defects and irregularity of the duct wall

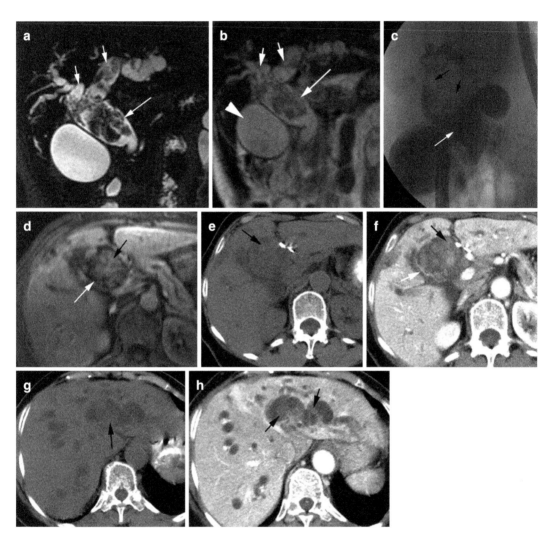

Fig. 12.17 Biliary papillomatosis. (**a**, **b**) MRCP and T2W coronal images show multiple nodular lesions within the dilated CBD (*long arrow*) and right and left bile ducts (*short arrows*). The wall of the bile ducts shows irregular thickening. The gallbladder is distended (*arrowhead*). (**c**) ERCP shows dilated CBD (*white arrow*) with multiple filling defects (*black arrows*). (**d**) T1W postcontrast axial MRI shows dilated CBD (*white arrow*) with irregular enhancing soft tissue mass (*black arrow*). Axial precontrast and CECT (**e**, **f**) of CBD and (**g**, **h**) of the left lobe of the liver show dilated CBD (*white arrow*) and intrahepatic bile ducts with faintly enhancing nodules (*black arrows*)

Choledochal Cyst

Diagnosis

Types 1 and 2

Imaging Features

1. Rounded or fusiform cystic lesion in porta hepatis separate from the gallbladder
2. Cystic lesion communicates with dilated common hepatic duct, CBD, or intrahepatic duct

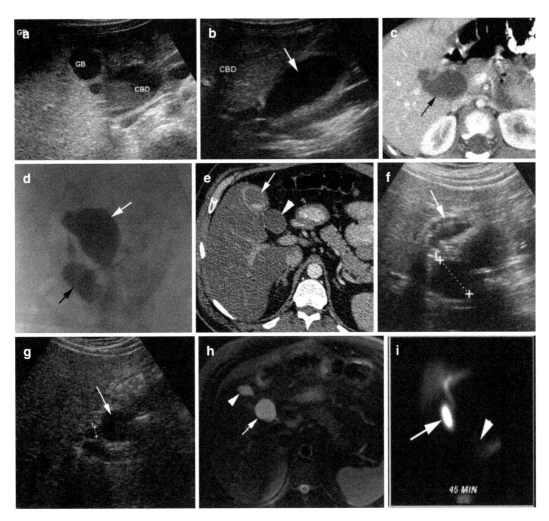

Fig. 12.18 Choledochal cyst. Type I. (**a**, **b**) Ultrasound shows the gallbladder to be separate from the dilated common bile duct (*arrow* in **b**) which contains sludge. (**c**) Axial CT again shows dilated CBD (*black arrow*) and no dilated intrahepatic bile ducts. (**d**) Intraoperative cholangiogram again shows contrast-filled dilated CBD (*white arrow*), and the contrast flows freely into the duodenum (*black arrow*) and intrahepatic ducts. At surgery the cyst was seen to be extending from the right common hepatic duct to the pancreas. Type II. (**e**) Axial CECT shows a cyst (*arrowhead*) in the region of CBD and separate from the contracted GB (*arrow*) with stones. Grayscale US shows (**f**) the cyst (*cursor*) separate from the stone-filled thick-walled GB. (**g**) The cyst (*arrow*) is arising from the CBD (*cursor*). (**h**) MRI axial T2W BH FS image shows a cyst adjacent to CBD (*arrow*) and separates from small GB (*arrowhead*). (**i**) HIDA scan 45 min after morphine injection shows radiotracer filling the choledochal cyst (*arrow*) and free flow into small bowel (*arrowhead*)

Diagnosis
Caroli Disease (Type 5)

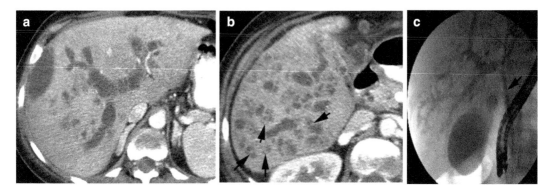

Fig. 12.19 Caroli disease. (**a**, **b**) Axial CT. (**c**) ERCP shows dilated intrahepatic biliary ducts with beaded appearance. The common bile duct in the ERCP study is not dilated (*arrow*). Central dot sign (*arrows* in **b**)

Biliary Cystadenoma

Imaging Features

1. Unilocular but commonly multilocular cystic lesion.
2. Internal septation may be seen which can enhance by CT study.
3. May have wall or septal calcification.
4. Mural nodules and papillary projections when present are echogenic and enhance with contrast.
5. Fluid may contain blood products, mucin, or protein.

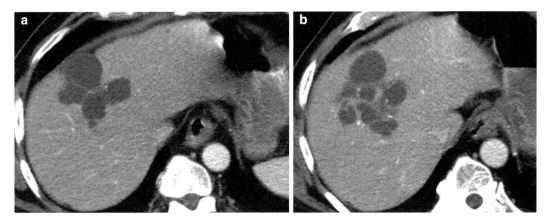

Fig. 12.20 Biliary cystadenoma. Axial CT (**a**, **b**) show multiloculated cystic lesion at the dome of the liver with multiple septations with prominent vessels

Gallbladder Wall Thickening

Diagnosis
Acute Cholecystitis

Imaging Features
1. Wall thickening (>3 mm) by ultrasound and pericholecystic fluid, nonspecific findings
2. Impacted stone in the gallbladder neck and gallbladder distension and wall edema
3. Presence of Murphy sign
4. Enhancement of the gallbladder bed and pericholecystic edema by CT

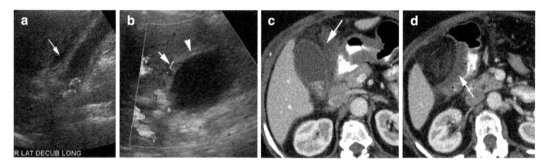

Fig. 12.21 Acute cholecystitis. Ultrasound examination shows (**a**) gallbladder wall thickening and impacted stones (*cursors*) at the neck with pericholecystic fluid (*white arrow*). (**b**) Color Doppler study shows increased vascularity of the gallbladder wall (*white arrow*) and lin-ear sonolucent edema in the wall (*arrowhead*). CT axial (**c**) shows distended gallbladder with stones and inflammatory changes in the surrounding adipose tissue (*arrow*). (**d**) Shows reactive edema in the adjacent lateral wall of the hepatic flexure of the colon (*white arrow*)

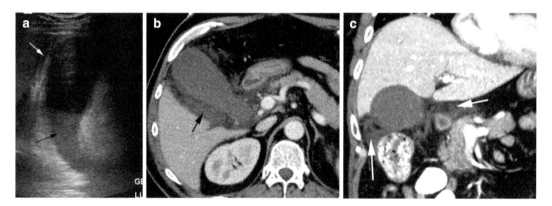

Fig. 12.22 Acalculous cholecystitis. History of thrombotic thrombocytopenic purpura. (**a**) Ultrasound shows distended gallbladder with thick wall having linear sonolucent edema (*white arrow*) and sludge (*black arrow*) but no stones. Murphy sign was positive. CT (**b**) axial and (**c**) coronal reformatted images show distended gallbladder with pericholecystic edema (*arrows*)

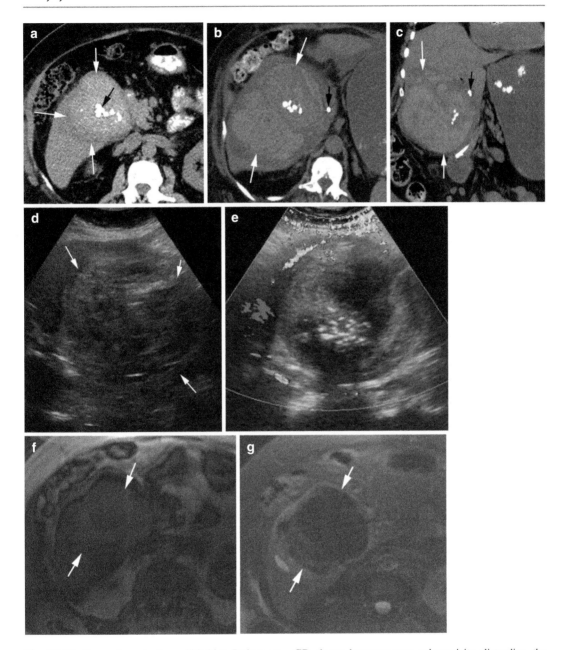

Fig. 12.23 Hemorrhage in the gallbladder. Patient on lifelong anticoagulation with dropping hemoglobin, supratherapeutic INR, and right upper quadrant pain. (**a**) Axial unenhanced CT shows distended gallbladder with uniform high-density hemorrhage (*white arrows*) surrounding the stones (*black arrow*) with no layering. (**b**, **c**) Axial and coronal noncontrast CT done 5 days later shows the hemorrhage to be heterogeneous (*white arrows*). A stone is seen in the cystic duct (*black arrow*). (**d**, **e**) US of GB shows heterogeneous echogenicity distending the gallbladder lumen (*white arrows*) and echogenic stones with echo shadow. No vascularity is seen in the wall or within the gallbladder. MRI study: (**f**) Axial T1W and (**g**) axial T2W fat-sat images show acute to early subacute hematoma in the gallbladder with mixed low/intermediate/high T1 signal and mixed low/intermediate T2 signal intensities (*white arrows*)

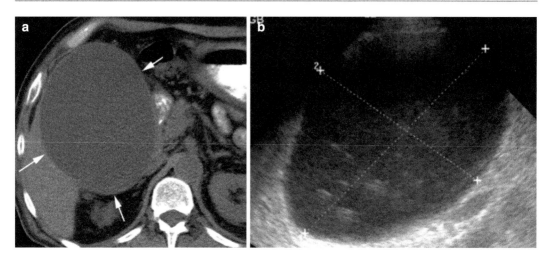

Fig. 12.24 Hydrops gallbladder. (**a**) Unenhanced axial CT shows markedly distended gallbladder (*arrows*) with no reaction in the surrounding adipose tissue. (**b**) Ultrasound of the gallbladder shows distended gallbladder (*calipers*) with sludge, no wall thickening, or edema

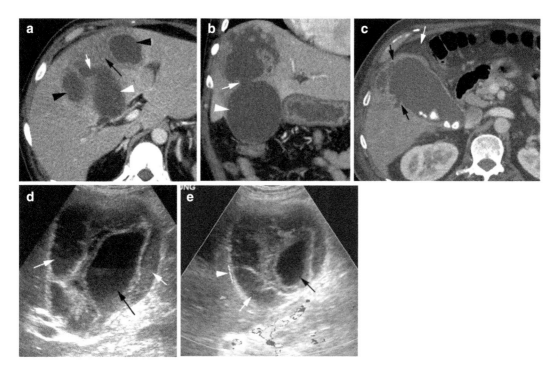

Fig. 12.25 Cholecystitis with perforation into the liver. Patient 1: (**a, b**) Axial and coronal reformatted CT shows distended gallbladder (*white arrowhead*) with perforation within the liver (*white arrow*), surrounding low-density edema of the liver (*black arrow*), and focal abscesses (*black arrowheads*). Patient 2: (**c**) Axial CT shows gallstone cholecystitis with perforation (*black arrows*) and pericholecystic edema (*white arrow*). (**d**) Grayscale ultrasound shows distended gallbladder (*black arrow* also in **e**) with surrounding intrahepatic abscesses as loculated fluid collections (*white arrows* also in **e**). (**e**) Color Doppler shows increased vascularity (*arrowhead*) in the abscess wall

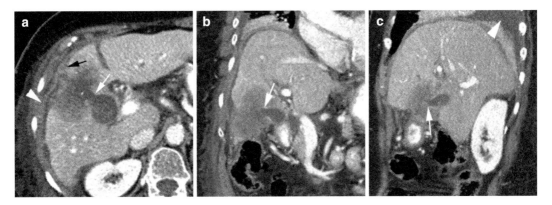

Fig. 12.26 Adenocarcinoma of the gallbladder with perforation into the liver. (**a**–**c**) Axial, coronal, and sagittal reformatted images show a nondistended gallbladder with perforation at the fundus (*thin white arrow*). The liver component shows low-density heterogeneous mass which is infiltrating through the liver capsule into the right subphrenic space (*black arrow*) and into the intercostal muscles (*arrowhead* in **a**) and with edema in the adjacent subcutaneous tissues. The pleural effusion (*arrowhead* in **c**) was malignant

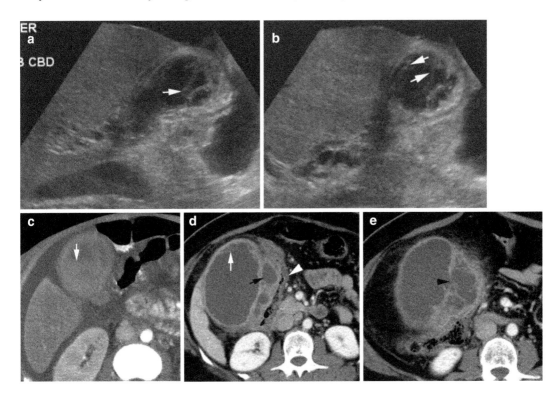

Fig. 12.27 Gangrenous cholecystitis in two patients. First patient, (**a**, **b**) ultrasound of the gallbladder shows irregular intraluminal sloughed membrane (*arrows*). (**c**) Axial CT also shows irregular thick intraluminal sloughed membrane (*arrow*). Second patient, (**d**, **e**) axial CT shows intraluminal sloughed membrane (*thin white arrow*) and perforation of the medial wall (*black arrowhead*) with contained abscesses (*black arrow*). The hepatic flexure is displaced (*white arrowhead*)

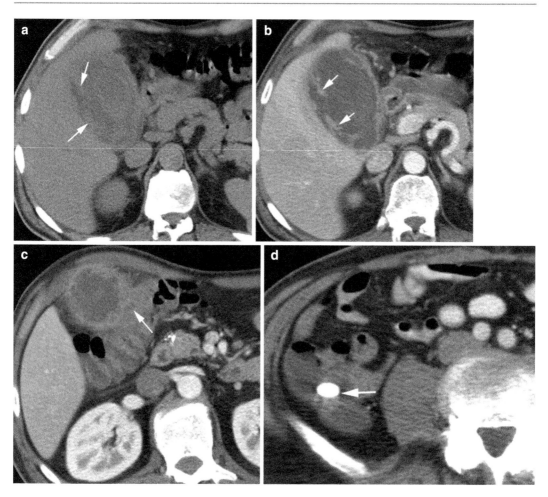

Fig. 12.28 Gangrenous cholecystitis with colonic fistula. Axial CT (**a**) precontrast and postcontrast axial CT (**b**, **c**) show sloughed membrane within the gallbladder (*arrows*). The hepatic flexure is displaced medially with wall thickening adjacent to the gallbladder with a faint fistulous tract (*arrow* in **c**). (**d**) Axial CT of the lower abdomen shows gallstone in the cecum (*arrow*). Fistula with colon was seen at surgery

Diagnosis

Xanthogranulomatous cholecystitis

Imaging Features

1. Focal or diffuse mass-like wall thickening of the gallbladder
2. Heterogeneous contrast enhancement
3. Extension into the adjacent soft tissues, liver, duodenum, or colon
4. Hypoechoic nodules or bands within thickened gallbladder wall
5. Disruption of mucosal line, pericholecystic fluid, and stones

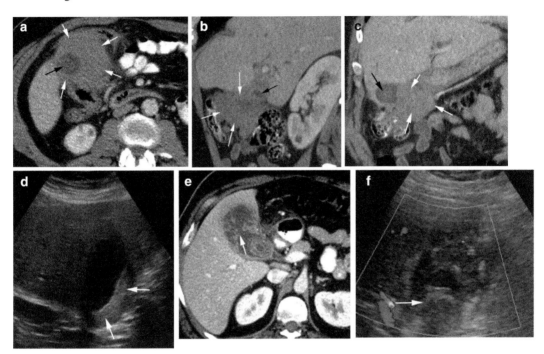

Fig. 12.29 Xanthogranulomatous cholecystitis (XGC). Postcontrast CT (**a–c**) axial, sagittal, and coronal reformatted images show marked lobulated wall thickening mostly medially (*white arrows*) of a nondistended stone-filled gallbladder (*black arrow*). (**d**) Ultrasound of the gallbladder shows wall thickening medially and inferiorly (*arrows*). (**e**) Axial CT of another patient shows mucosal disruption of the fundus of the gallbladder (*arrow*) and extension of XGC inflammation into the liver. (**f**) US shows heterogeneous density as seen in the CT with increased vascularity in the soft tissues at the fundus and large stone at the neck (*arrow*)

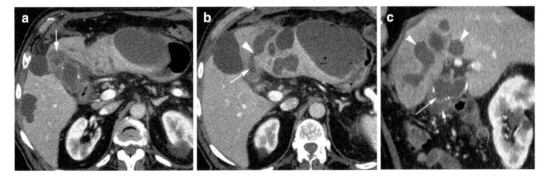

Fig. 12.30 Xanthogranulomatous cholecystitis with perforation and abscesses. CT axial (**a**) shows focal low-density nodule at fundus of GB (*arrow*) and focal calcifications in the GB wall. (**b**) Axial CT at higher plane shows perforation (*arrowhead*) of the fundus of the (*arrow*) gall-bladder into the liver with multiple abscesses, some with gas collections. (**c**) Sagittal reformatted image shows XGC with wall calcification (*long arrow*), nodule (*short arrow*) at the fundus, and multiple fluid pockets in the liver (*arrowheads*), all of which interconnected with one another

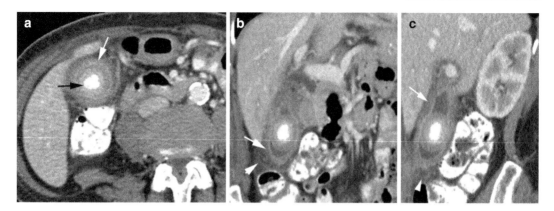

Fig. 12.31 Acute or chronic cholecystitis. History of chronic right upper quadrant pain. CT axial (**a**), coronal (**b**), and sagittal (**c**) reformatted views show markedly thick-walled (*white arrow*) nondistended GB with a large stone (*black arrow*). Mild pericholecystic edema is seen (*arrowhead*). Pathology showed mucosal erosion of the gallbladder

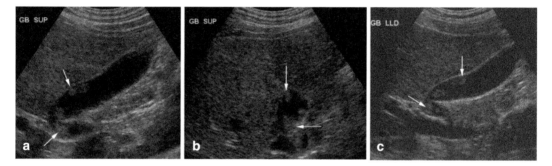

Fig. 12.32 Multiple gallbladder cholesterol polyps. (**a–c**) Multiple hypoechoic nodules involving the anterior and posterior walls and neck of the gallbladder which did not change position in decubitus position (*arrows*) and do not have posterior acoustic shadowing. The polyps are pedunculated and have a granular outline

Diagnosis
Gallbladder Carcinoma

Imaging Features

1. Mass replacing the gallbladder.
2. Focal or diffuse gallbladder wall thickening.
3. Intraluminal polypoid mass.
4. Calcifications can be from gallstones, gallbladder wall calcification, or tumoral calcification.
5. Direct extension into the liver or biliary tree.
6. Contrast-enhanced CT can show hypo- or isoattenuation.

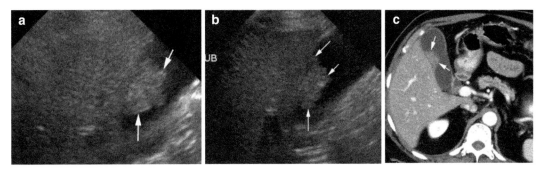

Fig. 12.33 Adenocarcinoma of the gallbladder. Ultrasound in supine (**a**) and decubitus (**b**) positions shows fixed mass in the anterior wall of the gallbladder (*arrows*). (**c**) Axial CT again shows the mass (*arrows*) with no extension outside the gallbladder

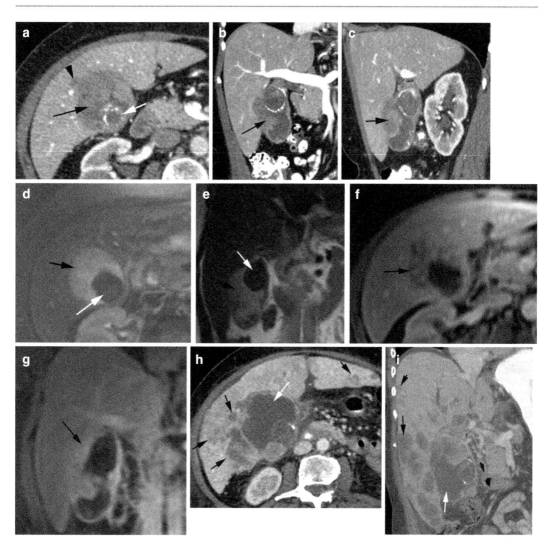

Fig. 12.34 Poorly differentiated gallbladder carcinoma. (a–c) CECT, axial, coronal, and sagittal reformatted images show soft tissue mass in the gallbladder (*thin black arrow*) with poor enhancement around a gall stone (*white arrow*). Liver invasion (*arrowhead*) is seen in axial view. (d, e) MRI axial (with FS) and coronal (without FS) T2W views show mixed intermediate/high signal in the mass (*black arrow*) with low-signal stone (*white arrow*). Postcontrast MRI (f, g) and axial and coronal views show enhancement of mass (*arrow*). (h, i) Axial and coronal reformatted CT 1 year later after treatment show increased liver invasion and multiple hepatic metastases (*black arrows*). Most of the gallbladder is distended with necrotic low-attenuating mass (*white arrow*)

Cholangiocarcinoma

Imaging Features
1. Mass-forming
   (a) Homogeneous attenuation with distinct borders
   (b) Irregular peripheral attenuation with gradual centripetal enhancement
   (c) Capsular retraction
   (d) Satellite nodules
   (e) Vascular encasement

2. Periductal infiltration
   (a) Diffuse periductal thickening
   (b) Common in hilar but rare in intrahepatic lesions

3. Intraductal type
   (a) Diffuse duct ectasia with or without papillary mass
   (b) Localized duct ectasia with polypoid mass
   (c) Mildly dilated duct with cast-like lesion
   (d) Focal stricture-like lesion with mild proximal duct dilatation

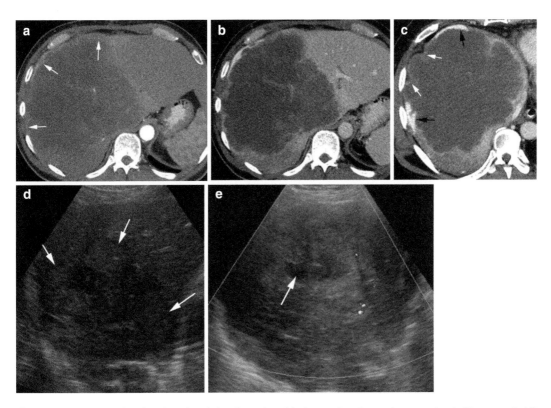

Fig. 12.35 Mass-forming intrahepatic cholangiocarcinoma. CT axial (**a**) in early arterial phase shows a large low-density mass with faint peripheral enhancement (*arrows*). (**b**) Portal venous phase shows increased centripetal enhancement. (**c**) Dilated subphrenic veins (*thin black arrow*) and capsular retraction (*white arrows*). (**d**) Ultrasound of the mass shows a well-marginated heteroechoic mass (*arrows*). (**e**) Color Doppler US shows peripheral vascularity and central necrosis (*arrow*)

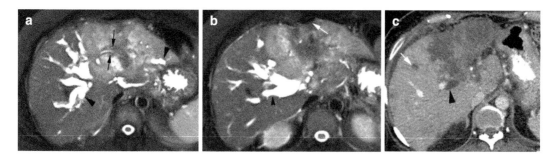

Fig. 12.36 Peptidal infiltrating intrahepatic cholangiocarcinoma. (**a**, **b**) T2W FS MRI images of the liver show low-signal tumor around the left lobe duct (*thin arrows*) with dilatation of ducts at the periphery of mass (*arrowheads*). Mass is infiltrating the liver parenchyma with cap-sular retraction (*white arrow*). (**c**) CT shows low-density mass in the left lobe of the liver with peripheral duct dilatation (*arrowhead*). Multiple metastases are seen in the right lobe (*white arrow*)

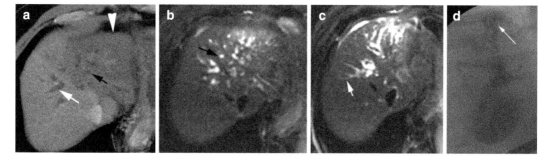

Fig. 12.37 Peptidal infiltrating intrahepatic cholangiocarcinoma. (**a**) Axial CT shows infiltrating mass in the left lobe of the liver with subcapsular retraction (*arrowhead*). Duct dilatation is seen within the lesion (*black arrow*) and at the periphery (*white arrow*). (**b**, **c**) T2W FS MRI again shows dilated ducts within and at the periphery of the lesion (*arrows*). (**d**) ERCP shows beaded appearance of the dilated ducts in the left lobe of the liver (*arrow*)

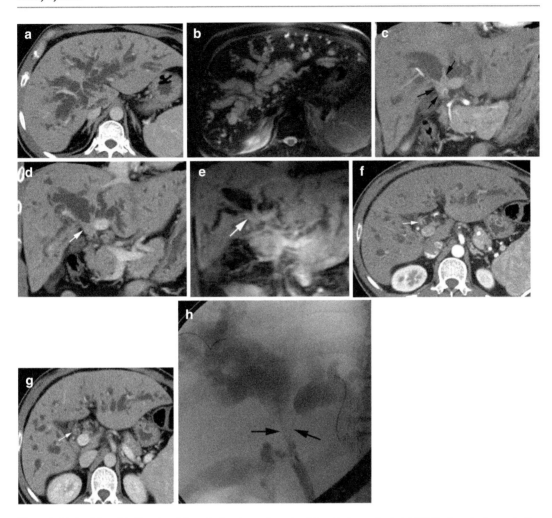

Fig. 12.38 Periductal-infiltrating hilar cholangiocarcinoma. (**a, b**) Axial CT and MRI T2W FS images show dilated biliary ducts in the right and left liver lobes. (**c, d**) CT coronal reformatted CT (**e**) coronal postcontrast MRI T1 FAME image shows enhancement (more in arterial **c** than portal phase **d**) of the obstructing soft tissue around both the common hepatic ducts with tapered narrowing on the right side (*arrow*). Axial CT (**f, g**) again shows similar enhancing soft tissues surrounding the constricted CBD more in the arterial phase (**e**) than the portal venous phases (**f**). (**h**) ERCP examination shows Bismuth type II obstruction of distal common hepatic ducts (*arrow*) and origin of the common bile duct

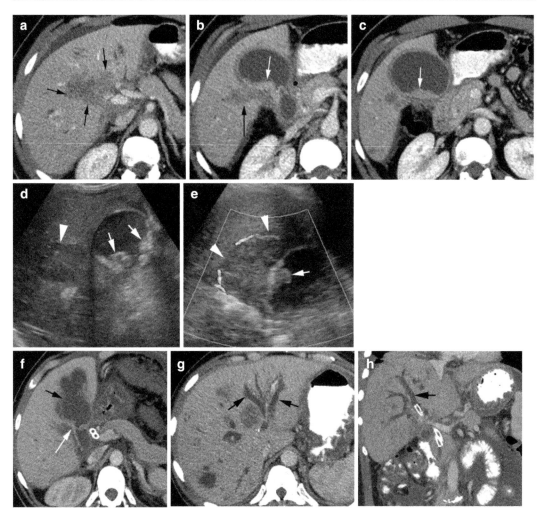

Fig. 12.39 Combined periductal infiltrating and intraductal growth-type cholangiocarcinoma. Axial CT (**a**) shows low-density mass at the hilum with faint peripheral enhancement (*thin black arrows*). (**b**) The gallbladder wall is thickened adjacent to the tumor (*white arrows*) from periductal infiltration. (**c**) Polypoid growth within the gallbladder (*white arrow*). (**d**, **e**) Ultrasound shows multiple echogenic polypoid masses with localized all thickening of GB (*white arrows*). Heteroechoic well-marginated mass adjacent to the gallbladder with peripheral vascularity (*arrow heads*). Axial CT (**f**) 2 months later shows constriction of the body of the gallbladder by the polypoid growth (*white arrow*) with intrahepatic rupture of the fundus of the gallbladder (*black arrow*). (**g**, **h**) Axial and coronal reformatted CT show dilated intrahepatic biliary ducts (*thick black arrows*) from mucin secretion in spite of two stents

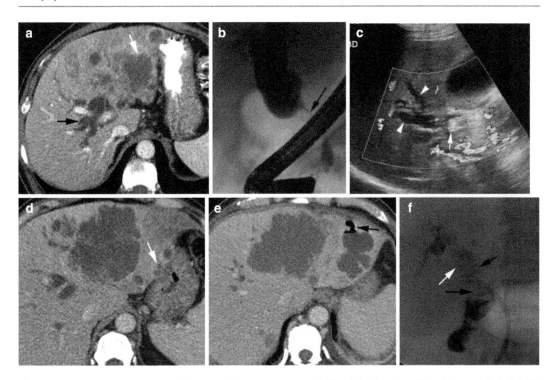

Fig. 12.40 Polypoid cholangiocarcinoma of the common bile duct with stomach invasion. (**a**) Axial CT in portal venous phase shows dilated intrahepatic biliary ducts (*black arrow*) and multiple low-density metastases to the left liver lobe (*white arrow*). (**b**) ERCP shows stricture of mid-CBD (*arrow*) with dilated ducts proximally. (**c**) Ultrasound shows dilated common bile duct and intrahepatic ducts (*arrowhead*). Echogenic mass (*white arrow*) is seen within CBD distal to dilated ducts. (**d**) Axial CT done 1 month later shows low-density metastasis at the margin of the left liver lobe continuous with the stomach (*arrow*). (**e**) Higher section than **d** shows gas within the metastasis (*arrow*) which is continuous metastasis in **d**. (**f**) Upper GI swallow study shows contrast within the left lobe of the liver from the distal stomach (*black arrows*) and separate from the biliary stent (*white arrow*)

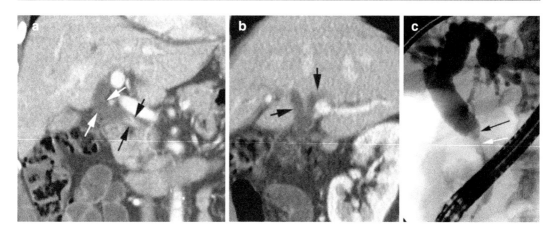

Fig. 12.41 Cholangiocarcinoma sclerosing-type mid-common bile duct. (**a**) Coronal reformatted CT shows dilated CBD (*white arrows*) with tapering of mid-CBD. The tapered area is thick walled (*black arrows*). (**b**) Sagittal reformatted CT shows dilated common hepatic ducts (*arrows*). (**c**) ERCP shows tapered narrowing of dilated CBD (*black arrow*) proximal to the complete obstruction (*white arrow*)

Diseases of Extrabiliary Liver

Infection

Diagnosis
Pyogenic Liver Abscess

Imaging Features
1. Single or cluster of small abscesses
2. (a) US—variable appearance from cystic (anechoic or echogenic fluid) to solid lesions
   (b) CECT—uni- or multilocular cystic lesions, with rim enhancement and surrounding edema, may appear solid
3. May have gas within the abscess

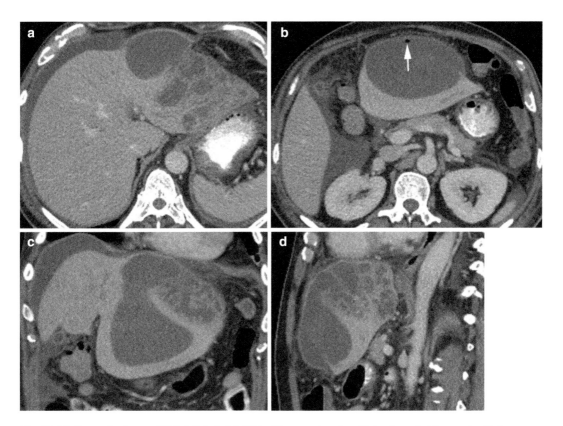

Fig. 12.42 Pyogenic abscess (*Klebsiella*). Axial CT (**a**, **b**), coronal, and sagittal reformatted images (**c**, **d**) show complex abscess in the left lobe of the liver. (**b**) At lower level than (**a**) shows the unilocular component with air (*arrow*)

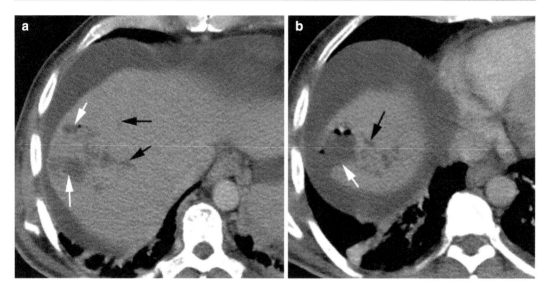

Fig. 12.43 Ascending cholangitis forming abscess with rupture into peritoneal space. Patient with cholecystoduodenal fistula (surgically proven). (**a**, **b**) Axial CT shows fluid-filled bile ducts (*black arrows*) and abscesses with gas in the periphery of the liver extending to the capsule (*white arrows*). (**b**) Higher section than (**a**) shows rupture of abscess into the right subphrenic space (*white arrow*)

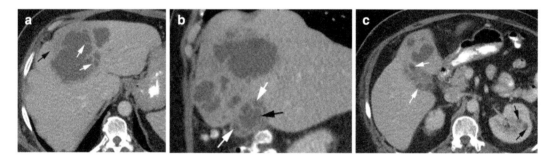

Fig. 12.44 Complex pyogenic liver abscess extending to the gallbladder wall. Patient with history of diabetes mellitus. Axial CT (**a**) of large liver abscess with septations (*white arrows*) and surrounding edema (*black arrow*). (**b**) Sagittal reformatted image shows extension of abscess to the gallbladder with multiple small low-density abscesses (*white arrows*) in the wall surrounding the lumen (*black arrow*). (**c**) Axial CT shows multiple small abscesses in the gallbladder wall (*white arrows*) and abscesses in the left kidney (*black arrows*)

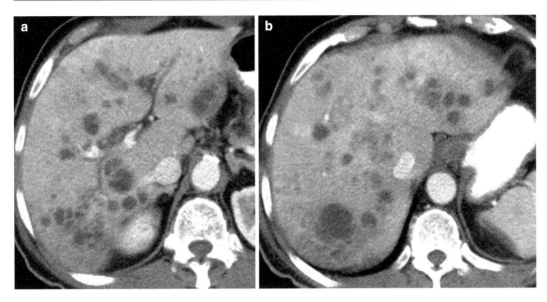

Fig. 12.45 Multiple pyogenic abscesses. History of mental status change and failure to thrive. (**a, b**) Postcontrast axial images show multiple low-density abscesses scattered throughout the liver with faint surrounding edema

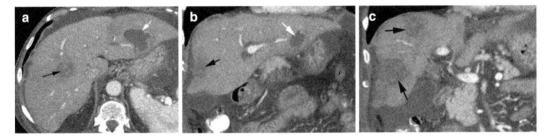

Fig. 12.46 Abscess and liver metastasis in patient with gastric cancer. (**a, b**) Axial and coronal reformatted CT shows a well-marginated abscess in the left lobe of the liver with enhancing rim and surrounding edema (*white arrow*). Metastasis in the right lobe (*black arrow*) is less well marginated and the center of metastasis is of higher density than the abscess cavity. (**c**) Coronal reformatted image shows two large metastases (*arrows*)

Diagnosis
Amebic Abscess

Imaging Features
Similar to pyogenic abscesses

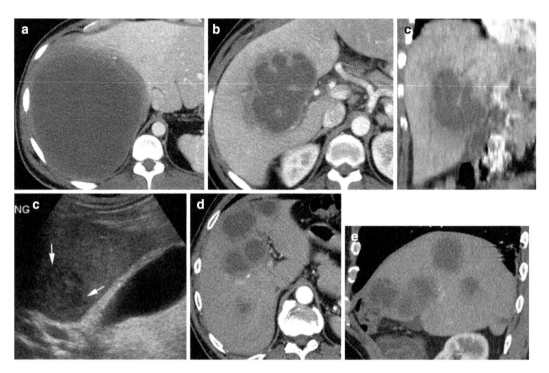

Fig. 12.47 Amebic liver abscess in three patients. Patient 1: (**a**) Axial CT shows large abscess in the right lobe of the liver, with thick stratified wall and surrounding edema. Patient 2: (**b**, **c**) Axial and coronal reformatted images show thick-walled lobulated abscess at hilum of the liver.

(**d**) Ultrasound shows focal area of low echogenicity with internal heterogeneous echo and no echogenic wall (*arrows*). Patient 3: (**e**, **f**) Axial and sagittal reformatted images show multiple thick-walled amebic abscesses

Fig. 12.48 Hydatid cyst of three patients. Patient 1: (**a**) Axial CT of the liver shows a cyst with thin wall, linear septation (*white arrow*), and low-density daughter cysts (*black arrows*). (**b**, **c**) Axial MRI study, T1W FSE, and T2W FS images show thin hypointense rim of pericyst (*white arrow*). The daughter cyst is of low signal in T1W and high signal in T2W images (*arrowheads*). (**d**) Coronal MRCP image shows thin black line (*white arrow*) of peri-cyst in the wall and multiple high-signal daughter cysts (*black arrow*). (**e**) Ultrasound of the same patient shows large cyst with central septation (*arrow*). Patient 2: (**f**) Axial CT shows linear low density between the two layers of the split wall (*black arrows*). (**g**) Ultrasound shows thick wall of the cyst with no vascularity. Patient 3: (**h**) Axial CT shows coarse calcification of the wall

Diagnosis

Hydatid Cyst

Imaging Features

CT:

1. Well-marginated, hypoattenuating lesions
2. Coarse wall calcifications in 50 % of cases and daughter cysts in 75 % cases

MRI:

1. Pericyst is hypointense in both T1W and T2W images.
2. Cyst matrix is hypointense on T1W and markedly hyperintense on T2W images.
3. Daughter cysts are hypointense relative to matrix on both T1W and T2W images.

US:

1. Variable from purely cystic to solid.
2. Wavy bands of endocyst may be seen.

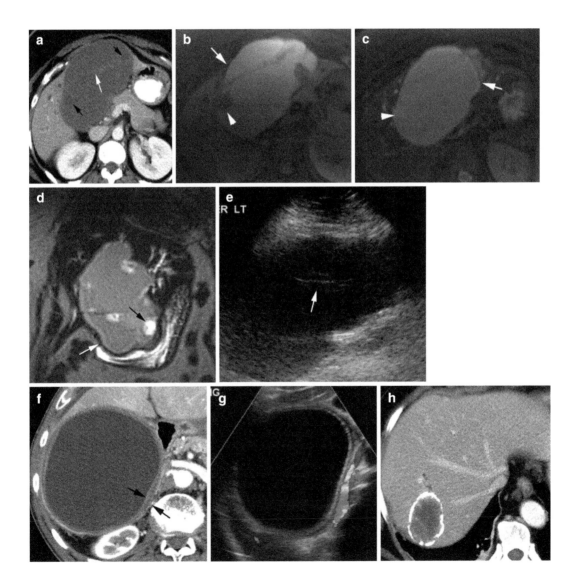

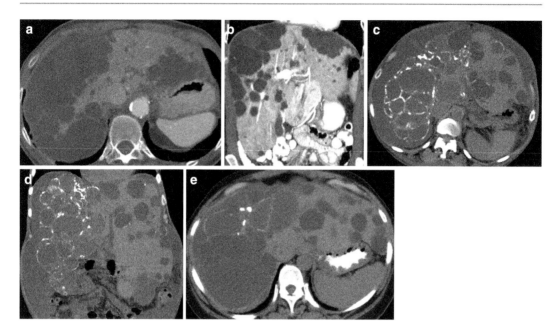

Fig. 12.49 Polycystic liver disease in two patients. Patient 1: (**a, b**) Axial and coronal reformatted CT images show hepatomegaly with multiple simple cysts of varying sizes in both lobes. Patient 2 with right upper quadrant pain: CT axial (**c**) and coronal reformatted images (**d**) show rim calcification of many of the cysts in both the liver lobes. Drainage of some of the cysts showed MRSA infection. (**e**) Axial CT done 10 years prior shows fewer calcified cysts

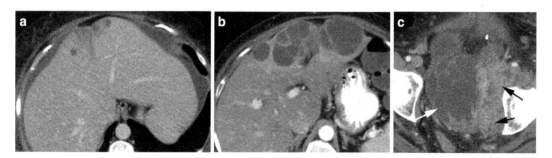

Fig. 12.50 Cystic metastasis from ovarian carcinoma. Postcontrast axial CT (**a**) shows small cystic metastasis around the falciform ligament. (**b**) A few months later, the metastases have grown in size and number. (**c**) Axial CT through the pelvis shows complex ovarian mass with cystic (*white arrow*) and more solid component (*black arrows*)

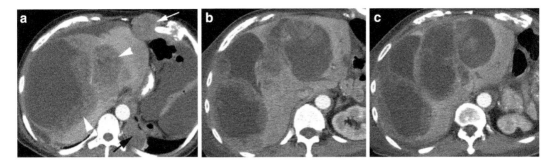

Fig. 12.51 Complex cystic metastases from stromal tumor of the stomach. Postcontrast axial CT (**a**) shows multiple metastases to the liver (*arrow head*), anterior abdominal wall (*white arrow*), and left lung base (*black arrow*). The larger liver lesion has a large cystic component with rim of solid tissue. (**b**, **c**) Post-treatment shows increase in metastasis which had a larger cystic component

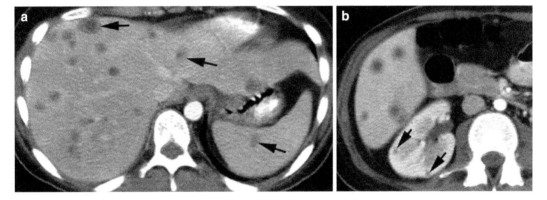

Fig. 12.52 Candidiasis. History of acute lymphoblastic leukemia and systemic candidiasis. (**a**, **b**) Axial CT images of the upper abdomen show multiple focal liver microabscesses with beveled margins. Small abscesses are also seen in the spleen and right kidney (*arrows*)

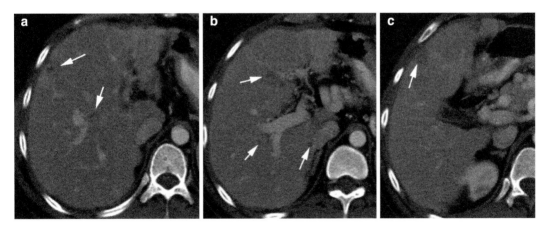

Fig. 12.53 Yellow fever. (**a–c**) Axial CECT shows multiple very small low-density areas of necrosis which have thick walls mostly in the right lobe of the liver (*arrows*)

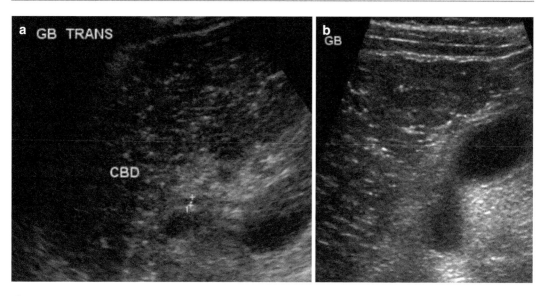

Fig. 12.54 Hepatitis, pneumocystis infection. Ultrasound of the liver (**a**, **b**) shows diffuse decreased parenchymal echogenicity from intralobular edematous swelling of hepatocytes and change in acoustic properties between portal vein radicals and hepatic lobules, giving the starry night pattern

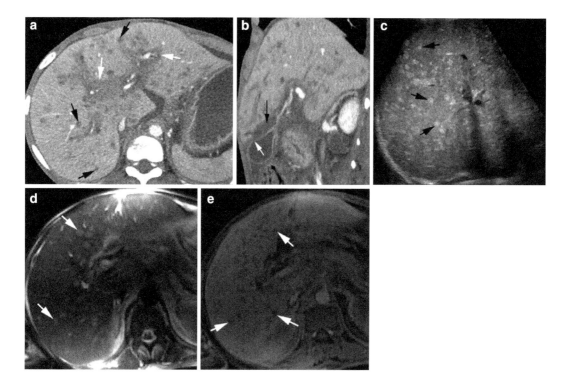

Fig. 12.55 Drug-induced hepatitis. Patient on treatment for TB and candida with right upper abdomen pain. Biopsy was negative for fungus and acid-fast bacillus. (**a**) Axial CT shows multiple low-density nodules (*black arrow*) and diffuse periportal edema (*white arrows*). (**b**) Sagittal reformatted image shows gallbladder wall thickening (*white arrow*) and pericholecystic edema (*black arrow*). (**c**) US shows diffuse small echogenic foci scattered throughout the liver (*arrows*). (**d**) MRI T2W images show multiple nodules of intermediate signal (*arrows*), and (**e**) post-gad T1W shows multiple low-signal nonenhancing nodules (*arrows*)

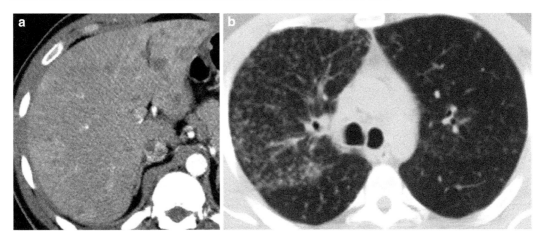

Fig. 12.56 Tuberculosis. (**a**) Contrast-enhanced axial CT of the liver shows multiple low-density foci of varying sizes throughout the liver with mild enhancement around the lesions. (**b**) Axial CT of the chest shows miliary pulmonary nodules more in the right upper lobe from TB infection

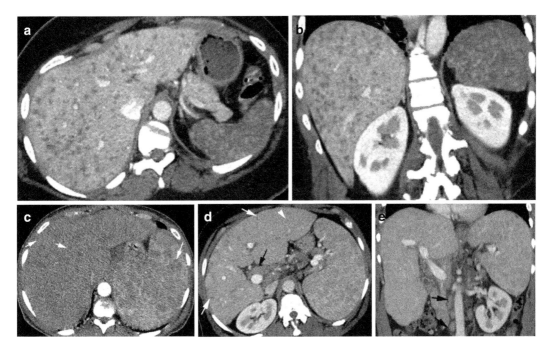

Fig. 12.57 Sarcoidosis in two patients, biopsy proven. Patient 1: (**a**, **b**) Axial CT shows diffuse low-density nodules in the liver. The nodules in the atrophic spleen are seen as higher density due to decrease density of the spleen. Patient 2: Axial CT (**c**) shows hepatosplenomegaly with multiple low-density nodules in both the liver and spleen (*arrows*). (**d**, **e**) Axial and coronal reformatted CT 2 year later show decrease in nodules especially in the liver (*arrowhead*) with diffuse scar tissue (*white arrows*). Hepatosplenomegaly, lymphadenopathy in porta hepatis, and para-aortic region (*arrows*) are stable

Cirrhosis

Imaging Features

1. Irreversible remodeled liver architecture with bridging fibrosis
2. Hepatocellular nodules—regenerative, dysplastic, or neoplastic
3. Surface and parenchymal nodularity
4. Hypertrophy of segments I, II, and III and atrophy of posterior segments VI and VII
5. Heterogeneous coarse parenchyma
6. Portal vein thrombosis and cavernous transformation

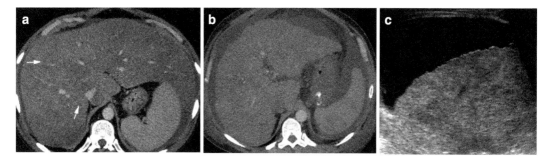

Fig. 12.58 Cirrhosis. (**a**, **b**) Axial CT shows enlarged liver with diffuse fine low-density granularity of regenerating nodules (*arrows*). Larger patchy ill-marginated scattered fatty change throughout the liver. (**b**, **c**) Axial CT and ultrasound of the cirrhotic liver on different patients show surface nodularity and ascites. US shows diffuse coarse and heterogeneous echotexture

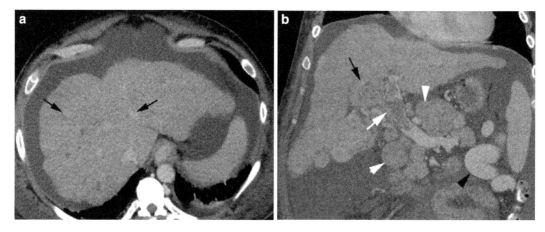

Fig. 12.59 Cirrhosis with multifocal hepatocellular carcinoma. (**a**) Axial CT in portal phase shows multiple enhancing nodules of various sizes (*black arrows*) throughout the liver. The liver surface is nodular, and the liver is contracted. (**b**) Coronal reformatted image shows enhancing tumor thrombus (*white arrow*) surrounded by low-density bland thrombus distending the portal vein extending from HCC at the liver hilum (*black arrow*). The splenic vein is dilated (*black arrowhead*) and enlarged lymph nodes (*white arrowheads*) around the portal vein

Diagnosis
HCC

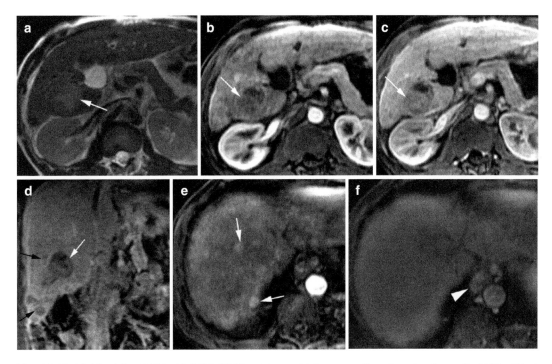

Fig. 12.60 Multinodular HCC. (**a**) MRI T2W axial image shows slightly increased signal in an HCC (*arrow*) than the rest of the liver. Postinfusion T1W axial images (**b**) in the arterial phase and (**c**) in portal venous phase show heterogeneous enhancement of the HCC (*white arrow* also in **d**), but the enhancement is less than the adjacent liver. (**d**) Coronal postcontrast T1W image shows multiple-surrounding low-signal small HCC (*black arrows*). (**e**) Axial MRI postcontrast of the liver dome shows multiple-enhancing small HCC (*arrows*) in the arterial phase. (**f**) Portal venous phase of the same area of the liver shows complete washout of the nodules. The esophageal varices (*arrowhead*) are better seen in this phase

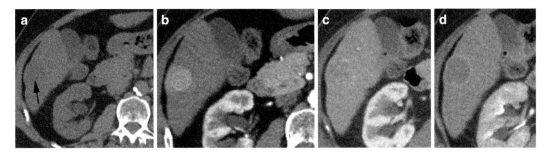

Fig. 12.61 Hepatocellular carcinoma with a typical enhancement pattern. Axial CT (**a**) noncontrast study shows low-density focus with surface bulging in the right liver lobe (*arrow*). (**b**) Arterial phase shows hyperenhancement of the same nodule, more than 1 cm in size. (**c**) Portal phase shows hypoenhancement of the nodule relative to the rest of the liver parenchyma. (**d**) Delayed phase shows delayed-enhancing capsule or pseudocapsule

Diagnosis

HCC with Vascular Invasion

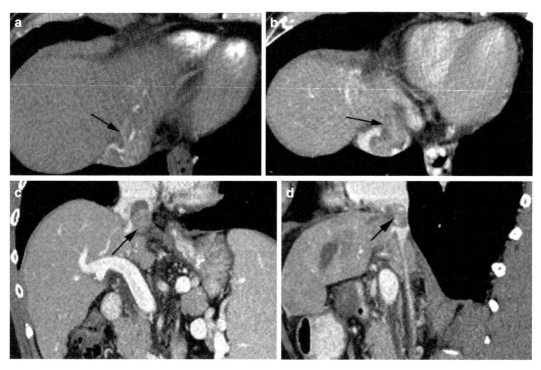

Fig.   12.62 Hepatocellular   carcinoma   invading IVC. Axial CT in arterial (**a**) and portal venous (**b**) phases show enhancing mass invading IVC (*arrow*). (**c**) Coronal and (**d**) sagittal reformatted images show tumor thrombus (*black arrow*) in suprahepatic IVC capped by nonenhancing bland thrombus

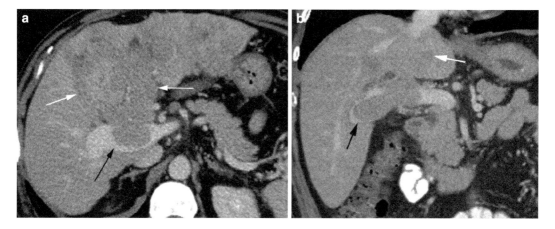

Fig. 12.63 Hepatocellular carcinoma invading the portal vein. Postcontrast portal phase CT (**a**) axial and (**b**) coronal reformatted images show large heterogeneously enhancing low-density mass (*white arrows*) invading into the portal vein (*black arrow*)

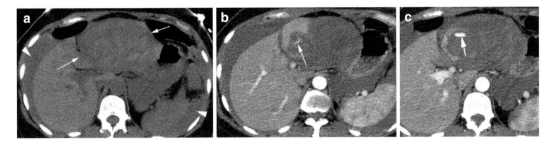

Fig. 12.64 Rupture of poorly differentiated HCC into the peritoneum. History of upper abdominal pain. Axial CT (**a**) precontrast shows heterogeneous high-density acute hemorrhage in the left lobe (*arrows*) of the liver and hemoperitoneum (*arrowheads*). (**b**) Arterial phase shows active extravasation into the tumor (*arrow*). (**c**) Venous phase shows pooling of contrast within the tumor (*arrow*)

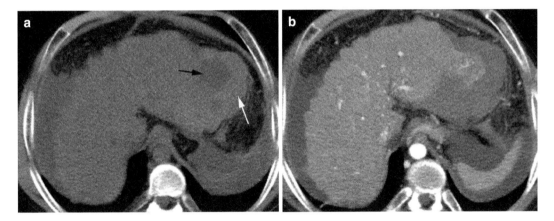

Fig. 12.65 Subcapsular rupture of HCC. History of HIV infection and hepatitis in a 20-year-old patient comes with left upper quadrant pain and vomiting. Axial CT (**a**) unenhanced CT shows focal low-density lesion in the left lobe of the liver (*black arrow*) surrounded by well-marginated high-density hemorrhage (*white arrow*). (**b**) Arterial phase CT shows poorly enhancing HCC in the left lobe surrounded by hemorrhage which was in the subcapsular space at surgery. The liver is cirrhotic with nodularity of surface

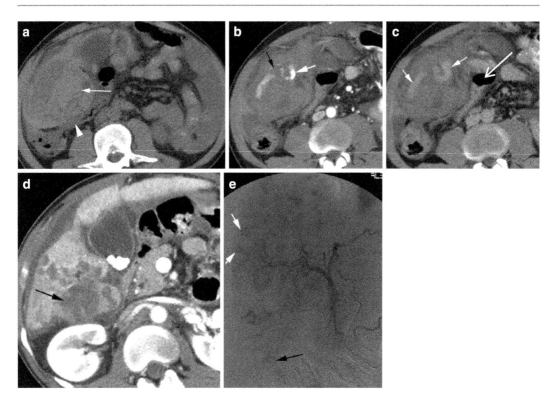

Fig. 12.66 Intraperitoneal rupture of HCC. History of chronic hepatitis C and right upper quadrant pain. Axial CT (**a**) precontrast study shows heterogeneous hemorrhage in the subhepatic space (*white arrow*) displacing the hepatic flexure (*arrowhead*). (**b**, **c**) Arterial and venous phases show active bleeding (*white arrow*) from a necrotic HCC (*black arrow*). (**d**) At a higher plane axial CT in portal venous phase shows multiple necrotic HCC in the right lobe (*arrow* in the larger mass). (**e**) Angiogram shows faint blush of extravasated contrast in the inferior right lobe of the liver (*black arrow*). The rest of the liver shows multiple-enhancing HCC nodules (*white arrows*)

Diagnosis
Fibrolamellar HCC

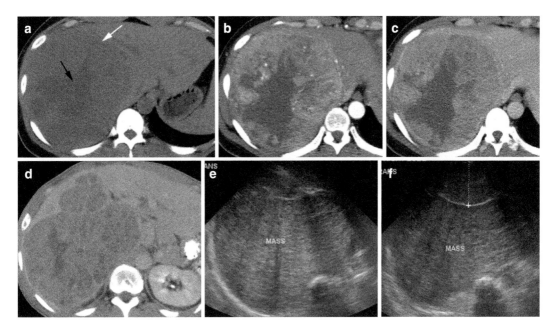

Fig. 12.67 Fibrolamellar HCC. Axial precontrast CT (**a**) shows a large mass of the right lobe of the liver (*white arrow*) with central low-density scar (*black arrow*) and minimal decreased density compared to the adjacent liver. (**b**) Arterial phase shows heterogeneous enhancement of mass greater than the liver with prominent arteries throughout the mass. (**c**) Portal venous phase shows faster clearing of contrast than the rest of the liver and is still heterogeneous. The central scar remains unchanged, and the rest of the liver has a normal appearance. Different patient: (**d**) Portal venous phase shows less enhancement of the heterogeneous mass relative to the surrounding normal-appearing liver. (**e, f**) Ultrasound of the liver shows large mass as seen in (**d**) which is marginated with echogenicity very similar to the liver (*caliper*) but is heterogeneous

Liver Mass

Diagnosis
Giant Hemangioma

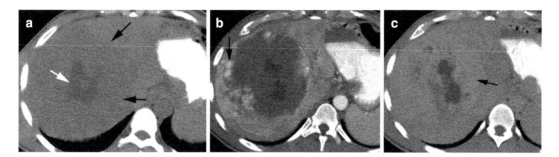

Fig. 12.68 Giant liver hemangioma. Axial CT: (**a**) Unenhanced CT shows a low-density mass in the right lobe of the liver (*black arrows*) with central scar (*white arrow*). (**b**) Arterial phase shows peripheral nodular bright enhancement (*arrow*). Central scar shows no enhance-ment. (**c**) Delayed image shows centripetal enhancement with complete filling of the hemangioma except the scar and is of higher density (*arrow*) than the liver parenchyma

Diagnosis

Lymphoma

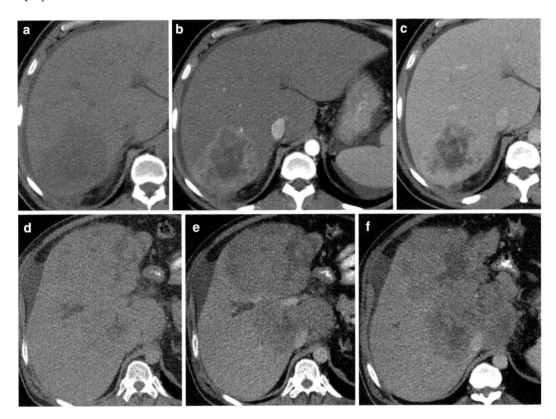

Fig. 12.69 Primary lymphoma of the liver in two patients. Patient 1 with anaplastic large cell lymphoma with underlying cirrhosis: (**a–c**) Axial CT precontrast phase shows a low-attenuating mass in the right lobe of the liver. Postcontrast study shows peripheral enhancement of the solid component around the central necrosis in the arterial phase. The enhancement decreases in the venous phase but is of higher attenuation than the liver. Patient 2 with diffuse large B-cell lymphoma: (**d**) Precontrast axial CT shows a large mass in the right lobe with dilated biliary duct lateral to it and areas of necrosis. CECT (**e, f**) shows poor enhancement of the mass which is less than the liver with necrotic areas better seen in (**f**) which is at a lower plane

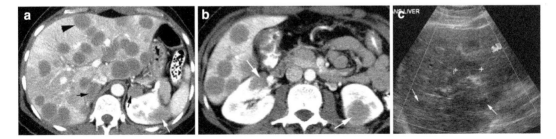

Fig. 12.70 Diffuse large B-cell lymphoma of multiple organs. Postcontrast axial CT (**a, b**) shows multiple poorly enhancing well-marginated discrete nodules throughout the liver (*arrowhead*). Similar nodules are seen in both the adrenal glands (*black arrows*) and kidneys (*white arrows*). (**c**) Color Doppler ultrasound of the liver shows multiple low echogenic nodules without increase in vascularity (*white arrows*)

Diseases of the Pancreas

Contents

R. Agarwala, *Atlas of Emergency Radiology:*
Vascular System, Chest, Abdomen and Pelvis, and Reproductive System,
DOI 10.1007/978-3-319-13042-2_13, © Springer International Publishing Switzerland 2015

Pancreatitis

Imaging Features

A. Less than 4 weeks after onset
 1. Interstitial edematous pancreatitis—acute peripancreatic fluid collection, sterile or infected
 2. Necrotizing pancreatitis
    (a) Parenchymal necrosis alone
    (b) Peripancreatic necrosis alone
    (c) Pancreatic and peripancreatic necrosis

B. More or equal to 4 weeks
    (a) Interstitial edematous pancreatitis with pseudocyst (sterile or infected)
    (b) Necrotizing pancreatitis with walled-off necrosis (sterile or infected)

Diagnosis

Interstitial Edematous Pancreatitis

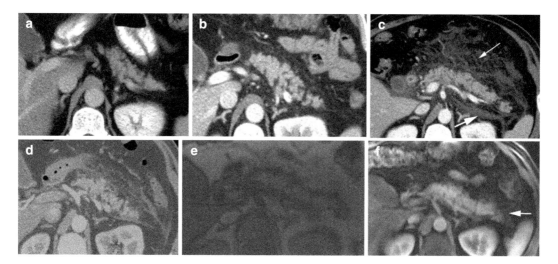

Fig. 13.1 Interstitial edematous pancreatitis. Axial post-contrast CT (**a**) examination done a few years earlier shows normal pancreas. (**b**) CT done for suspicion of pancreatitis shows pancreatitis with diffuse increased enhancement of the pancreas with mild increase in size and minimal peripancreatic inflammation. (**c**) Examination done 5 months later shows increase in inflammation involving the transverse mesocolon (*thin arrow*) and peripancreatic fluid collection in the anterior pararenal space (*thick arrow*). (**d**) Axial CT done 2 weeks later shows improved peripancreatic inflammation and fluid collection. (**e**) T1W MRI and (**f**) postcontrast fat-saturated T1 MRI done at the same time as (**d**) show improved pancreatitis with minimal mistiness of surrounding fat (*arrow*)

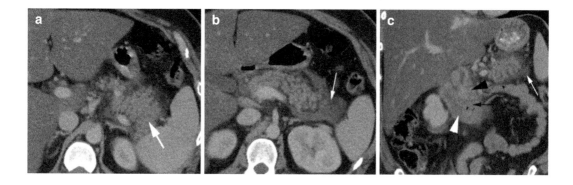

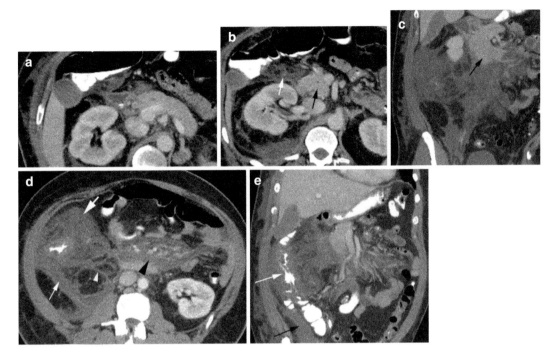

Fig. 13.3 Peripancreatic necrosis alone. Postcontrast CT (**a**) axial image shows normal homogeneous pancreatic enhancement. (**b**, **c**) Axial CT and coronal reformatted images show normal size of the head and uncinate process (*black arrow*). Extensive acute heterogeneous nonliquified inflammation in the right anterior pararenal space (*white arrow*), root of mesentery, and transverse mesocolon with edema in right-sided subcutaneous tissue. (**d**, **e**) Axial and coronal reformatted CTs show diffuse inflammation around the root of the mesentery (*black arrowhead*) and transverse mesocolon (*thick white arrow*) causing luminal narrowing of the right colon with wall edema, extending inferiorly to the perirenal space (*white arrowhead*) and APS laterally (*thin head*). Fluid is tracking down to the pelvis in the APS (*black arrow*)

Fig. 13.2 Interstitial edematous pancreatitis. Axial postcontrast CT (**a**, **b**) shows localized enlargement of the pancreatic tail (*thick arrow*) with diffuse enhancement of the body and tail and surrounding acute peripancreatic fluid collection (*thin arrow*). (**c**) Coronal reformatted image shows increased enhancement of the head of the pancreas (*black arrowhead*) and edema of the adjacent duodenum (*white arrowhead*), fluid in the pancreaticoduodenal groove (*black arrow*), and around the tail of the pancreas (*white arrow*)

Diagnosis
Necrotizing Pancreatitis

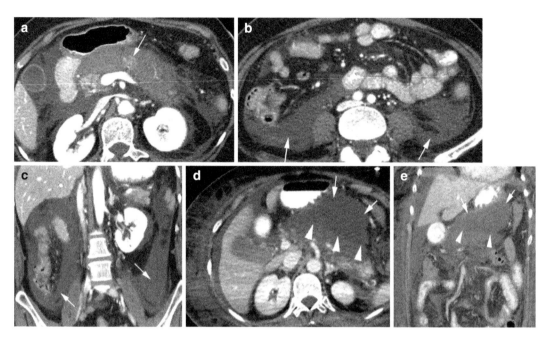

Fig. 13.4 Necrotizing pancreatitis with acute necrotic collections. (**a**) Axial CT image shows a diffusely enlarged nonenhancing body and tail of the pancreas with patchy areas of enhancing pancreatic tissue (*arrow*) and diffuse surrounding peripancreatic necrotic collection. Axial CT (**b**) and (**c**) coronal reformatted images show acute peripancreatic necrotic collection which is faintly heterogeneous, in bilateral anterior pararenal spaces (*arrow*). (**d**, **e**) Axial and coronal reformatted CTs 3 weeks later show large necrotic collection in the lesser sac (*arrows*) between the necrotic pancreas (*arrowheads*) and contrast-filled stomach

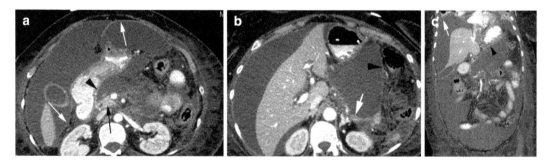

Fig. 13.5 Necrotizing pancreatitis with peritonitis. Same patients as in Fig. 13.4 about 5 weeks later. CECT axial (**a**, **b**) and coronal reformatted images (**c**) show nearly complete necrosis of the body and small residual tail of the pancreas (*short white arrow*). Large pseudocyst in the lesser sac with enhancing wall (*black arrowhead*) adjacent to the head (*black arrow*) and tail of the pancreas and diffuse reactive peritonitis with enhancement of the peritoneum (*long white arrows*) and large ascites. The abdominal wall shows diffuse edema

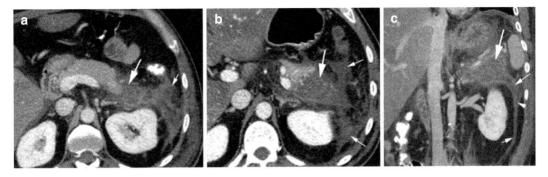

Fig. 13.6 Acute necrotizing pancreatitis. Contrast-enhanced CT axial (**a**, **b**) and coronal reformatted images show necrosis of the tail of the pancreas (*thick white arrow*) with surrounding heterogeneous acute necrotic collection (*thin white arrows* in **a**, **b**) with fluid and necrotic material in the left anterior pararenal space (*long thin arrow*), causing thickening of the lateroconal fascia (*arrowhead*) and posterior renal fascia (*short thin arrow* in **c**)

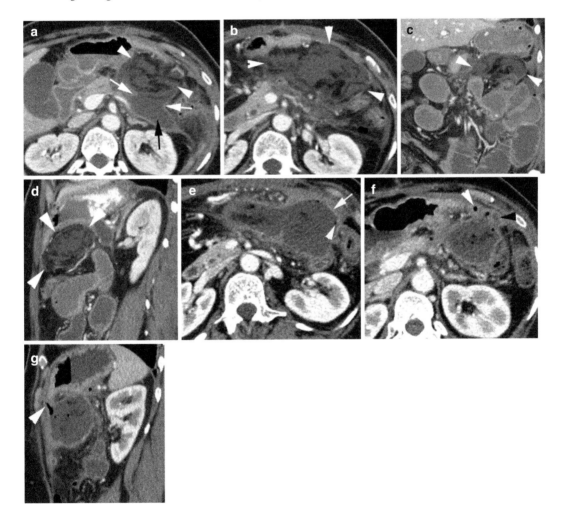

Fig. 13.7 Walled-off necrosis. History of recent resection of the body and tail of the pancreas. CECT (**a**, **b**) axial CT, (**c**) coronal, and (**d**) sagittal reformatted images show loculated fluid collection in the region of the resected body and tail of the pancreas (*black arrow*) which has ruptured (*white arrows*) into the lesser sac. The lesser sac collection (*arrowheads*) shows areas of low-density fat necrosis and areas of higher density and with faint surrounding rim of loculation. About 8 weeks later, (**e**) axial CT shows pseudocyst formation of the WON (*arrow*) with wall enhancement and superimposed infection with gas collections (*arrowhead*). (**f**, **g**) Axial and sagittal reformatted images show focal perforation (*black arrowhead*) of the pseudocyst wall with gas (*white arrowhead*) and fluid (*black arrowhead*) extending into the abdominal wall

Diagnosis
Gallstone Pancreatitis

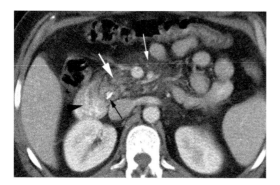

Fig. 13.8 Gallstone pancreatitis. Axial contrast-enhanced CT shows calcified stone in the distal common bile duct at the head of the pancreas (*thin black arrow*). The head of the pancreas is enlarged with heterogeneous enhancement (*long thick white arrow*) with diffuse peri-pancreatic inflammatory changes (*thin white arrow*). The second part of the duodenum shows reactive dilatation and wall thickening (*black arrowhead*)

Diagnosis
Groove Pancreatitis

Imaging Features
1. Soft tissues or fluid within the pancreaticodu-odenal groove.
2. Small cystic lesions may be seen along the medial wall of the duodenum.

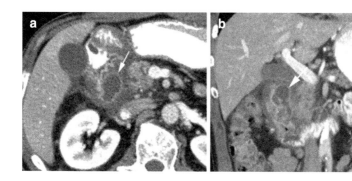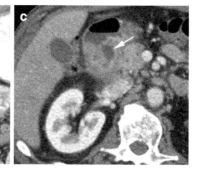

Fig. 13.9 Groove pancreatitis in a patient with a history of alcohol abuse. Axial (**a**) and coronal reformatted (**b**) CT show fluid in the pancreaticoduodenal groove. The second part of the duodenal sweep shows mucosal enhancement. Cystic lesions are attached to the medial wall of the duodenum (*arrow*). (**c**) Axial CT done 5 months later shows dense scar tissue in the groove with decreased size of the cystic lesions (*arrow*). Endoscopic study showed periampullary mass, biopsy of which showed acute and chronic inflammation

Diagnosis
Infected Necrotizing Pancreatitis

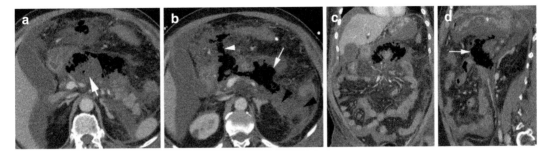

Fig. 13.10 Infected necrotizing pancreatitis. CECT (**a**) axial shows necrosis of the head and body of the pancreas (*arrow*) surrounded by gas, diffuse peripancreatic inflammation, and small ascites. (**b**) Axial CT shows acute necrotic collection in the left anterior pararenal space with fluid and necrotic (*black arrowheads*) material. Gas (*arrow*) from the infected necrotic pancreas is extending to the transverse mesocolon (*arrowhead*). (**c, d**) Coronal and sagittal reformatted images show a large amount of gas in the region of the pancreas (*arrow*) surrounding the superior mesenteric vessels

Diagnosis
Infected WON

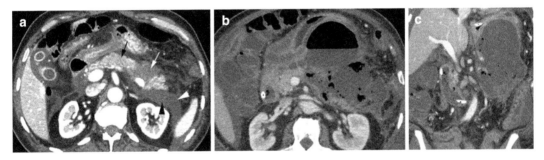

Fig. 13.11 Infected walled-off necrosis. Patient 1 with interstitial pancreatitis and focal necrosis: CECT (**a**) axial image shows diffuse enlargement of the pancreas with slightly heterogeneous enhancement (*black arrow*) and with focal area of necrosis at the tail (*white arrow*). Acute necrotic collection is seen in the anterior pararenal space with mild heterogeneous density (*black* and *white arrowheads*). Large pericholecystic fluid is seen around the gallbladder. Axial (**b**) and coronal reformatted images (**c**) 12 days later show infected WON necrosis with large gas collection in inhomogeneous fluid collection in the lesser sac

Diagnosis
Pseudocyst

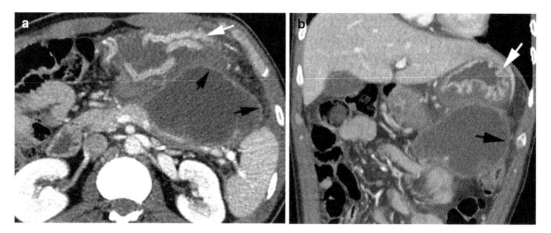

Fig. 13.12 Pseudocyst from alcoholic pancreatitis. Postcontrast axial (**a**) and coronal reformatted (**b**) CT images show a large low-density fluid collection with enhancing wall (*black arrows*) in the lesser sac. The adjacent stomach shows wall edema and thick rugal folds (*white arrow*)

Diagnosis
Infected Pseudocyst

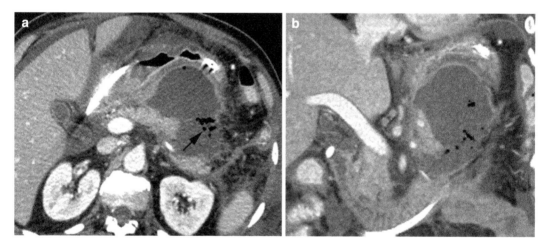

Fig. 13.13 Pseudocyst with infection. (**a**) Axial and coronal reformatted (**b**) CTs show pseudocyst with enhancing wall around the tail of the pancreas causing mass effect on the stomach and with small gas collections (*arrow*)

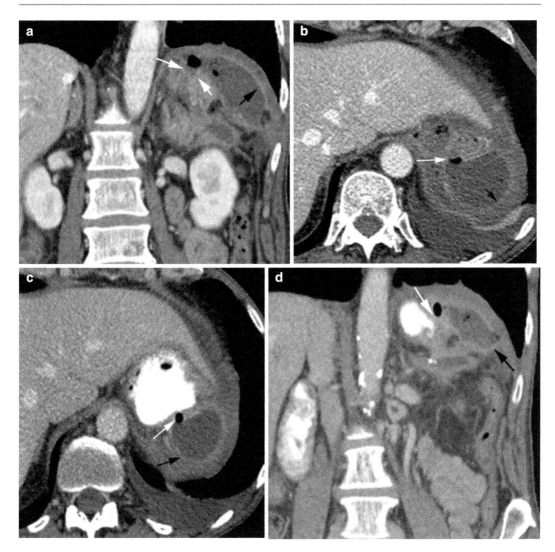

Fig. 13.14 Pseudocyst spontaneously decompressing into the stomach. History of trauma in the left upper abdomen with splenectomy and resection of the pancreatic tail 1 month prior comes in with left upper quadrant pain. CT (**a**) coronal reformatted image and (**b**) axial image show pseudocyst with enhancing wall (*black arrow*) communi-cating with the stomach (*white arrows*) with gas in the tract. One week later, CT (**c**) axial and (**d**) coronal refor-matted images show smaller size of the pseudocyst (*black arrow*) with the tract filled with gas (*white arrow*) com-municating with the contrast-filled stomach

Diagnosis

Hemorrhage in Pseudocyst

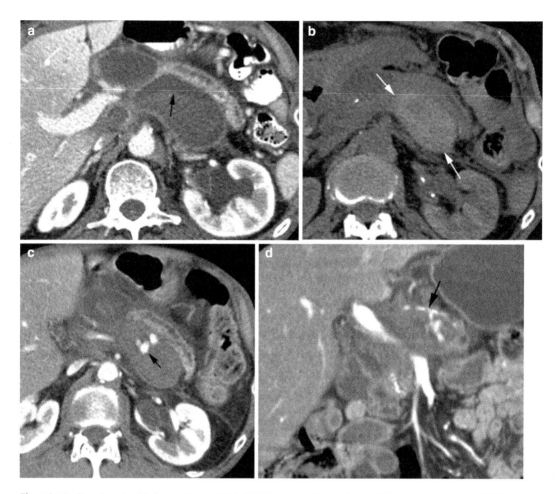

Fig. 13.15 Pseudocyst with hemorrhage. Axial CECT (**a**) shows large pseudocyst posterior to the pancreas with subacute hemorrhage having fluid/fluid level (*arrow*). (**b**) Later precontrast axial CT done for abdominal pain shows acute hemorrhage within the pseudocyst with increased attenuation of the hemorrhage (*arrow*). (**c, d**) Postcontrast axial and coronal reformatted CTs show active bleeding within the pseudocyst from the splenic artery (*arrow*)

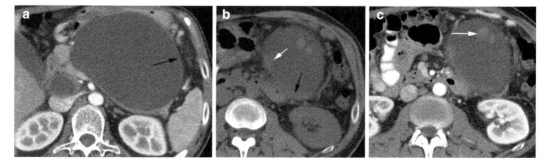

Fig. 13.16 Pseudocyst with hematoma. Axial CECT (**a**) shows a large low-density pseudocyst with enhancing wall (*arrow*). At lower level noncontrast (**b**) and postcontrast (**c**) axial CTs show high-density focal hematomas (*white arrow*) and layering hemorrhage (*black arrow*) in the dependent portion of the pseudocyst in unenhanced CT which does not enhance with contrast. Hemorrhagic fluid was drained

Pancreatic Neoplasms

Cystic Neoplasms

Imaging Features
1. Serous cystadenoma or microcystic cystadenoma
    (a) Cluster of small cysts <2 cm with honeycomb appearance.
    (b) Central stellate scar with calcification may be seen.
    (c) Can appear solid by US and CT depending on cyst size.
    (d) High signal in T2W image and can have delayed enhancement of central scar.
2. Mucinous cystic neoplasm or macrocystic cystadenoma
    (a) Cluster of cysts >2 cm.
    (b) Thick-walled septation with peripheral calcification.
    (c) High signal on T2W image and low signal on T1W image.
    (d) Walls of cyst can show nodular enhancement.
    (e) Located mostly at the body and tail of the pancreas.
3. Intraductal papillary mucinous tumor (IPMT)
    (a) Subtype of mucinous cystic neoplasm
    (b) Main duct or side branch type
    (c) Dilated main duct or cluster of small cysts in side branch type

Diagnosis
Microcystic Adenoma

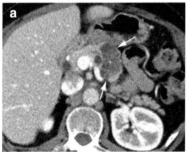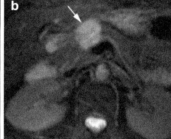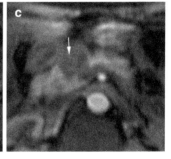

Fig. 13.17 Microcystic adenoma. (**a**) Axial CECT shows well-circumscribed lobulated cystic mass (*arrows*) at the body of the pancreas with central stellate scar with calci-fication. (**b**) MRI T2 FS shows the same lesion (*arrow*) with high-signal and central low-density scar. (**c**) Post-gad T1 shows enhancement of septations of the lesion (*arrow*)

Diagnosis
Macrocystic Adenoma

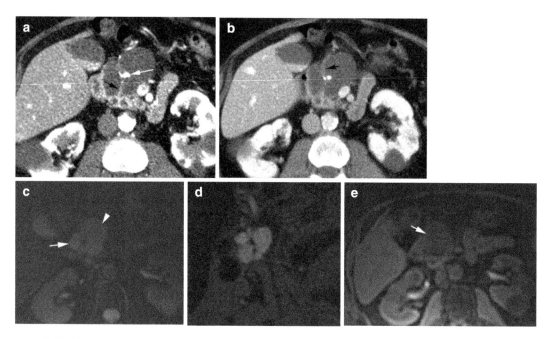

Fig. 13.18 Macrocystic adenoma. Axial CT in arterial phase (**a**) shows multiseptated cystic lesion divided by enhancing septa (*black arrow*) and central calcification (*white arrow*). (**b**) Portal phase shows decrease in septal enhancement (*black arrow*). MRI study (**c**) T2 BH FS image shows hyperintense signal in one lobule (*thin arrow*) and lower signal in another lobule (*arrowhead*) due to different protein contents of the mucin. (**d**) MRCP thin-slice coronal image again shows septated cyst with high signal. (**e**) T1 post-gad FS image shows low signal in the cyst (*arrow*). Enhancement of septa is better seen by CT

Diagnosis
Solid and Papillary Epithelial Neoplasm

Imaging Features

1. Mass usually large >10 cm with thick well-defined rim.
2. Mostly solid mass with cystic areas, necrosis, and hemorrhage.
3. T1- and T2-weighted images have heterogeneous signal.

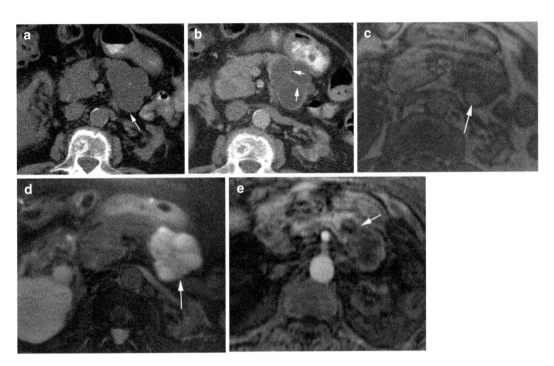

Fig. 13.19 Solid and papillary epithelial neoplasm, biopsy proven. (**a**, **b**) Axial CT pre- and postcontrast images show lobulated lesion at the pancreatic tail with central calcification and with enhancement of rim and multiple septa (*arrow*). (**c**) MRI T1W FSPGR dual-echo axial image shows high signal in the hemorrhagic component of mass (*arrow*). (**d**) MRI axial T2W FSE fat-sat image shows high signal in the mass with low-signal septa (*arrow*). (**e**) Postcontrast axial MRI shows enhancement of the soft tissue rim and septa (*arrow*)

Diagnosis
Intraductal Papillary Mucinous Neoplasm

Imaging Features

1. Mucin-producing tumor in the main duct or branch duct.
2. Main-duct type shows marked dilatation of the main duct, diffuse or multifocal involvement, large mural nodule or solid mass, and CBD obstruction.
3. Side-branch type looks like other cystic neoplasms.

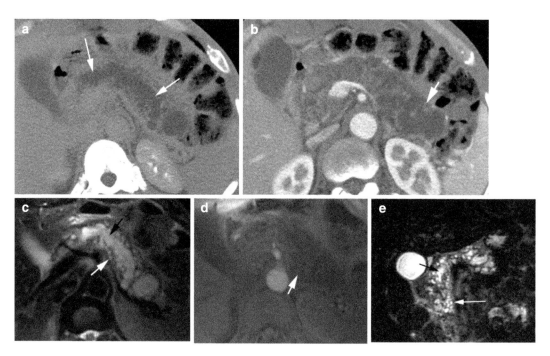

Fig. 13.20 Intraductal papillary mucinous adenocarcinoma combined type. Axial CT (**a**) noncontrast and (**b**) late arterial phase shows marked lobulated dilatation of the main pancreatic duct (*arrows*) with minimal enhancement. Axial MRI (**c**) T2W fat-sat shows high signal in the dilated main duct (*black arrow*) and the smaller side branches (*white arrow*). (**d**) Axial postcontrast T1W shows low signal with no significant enhancement. (**e**) MRCP thin-slice coronal image shows clustered cystic dilated branch ducts (*white arrow*) and dilated main duct (*black arrow*)

Solid Neoplasms

Diagnosis
Neuroendocrine Tumor, Nonfunctioning

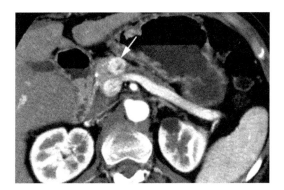

Fig. 13.21 Neuroendocrine tumor, nonfunctioning. Axial contrast-enhanced CT shows small enhancing nodule at the head of the pancreas (*arrow*)

Diagnosis
Carcinoid

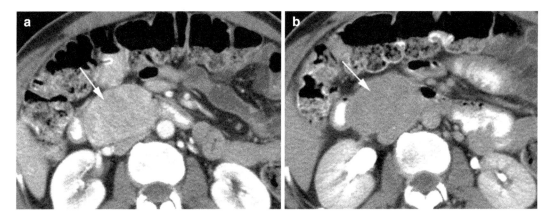

Fig. 13.22 Carcinoid at the uncinate process of the pancreas. Axial CT in portal venous phase (**a**) and delayed phase (**b**) shows large solid mass at the uncinate process of the pancreas with minimal enhancement (*arrow*)

Diagnosis
Pheochromocytoma

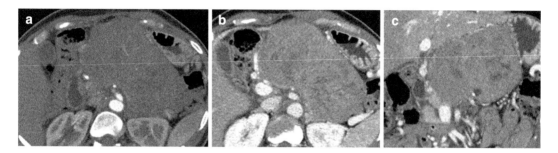

Fig. 13.23 Pheochromocytoma of the pancreas. Axial CT in arterial (**a**) and portal venous (**b**) phase and (**c**) coronal reformatted images show a large solid poorly enhancing mass in the body and tail of the pancreas with focal areas of necrosis

Diagnosis
Neuroendocrine Carcinoma

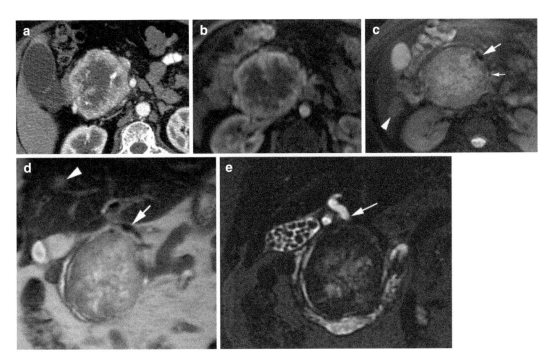

Fig. 13.24 Neuroendocrine carcinoma, well differentiated. (**a**) Axial CECT and (**b**) axial post-gad T1 MRI show a large mass with peripheral enhancement and central necrosis at the head of the pancreas. (**c**) Axial and (**d**) coronal T2W MRIs show high signal in the central necrosis. Metastasis with intermediate signal is seen in the liver (*arrowhead*). Portal (*thick arrow*) and superior mesenteric veins (*thin arrow*) show extrinsic compression by the mass. (**e**) MRCP shows dilated common bile duct by mass compression (*arrow*)

Diagnosis
Adenocarcinoma

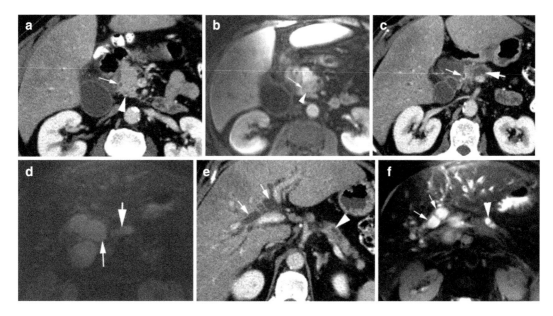

Fig. 13.25 Adenocarcinoma of the head of the pancreas obstructing the CBD and PD. (**a**) Axial CECT and (**b**) axial post-gad T1W MRI images show adenocarcinoma at the head of the pancreas (*arrowheads*) encasing the distal CBD (*arrows*). (**c**) Axial CT and (**d**) MRI T2W FS show constriction of dilated CBD (*thin arrow*) and dilated PD (*thick arrow*) adjacent to the mass (mass not seen at this level). (**e**) Axial CT and (**f**) MRI T2W fat-sat show intrahepatic biliary duct dilatation (*arrows*) and dilated PD (*arrowhead*)

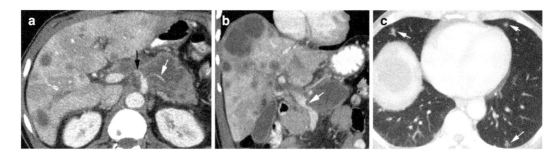

Fig. 13.26 Adenocarcinoma in the pancreas encasing vessels and invading the portal vein. (**a**) Axial CECT shows necrotic mass body of the pancreas encasing the splenic artery (*white arrow*) and the hepatic artery (*black arrow*). (**b**) Coronal reformatted image shows invasion of mass into the portal vein (*arrow*). The liver shows multiple metastases. (**c**) Axial CT of lung bases shows nodular metastasis (*arrows*)

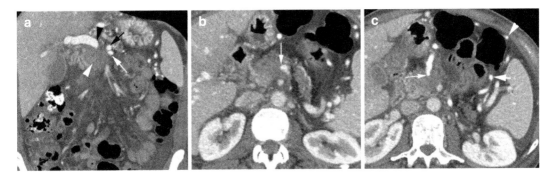

Fig. 13.27 Adenocarcinoma of the head of the pancreas encasing veins. CECT (**a**) coronal reformatted image shows a low-density mass at the head and uncinate process of the pancreas (*white arrowhead*) obstructing the confluence of the splenic vein (*black arrow*), superior mesenteric vein (*thin white arrow*), and portal vein (*black arrowhead*). (**b**) Axial image shows encasement and obstruction of the confluence of the superior mesenteric vein and splenic vein (*white arrow*) by mass. (**c**) Axial image shows obstruction of the left gastric vein (*thin white arrow*) resulting in a dilated short gastric vein (*thick white arrow*) and epiploic veins (*arrowhead*)

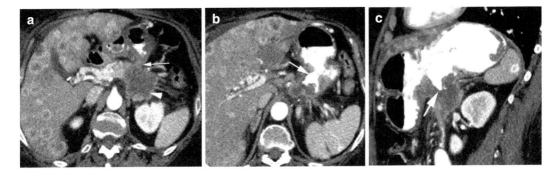

Fig. 13.28 Pancreatic adenocarcinoma eroding into the stomach. Axial CT (**a**) shows necrotic mass at the tail of the pancreas (*arrowhead*) extending to the wall of stomach (*white arrow*). The liver shows diffuse metastasis. Axial CT (**b**) at higher level and sagittal reformatted (**c**) images show protrusion of gastric enteric contrast (*white arrow*) into the necrotic mass

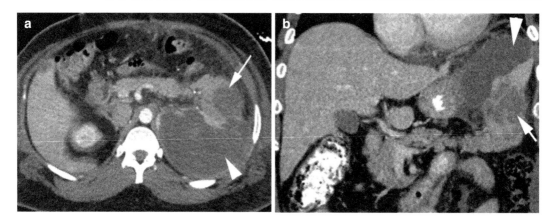

Fig. 13.29 Adenocarcinoma at the tail of the pancreas with splenic infarction. (**a**) Axial and (**b**) coronal reformatted postcontrast CT images show low-density adenocarcinoma at the tail of the pancreas (*arrow*) causing splenic infarction (*arrowhead*) from mass effect at the splenic hilum

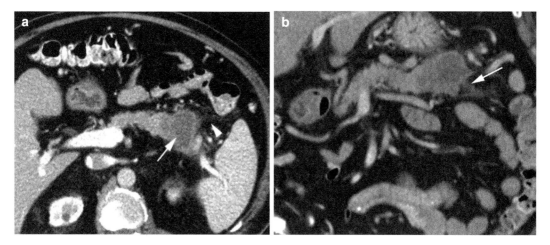

Fig. 13.30 Squamous cell carcinoma of the pancreas. Postcontrast CT (**a**) axial and (**b**) coronal reformatted images show low-density mass at the tail of the pancreas (*arrow*) with infiltrations into surrounding adipose tissue (*arrowhead*). Lesion was surgically resected

Diagnosis
Wermer Syndrome (MEN 1)

Imaging Features
1. Parathyroid disease is often multiglandular and hyperparathyroidism is common.
2. In pancreas, functional NET are common, mostly gastrinomas, and less common are insulinomas.
3. Anterior pituitary adenomas are usually functioning.
4. Adrenal adenomas may be functioning or nonfunctioning and can rarely be adrenal carcinomas.
5. Carcinoids are common in MEN 1, usually from the foregut affecting the thymus, bronchus, stomach, and duodenum.

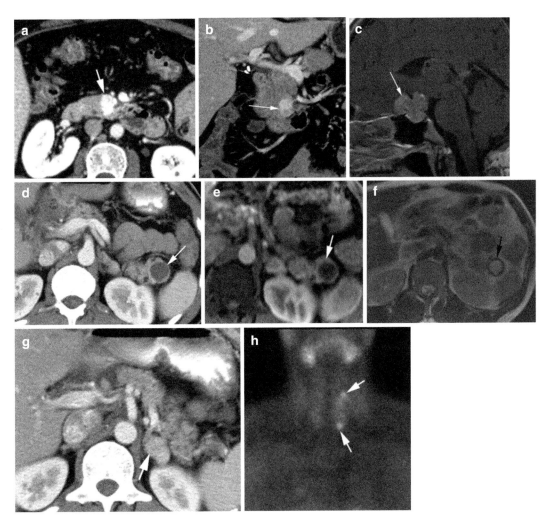

Fig. 13.31 MEN 1 in two patients. Patient 1: CECT axial (**a**) and coronal reformatted (**b**) images show small enhancing neuroendocrine tumor at the head of the pancreas (*arrow*). (**c**) Sagittal post-gad T1W brain MRI shows enhancing anterior pituitary macroadenoma (*arrow*). Patient 2: CECT axial (**d**) CT and (**e**) post-gad T1W MRI show rim enhancing cystic glucagonoma at the tail of the pancreas (*arrow*). (**f**) T2W MR image shows hyperintense cyst with low-signal rim (*arrow*). (**g**) CT axial shows adenoma in the left adrenal gland (*arrow*). (**h**) Nuclear medicine parathyroid scan shows increased uptake at two sites (*arrows*) in the left parathyroid gland

Diseases of the Urinary System

14

Contents

R. Agarwala, *Atlas of Emergency Radiology:*
Vascular System, Chest, Abdomen and Pelvis, and Reproductive System,
DOI 10.1007/978-3-319-13042-2_14, © Springer International Publishing Switzerland 2015

Urinary Stones

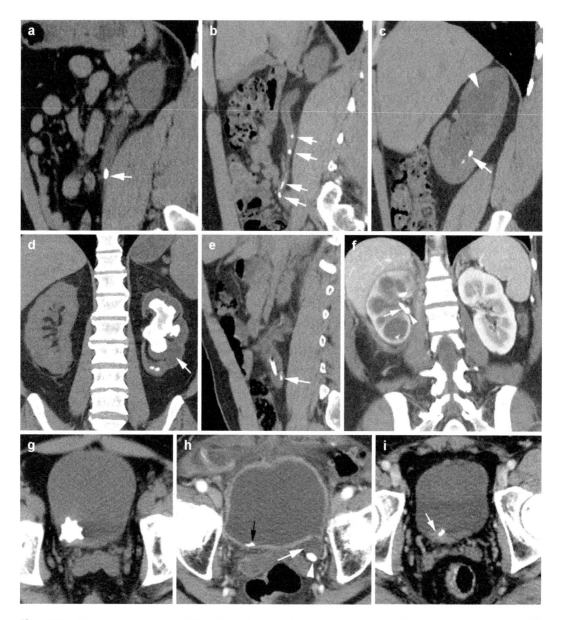

Fig. 14.1 Urinary stones in different patients. Noncontrast sagittal reformatted CT (**a**) shows a single stone (*arrow*) in the ureter which is dilated proximal to the stone. (**b, c**) Multiple stones in the right ureter (*arrows*) with hydronephrosis (*arrowhead*) and stones in lower pole calyces (*arrow*). (**d**) Coronal reformatted image shows large staghorn stone in the left kidney with hydronephrosis. The calyces distal to the stone are dilated and fluid filled (*arrow*). (**e**) Sagittal reformatted image shows stone (*arrow*) along with stent and hydroureter. (**f**) Postcontrast coronal reformatted image shows a stone (*arrowhead*) with stent (*white arrow*) at UPJ causing hydronephrosis. Axial CT (**g**) shows a jackstone urinary bladder. Axial CT shows (**h**) a stone (*arrowhead*) in Hutch diverticulum (*white arrow*) and a small stone within the bladder (*black arrow*). (**i**) Stone at ureterovesical junction with surrounding soft tissue (*arrow*) of the bladder wall

Urinoma

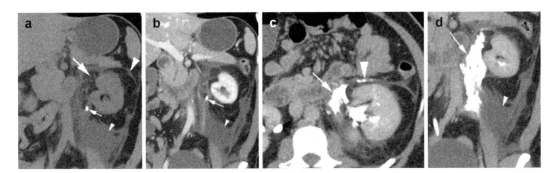

Fig. 14.2 Urinoma from ureteral stone. CT coronal reformatted images in precontrast (**a**) and arterial phase (**b**) show a stone (*thin arrow*) in the proximal ureter with stranding in the perirenal space medially (*thick arrow*), large fluid collection (*small arrowhead*) in the inferior perirenal cone-shaped space, and thick anterior renal fascia (*thick arrowhead*). Excretory phase, axial CT (**c**), and coronal reformatted (**d**) images show contrast in the perirenal space (*thin arrow*), in the anterior interfascial space (*thick arrowhead*), and extending inferiorly around the ureter (*arrow* in **d**)

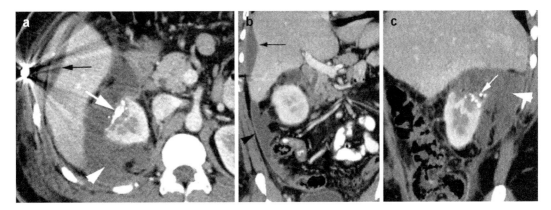

Fig. 14.3 Urinoma post gunshot injury and renal embolization. Postcontrast axial CT (**a**), coronal (**b**), and sagittal (**c**) reformatted images show truncated right kidney upper pole from GSW. Radio-opaque densities in the upper pole are from glue (*thick white arrow*) used to embolize the pseudoaneurysms of the renal artery branches. A large fluid (*arrowhead*) which was tested to be urine surrounds the upper pole of the kidney and is spilling into the peritoneal cavity. The peritoneum shows mild thickening from reactive changes (*black arrowhead*). Fluid in subcapsular region at the right lobe of the liver (*black arrow*) is due to resolving hematoma from liver laceration

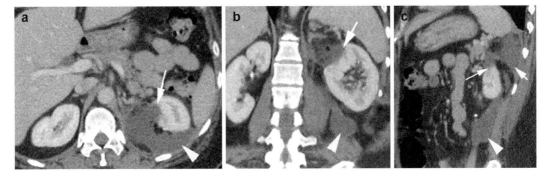

Fig. 14.4 Urinoma or chyle. Old resection of the upper pole of the left kidney for MRSA abscess. Postcontrast CT, axial (**a**), coronal (**b**), and sagittal (**c**) reformatted images show deformity of the upper pole of the left kidney with fluid extending from the defect (*long arrow*) to the perirenal space and then to the posterior (*arrowhead*) and anterior pararenal (*short arrow*) spaces

Tubulointerstitial Nephritis

Diagnosis
Bacterial Pyelonephritis

Imaging Features:
1. Renal enlargement
2. Striated nephrogram with one or multiple wedge-shaped areas of decreased enhancement involving the cortex

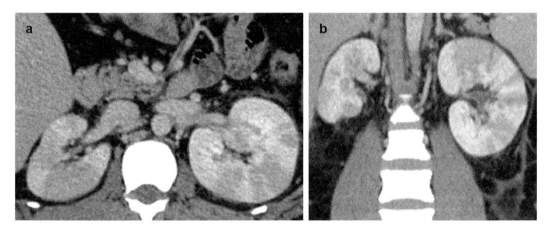

Fig. 14.5 Bacterial pyelonephritis. (**a**) Postcontrast axial CT and coronal reformatted CT images (**b**) show bilateral renal low-density striations

Diagnosis
Postobstructive Striated Nephrogram

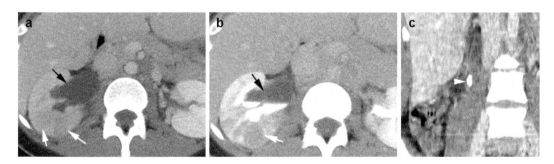

Fig. 14.6 Postobstructive striated nephrogram. No systemic or urinary infection. Postcontrast axial CT in nephrographic phase (**a**), delayed excretory phase CT (**b**), and coronal reformatted images (**c**) show hydronephrosis of the right kidney (*black arrow*) with renal parenchymal striations (*white arrows*). Large stone is seen in the proximal right ureter (*arrowhead*)

Diagnosis
Sarcoidosis

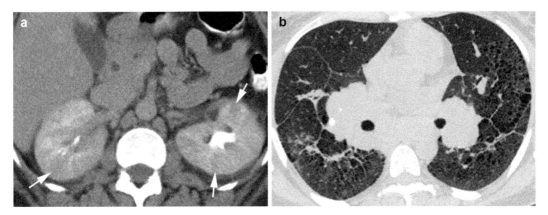

Fig. 14.7 Sarcoidosis. Postcontrast axial CT (**a**) shows multiple linear hypoattenuating striations (*arrows*) in both kidneys related to sarcoidosis with no clinical evidence of infection. (**b**) Chest of the same patients shows bilateral hilar lymphadenopathy and interstitial fibrotic changes

Diagnosis
Tumor Lysis Syndrome

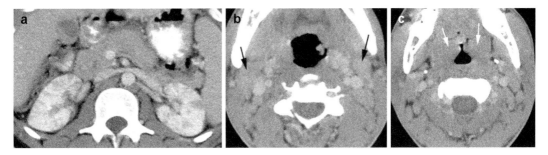

Fig. 14.8 Tumor lysis syndrome. Patient with Burkitt's lymphoma on chemotherapy. Axial CT (**a**) of the kidneys shows multiple focal striations from acute kidney injury with no evidence of infection. (**b**, **c**) CT of the neck shows enlarged lymph nodes (*black arrows*) and palatine tonsils (*white arrows*)

Diagnosis
Allergic Nephritis

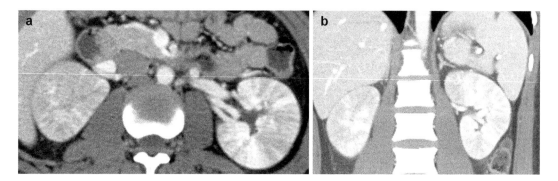

Fig. 14.9 Acute interstitial (allergic) nephritis. Patient with ALL on methotrexate. Postcontrast axial (**a**) and coronal reformatted (**b**) CTs show diffuse low-attenuated renal striation bilaterally

Diagnosis
Acute Kidney Injury

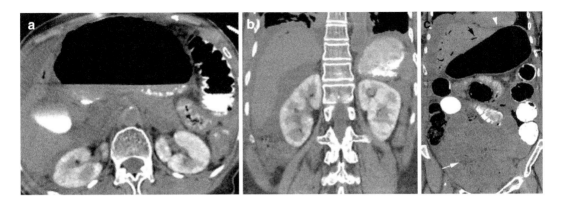

Fig. 14.10 Acute kidney injury with diffuse ischemic changes in bowels. (**a**) Noncontrast axial CT and (**b, c**) coronal reformatted image show retained contrast in renal cortex from CECT done the previous day. Bowel loops are dilated with gas in mesenteric veins (*white arrow*), portal veins (*black arrow*), and small pneumoperitoneum (*arrowhead*)

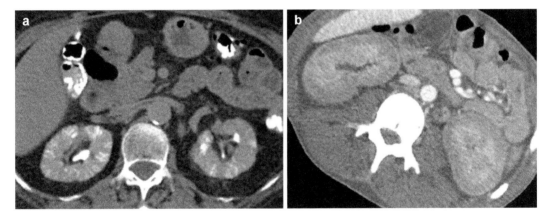

Fig. 14.11 Acute kidney injury. Patient 1: Axial CT (**a**) unenhanced study shows dense striations involving both the cortex and medulla in both kidneys from retained contrast in tubules. Patient soon recovered. Patient 2: (**b**) History of shortness of breath in a 30-year-old male with AIDS and end-stage renal disease. Postcontrast CT shows cortical necrosis with contrast only in the medullary portion of the kidneys

Diagnosis
Renal Infarction

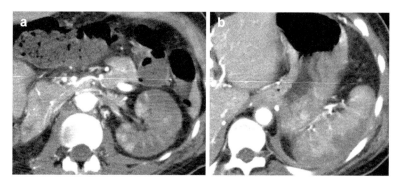

Fig. 14.12 Renal infarction. Patient with Takayasu arteritis with stenosis of the left renal artery. Postcontrast axial CT (**a**) shows multifocal, patchy wedge-shaped areas of decreased attenuation involving both the cortex and medulla involving the capsular surface. (**b**) Axial CT shows infarction of periphery of the spleen

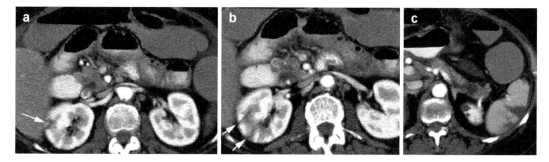

Fig. 14.13 Focal renal infarction in SLE. Axial CT images show (**a, b**) multifocal striated infarction of the right kidney (*arrows*) which were absent 10 days prior. (**c**) Infarction of lateral border of the spleen. Diffuse dilated bowel loops were found to be necrotic

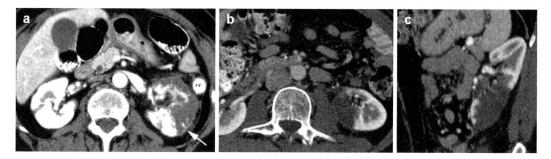

Fig. 14.14 Lobar renal infarction. Patient 1: (**a**) History of atrial fibrillation. Axial CT shows small focal infarction of the right kidney and large infarction of the left kidney with cortical rim sign (*arrow*). Patient 2: (**b, c**) History of marijuana use and sudden back pain with moderate heavy lifting. Axial and coronal CTs show large area of infarction at the lower pole of the left kidney

Nephritis

Diagnosis
Emphysematous Pyelitis

Imaging Features
1. Gas-fluid level in dilated calyces and ureters with no pyelonephritis

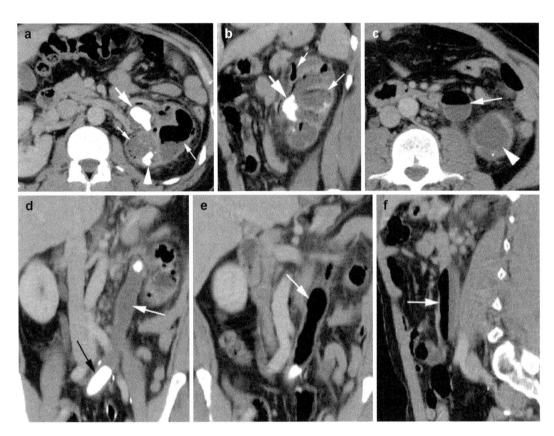

Fig. 14.15 Emphysematous pyelitis and ureteritis. History of bladder cancer, ileal conduit, left upper quadrant pain, and purulent discharge through left nephrostomy tube. CECT, axial (**a**), and sagittal reformatted (**b**) images show staghorn stone (*thick arrow*) in the renal pelvis and stone at the lower pole renal calyx (*arrowhead*). Emphysematous changes with fluid and gas in dilated calyces (*thin arrow*). Axial CT at lower level (**c**) shows gas and fluid in dilated left ureter (*arrow*) and fluid-filled lower pole left kidney (*arrowhead*). Coronal reformatted images (**d**, **e**) and sagittal reformatted image (**f**) show a second stone distal to the left ureter (*black arrow*) with air-fluid collection (*thin arrow*) in the ureter obstructed by the two stones

Diagnosis

Emphysematous Pyelonephritis

Imaging Features

1. Parenchymal enlargement and destruction with gas collections
2. Streaky or bubbly gas or gas-fluid level
3. Focal tissue necrosis with or without abscess

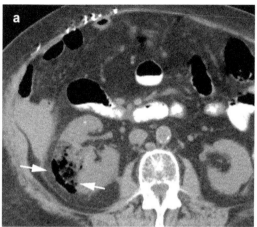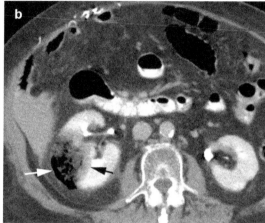

Fig. 14.16 Emphysematous pyelonephritis in an 82-year-old female. (**a**) Axial CT precontrast phase shows focal area of tissue necrosis midpole right kidney (*arrows*) with gas collection. (**b**) Postcontrast axial CT shows the gas to be contained within the capsule (*white arrow*). A thin rim of edema is seen surrounding the necrosis (*black arrow*). Urine culture grew *E. coli*

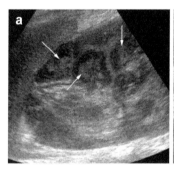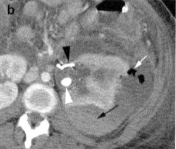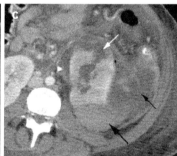

Fig. 14.17 Pyonephrosis with rupture. A pregnant 27-year-old patient with urosepsis. (**a**) US of the left kidney shows dilated calyces with debris (*arrows*). Patient had spontaneous abortion. CT done 5 days later. Axial CECT (**b**) shows a large stone in the renal pelvis (*white arrowhead*) with adjacent stent (*black arrowhead*). Gas bubbles extending into the subcapsular space from the renal parenchyma (*white arrow*) and also hematocrit level (*black arrow*). (**c**) Rupture of calyx into subcapsular space (*white arrow*) with fluid (*thin black arrow*) and hemorrhage (*thick black arrow*) in the subcapsular space. Patient had left nephrectomy, and urine grew *Acinetobacter baum annii/haemolyticus*

Diagnosis

Xanthogranulomatous Pyelonephritis

Imaging Features

1. Large staghorn calculus in most cases
2. Affected kidney is enlarged and nonfunctioning
3. Contracted renal pelvis, expansion of renal calyces, and inflammatory changes in perinephric fat
4. Extrarenal extension with formation of psoas abscess and fistula to the skin or colon

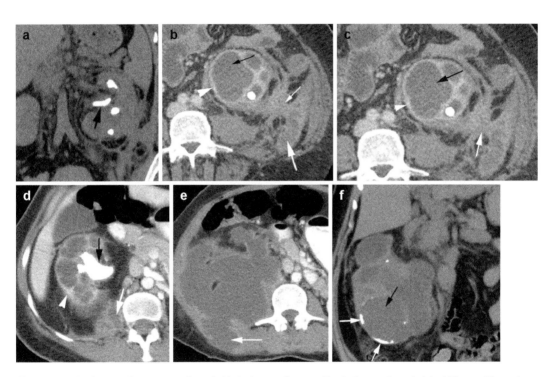

Fig. 14.18 Xanthogranulomatous pyelonephritis in three patients. Patient 1: (**a**) Noncontrast coronal reformatted (**b**, **c**) CECT shows enlarged left kidney with central staghorn stone (*thick black arrow*) and dilated calyces (*thin black arrow*). Inflammatory changes (*thin white arrow*) with fluid (*thick white arrow*) extend from the kidney to the peri- and pararenal spaces. Mild rim enhancement is seen of the calyces (*arrowhead*). Patient 2: CECT axial images (**d**, **e**) show enlarged right kidney with staghorn stone and dilated calyces with rim enhancement. A large collection of nonenhancing thick-rimmed fluid is extending from the lower pole of the kidney to the psoas muscle and posterior abdominal wall (*arrow*). Patient 3: (**f**) Coronal reformatted noncontrast CT shows dilated calyces (*black arrow*) with rim calcification (*short white arrows*)

Diagnosis

Abscess

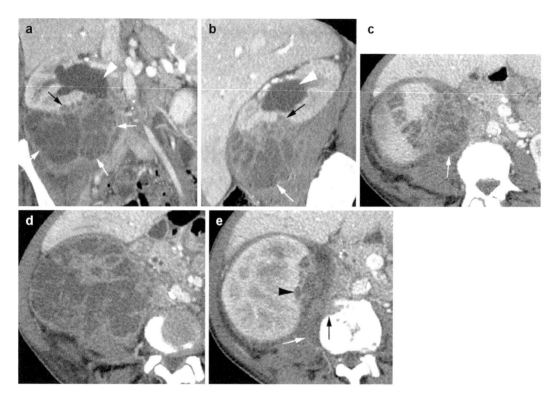

Fig. 14.19 Intrarenal abscess with perirenal extension and osteomyelitis. History of IV drug abuse and MRSA infection. CECT (**a**, **b**) coronal and sagittal reformatted images show multiple small abscesses in lower pole of the right renal parenchyma (*black arrow*) with large extension into perirenal space inferiorly (*white arrows*) and hydronephrosis (*arrowhead*) from obstruction of the ureter by the abscess. (**c**, **d**) Axial images show extension medially through the fascia muscularis (*arrow*) to the psoas muscle. (**e**) Axial CECT shows osteomyelitis of L3 vertebral body (*black arrow*) with paravertebral abscess (*white arrow*) from the lower pole abscess (*arrowhead*)

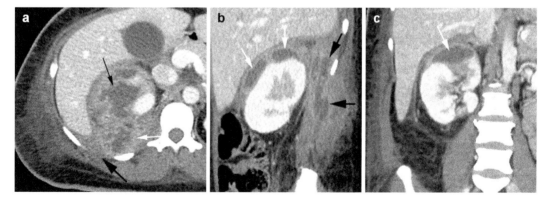

Fig. 14.20 Renal abscess extending to the posterior abdominal wall. CECT (**a**) axial, (**b**) sagittal, and (**c**) coronal reformatted images show parenchymal abscess (*thin black arrow*) in the upper pole of the right kidney is extending to the subcapsular and posterior pararenal space (*thin white arrow*) and then into the posterior abdominal wall (*thick black arrow*)

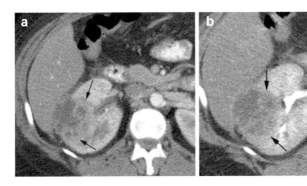

Fig. 14.21 Renal abscess compressing the liver. History of diabetes, fever, and hematuria. Axial postcontrast CT in (**a**) arterial (**b**) delayed phases show focal well-demarcated abscess with septations within the midpole of the right renal parenchyma (*arrows*) causing extrinsic compression on the liver

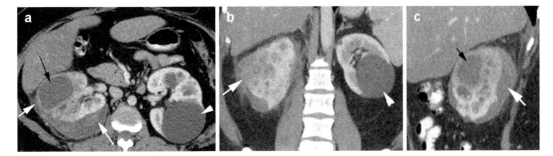

Fig. 14.22 Renal abscess involving the subcapsular space. Postcontrast CT (**a**) axial, (**b**) coronal, and (**c**) sagittal reformatted images show a large abscess of the right kidney (*thin black arrow* in **a** and **c**) and surrounding smaller abscesses (**b**) extending into the subcapsular space (*white arrow*) with edema of the surrounding renal parenchyma. Infected fluid collection is seen in the subcapsular space (*thick white arrow*), is of heterogeneous density causing extrinsic compression of the kidney, and was drained. The left kidney has a simple cyst (*arrowhead*)

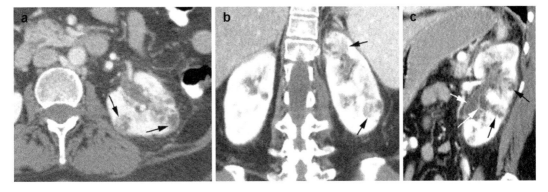

Fig. 14.23 Multifocal abscess. History of diabetes. CECT (**a**) axial, (**b**) coronal, and (**c**) sagittal reformatted images show multiple abscesses mainly in the left kidney (*black arrows*). Pyelitis is seen of the renal pelvis with enhancement of the wall of the renal pelvis (*white arrows*)

Diagnosis

Lobar Bacterial Nephritis

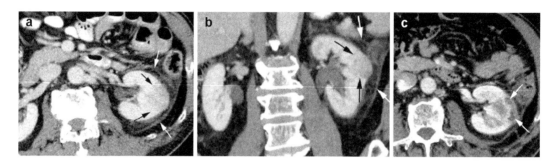

Fig. 14.24 Lobar bacterial nephritis. Patient with fever and left flank pain. CECT (**a**) axial and coronal reformatted (**b**) images show focal low-density area in the midpole of the left kidney with lateral bulge (*black arrows*), edema perirenal space, and thickening of anterior and posterior renal fascia (*white arrows*). (**c**) Postcontrast axial CT done 3 weeks later shows abscess formation (*arrow*) in the renal cortex in the same area

Diagnosis
Subcapsular Hemorrhage from Infection

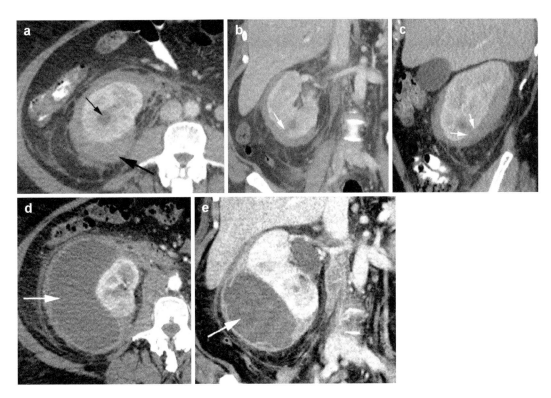

Fig. 14.25 Spontaneous subcapsular hemorrhage from infection. Patient with diabetes, right flank pain, and fever. Urine culture grew *E. coli*. Postcontrast axial CT (**a**) shows a small low-density abscess of the lower pole of the right kidney (*thin black arrow*), large subcapsular high-density hemorrhage (*thick black arrow*), and perinephric stranding. (**b**, **c**) Coronal and sagittal reformatted images show abscess tracking to the subcapsular space with cortical break (*white arrows*). (**d**, **e**) Axial and coronal reformatted CTs two months later show larger fluid collection in the subcapsular space which is now of low density with increased capsular thickening (*arrow*). This was drained and the fluid was seen to be infected

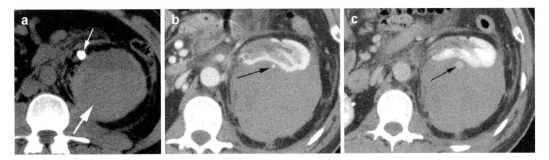

Fig. 14.26 Spontaneous subcapsular hemorrhage with ureteral stone and hypertension. Precontrast axial CT (**a**) shows large subcapsular high-density hemorrhage in the left kidney (*thick arrow*) with large stone in the proximal right ureter (*thin arrow*). (**b**) Postcontrast late arterial phase shows hemorrhage from a capsular vessel (*arrow*). (**c**) Excretory phase axial CT shows enlargement of the leaking contrast from the vessel (*arrow*)

Diagnosis

Pyelonephritis with Rupture

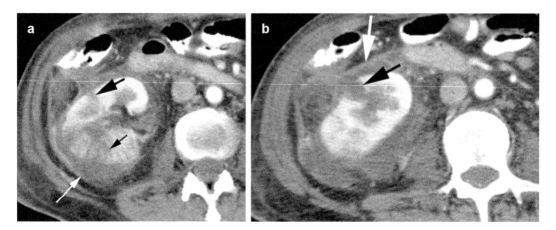

Fig. 14.27 Pyelonephritis with rupture. (**a**, **b**) Post-contrast axial CT of the right kidney shows striated nephrogram (*thin black arrow*) especially of the lower pole. Some of the striations have ruptured into the perirenal space (*thick black arrow*) which shows fluid collection and with thickening of the anterior (*thick white arrow*) and posterior renal fascia (*thin white arrow*)

Diagnosis
Tuberculosis

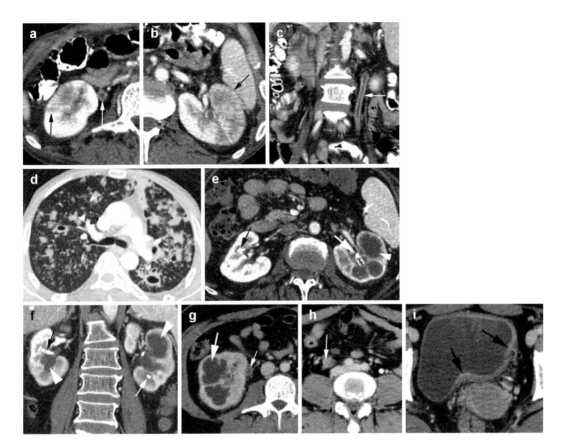

Fig. 14.28 TB infection of the urinary system. Axial postcontrast CT (**a**, **b**) of both kidneys at different levels show striated nephrogram (*black arrows*). The right ureter (*white arrow*) shows ureteritis with wall thickening. (**c**) Coronal reformatted image shows ureteritis of the left ureter (*arrow*). (**d**) Axial CT of the chest at the same time shows acute on chronic TB infection with nodules and thick-walled cavitation. (**e**, **f**) One year later axial and coronal reformatted images show medullary necrosis (*arrowheads*) with decreased density and increased size of the pyramids in both kidneys, calcification of the proximal left ureter (*thick white arrow*), focal calcification in the left kidney lower pole medulla (*thin white arrow*), and calcification of the right midpole infundibulum (*black arrow*). (**g–i**) Axial CT of a different patient shows medullary necrosis of the right kidney (*thick white arrow*) and ureteritis (*thin white arrow*) with bladder wall thickening (*black arrows*) from TB cystitis (biopsy proven)

Diagnosis
Candida Infection

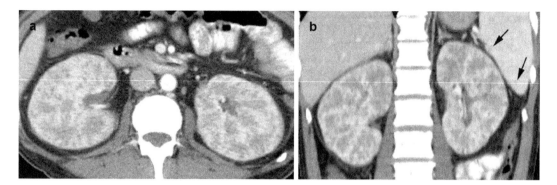

Fig. 14.29 *Candida* infection of the kidneys. A patient with B-cell ALL with systemic candidiasis. Postcontrast axial (**a**) and coronal reformatted (**b**) images show multiple punctate low-density foci throughout both kidneys. A few low-density foci are also seen in the spleen (*arrows*)

Emphysematous Cystitis

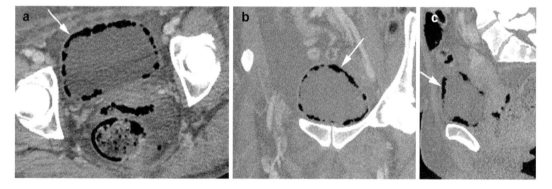

Fig. 14.30 Emphysematous cystitis. Postcontrast axial (**a**), oblique coronal (**b**), and sagittal reformatted (**c**) images show diffuse gas in bladder wall (*arrow*)

Prostate Abscess

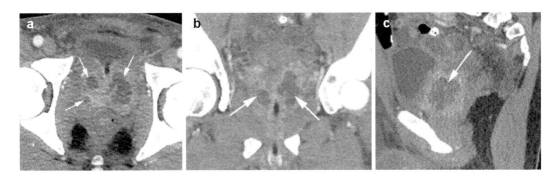

Fig. 14.31 Prostate abscess. Postcontrast CT axial (**a**), coronal (**b**), and sagittal (**c**) reformatted images show abscesses (*arrows*) in the prostate with multiple loculated rim-enhancing fluid collections

Hemorrhage

Diagnosis

Hemorrhage in the Bladder

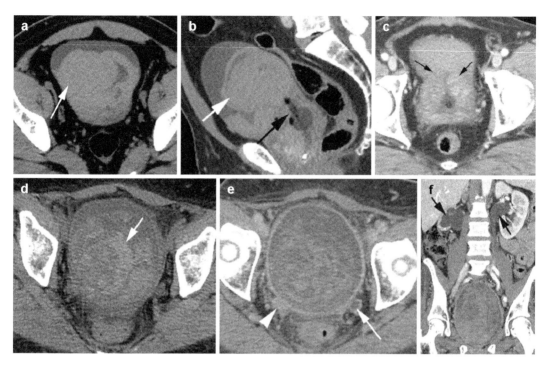

Fig. 14.32 Hemorrhage in the bladder in two patients. Patient 1: with enlarged prostate. Noncontrast axial CT (**a**) shows high-density lobulated hemorrhage (*arrow*) within the bladder. (**b**) Sagittal reformatted image shows Foley catheter in prostatic urethra (*black arrow*). Postcontrast axial CT (**c**) shows enlarged prostate (*arrows*) projecting into the hemorrhage-filled bladder base. Patient 2: hemorrhagic cystitis. (**d**) Axial noncontrast CT shows heterogeneous high-density hemorrhage distending the urinary bladder (*arrow*). (**e**) CECT axial image shows no enhancing lesions in the bladder. At the UVJ, the left ureter (*arrow*) is dilated and the right ureter (*arrowhead*) is filled with thrombus. (**f**) Coronal reformatted image shows bilateral hydronephrosis (*arrows*) with no enhancing urothelium

Diagnosis
Hemorrhagic Hydronephrosis

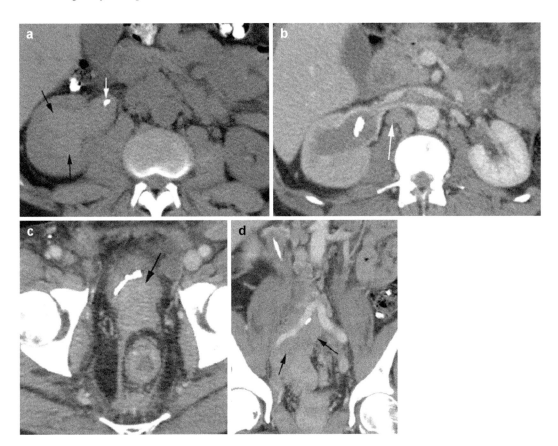

Fig. 14.33 Hemorrhagic hydronephrosis. A patient with prostate cancer with right ureteral obstruction and stent in place. Noncontrast axial CT (**a**) shows right-sided hydronephrosis with high-density hemorrhagic fluid (*black arrow*) and stent (*white arrow*). Axial postcontrast image (**b**) again shows hydronephrosis, but the hemorrhage is less obvious. Enlarged lymph nodes are seen posterior to the right renal artery (*arrow*). (**c**) Axial CT of the pelvis shows enlarged prostate (*arrow*) with stent in the bladder. (**d**) Coronal reformatted postcontrast image shows enlarged lymph nodes in the right common iliac chain (*arrows*) deforming the common iliac artery

Diagnosis
Hemorrhage in the Kidney, Liver, and Pararenal
Space

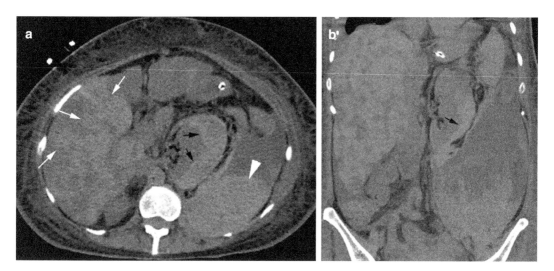

Fig. 14.34 Hemorrhage in the liver, kidney, and pararenal space. Patient with breast cancer on Lovenox. Noncontrast axial (**a**) and coronal reformatted (**b**) image shows diffuse high-density hemorrhage in the liver (*white arrows*). Hemorrhage is seen in the left renal subcapsular space (*black arrows*). The left pararenal space is distended with blood with hematocrit level (*arrowhead*)

Hamartoma

Diagnosis
Angiomyolipoma

Imaging Features

1. CT—well-marginated, cortical-based, heterogeneous mass predominantly of fat density and variable enhancement.
2. Angiogram—hypervascular mass and intralesional aneurysms and venous pooling.
3. Some are fat-poor especially those associated with tuberous sclerosis.
4. Spontaneous rupture and hemorrhage when the tumor is larger than 4 cm and intratumoral aneurysms larger than 5 mm.

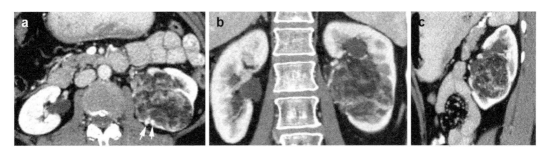

Fig. 14.35 Angiomyolipoma of the left kidney. Postcontrast axial (**a**), coronal (**b**), and sagittal (**c**) reformatted images show a large left renal mass predominantly of fatty tissue with interspersed soft tissue and dilated vessels (*arrow*)

Fig. 14.36 Hemorrhagic angiomyolipoma with large aneurysm. (**a**) Noncontrast axial CT shows large angiomyolipoma lower pole of the left kidney with surrounding high-density hemorrhage (*arrows*). (**b**, **c**) Coronal reformatted and axial CECT again show lower pole angiomyolipoma with surrounding hemorrhage (*thin white arrows*) in the subcapsular space, perirenal space, and posterior interfascial space (*black arrows*). (**d**) Angiogram of the left kidney shows large intratumoral aneurysm (*black arrow*)

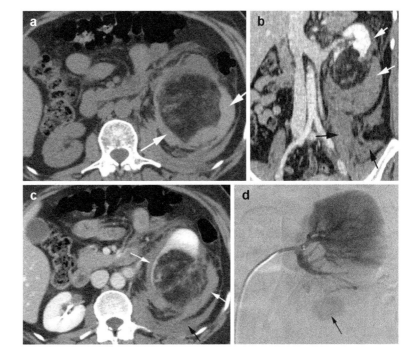

Diagnosis

Tuberous Sclerosis

Imaging Features

1. Subependymal tubers
2. Renal angiomyolipomas
3. Multiple lung cysts similar to lymphangiomyomatosis

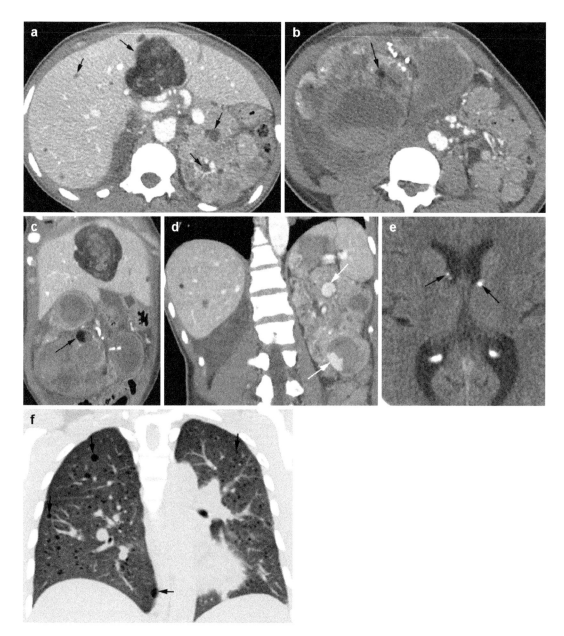

Fig. 14.37 Tuberous sclerosis. Axial CECT (**a**, **b**) and coronal reformatted (**c**, **d**) images show multiple angiomyolipomas in the liver (*arrows*). Both kidneys are deformed and enlarged by angiomyolipomas with small foci of fat collections (*black arrows*). Pockets of focal hemorrhage are seen in the left kidney (*white arrows*). (**e**) Axial CT of the head shows subependymomas adjacent to foramen of Monro bilaterally (*arrows*). (**f**) Coronal reformatted CT of the chest shows multiple small cysts in both lung fields (*arrows*)

Autosomal Dominant Polycystic Kidney Disease

Imaging Features
1. Bilateral enlarged kidneys with various size cysts.
2. Nonfunctioning kidneys.
3. Cysts may have hemorrhage and calcification.
4. Cysts in the liver and other organs.

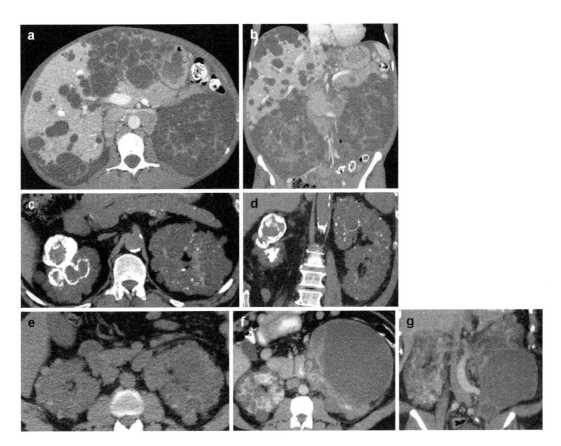

Fig. 14.38 Autosomal dominant polycystic kidney disease in three patients on dialysis. Patient 1: (**a, b**) Axial and coronal reformatted CT images show both kidneys entirely replaced by cysts with multiple cysts in the liver. Patient 2: (**c, d**) Axial and coronal reformatted CT images show multiple cysts in both kidneys. Left kidney is enlarged with multiple punctate calcifications. Right kidney smaller in size with coarse calcification in some of the cyst walls. Patient 3: (**e**) Axial CT shows multiple cysts of both kidneys with some cysts are hyperattenuating. (**f, g**) Postcontrast axial and coronal reformatted CT images at a later date show increased size of some cysts mostly on the left side with no internal flow in the cysts

Cystic Renal Masses

Diagnosis
Cystic Nephroma

Imaging Features
1. Multiloculated cystic mass; small locules may appear solid.
2. Locules are slightly hyperattenuating relative to water.
3. Septa enhance moderately.
4. No accumulation of contrast in cystic spaces.
5. Calcification is uncommon.

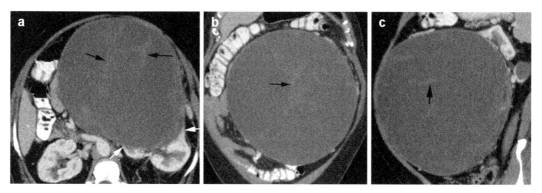

Fig. 14.39 Cystic nephroma. Postcontrast CT, axial (**a**), coronal (**b**), and (**c**) sagittal reformatted images show large septated cystic mass arising from the midpole of the left kidney with claw sign (*white arrows*). The septations show faint enhancement (*black arrows*)

Diagnosis
Multilocular Cystic RCC

Imaging Features

1. Variable imaging pattern from Bosniak category IIF to IV.
2. Septa enhance, may have irregular thickening or wall calcification.
3. The lesion is separated from the kidney by fibrous capsule.
4. The fluid may be serous or hemorrhagic.

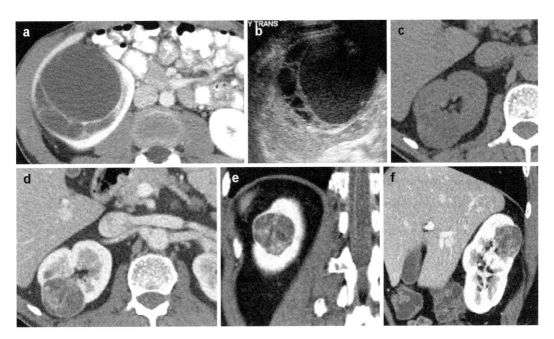

Fig. 14.40 Multilocular cystic RCC. Two patients. Patient 1: Axial CECT (**a**) and ultrasound (**b**) images show a large well-marginated cyst with multiple septa showing enhancement by CT. Patient 2: CT (**c**) precontrast study shows low-density protruding lesion of the right kidney. CECT (**d–f**) axial, coronal, and sagittal reformatted views show a well-marginated lesion with irregular enhancing septa

Solid Renal Masses

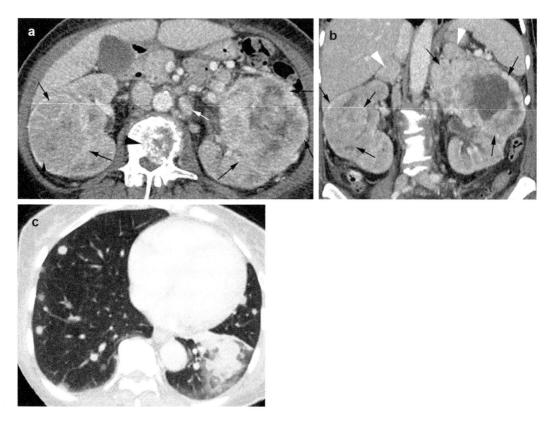

Fig. 14.41 Bilateral renal cell carcinoma, clear cell subtype with bilateral synchronous adrenal metastasis. CECT axial (**a**) and (**b**) coronal reformatted images show a large enhancing necrotic mass in the upper half of the left kidney and smaller tumor in the midpole of the right kidney (*black arrows*). Both adrenal glands are enlarged, with enhancing metastasis (*white arrowhead*). Enlarged lymph nodes are seen in the para-aortic region (*thin white arrows*). Lytic metastasis is seen in lumbar vertebra (*black arrowhead*). (**c**) Axial CT through lung bases shows multiple nodular metastases

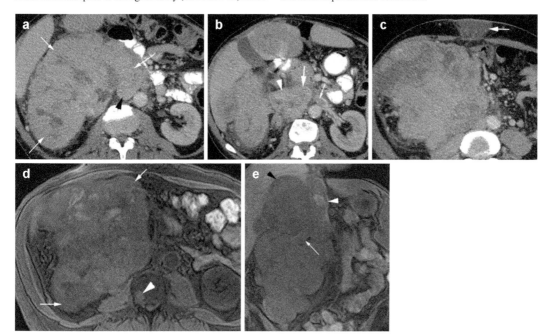

Diagnosis

Oncocytoma

Imaging Features

1. Homogeneous attenuation if less than 3 cm, heterogeneous if larger
2. Can have calcification
3. Can have central nonenhancing scar
4. Usually heterogeneous enhancement
5. Absent tumor thrombus in renal veins but it can have bland thrombus

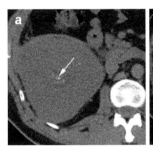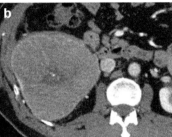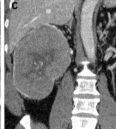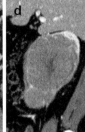

Fig. 14.43 Oncocytoma, biopsy proven. Precontrast CT (**a**) axial, CECT (**b**) axial, (**c**) coronal, and (**d**) sagittal reformatted images show a large mass at the lower pole right kidney having central stellate scar with calcification (*arrow*) and faint enhancement mostly at the periphery

Diagnosis

Leukemia

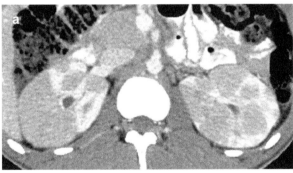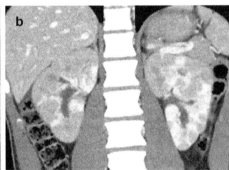

Fig. 14.44 Leukemic renal lesions in a patient with acute myeloid leukemia. Postcontrast axial (**a**) and coronal reformatted (**b**) images show multiple low-density nodules in both kidneys which retain their normal reniform shape

Fig. 14.42 Papillary renal cell carcinoma. CECT shows a large poorly enhancing mass with less enhancement than a clear cell RCC. Axial CT (**a**) shows a large mass in the right kidney (*arrows*) invading IVC (*arrowhead*). (**b**) Axial CECT shows mass invading the right renal vein (*arrowhead*), IVC (*thick arrow*), and left renal vein (*thin arrow*). (**c**) Axial CECT shows metastasis to Sister Mary Joseph umbilical lymph node (*arrow*). (**d**) Axial T1W spoiled gradient MRI shows large right renal mass (*arrows*) with vertebral metastasis (*arrowhead*). (**e**) Coronal T1W spoiled gradient MRI shows tumor extension into the right renal vein (*arrow*) and IVC (*white arrowhead*) and liver metastasis (*black arrowhead*)

Diagnosis
Lymphoma

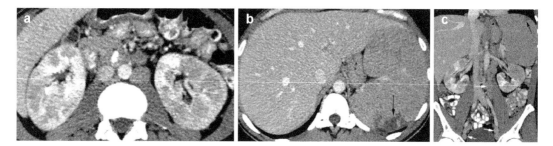

Fig. 14.45 Lymphoma of both kidneys in a patient with diffuse large B-cell lymphoma. CECT axial (**a**, **b**) and coronal reformatted (**c**) images show multiple solid low-density nodules in both kidneys which retain their reniform shape. Spleen is enlarged with focal infarction (*black arrow*). Lymphadenopathy is seen in the para-aortic and iliac chain (*white arrows*)

Diagnosis
Metastasis

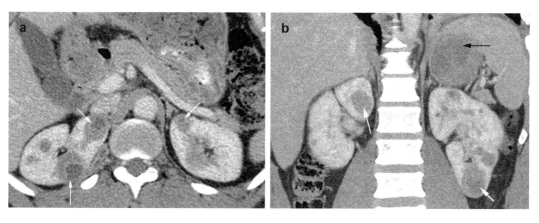

Fig. 14.46 Renal metastasis. History of adenoid cystic carcinoma of the salivary glands with metastasis. CECT (**a**) axial and (**b**) coronal reformatted images show multiple low-density nodules in both kidneys (*white arrows*) and in the spleen (*black arrow*)

Urothelial Carcinoma

Diagnosis
Renal Pelvis Transitional Cell Carcinoma

Imaging Features
1. On precontrast study TCC is hyperattenuating to urine but less than clot
2. Typically sessile
3. Enhance in urothelial phase

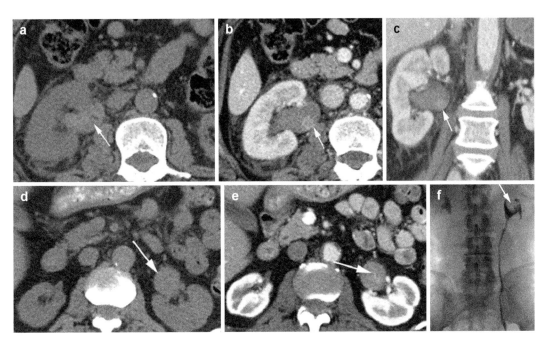

Fig. 14.47 Transitional cell carcinoma in two patients. Patient 1: TCC papillary subtype at renal pelvis with hemorrhage. (**a**) Precontrast study shows high-density hemorrhagic fluid in the right renal pelvis. Small focal low-density filling defect is seen (*arrow*). CECT (**b**) axial and (**c**) coronal reformatted images show enhancement of the same nodule with attenuation higher than surrounding blood (*arrow*). Patient 2: TCC low grade. (**d**) Noncontrast axial CT shows mass in the renal pelvis (*arrow*) with attenuation slightly more than the kidneys. (**e**) CECT axial image shows enhancement of the mass with a central vessel (*arrow*). (**f**) Retrograde cystogram shows filling defect in the contrast-filled renal pelvis (*arrow*)

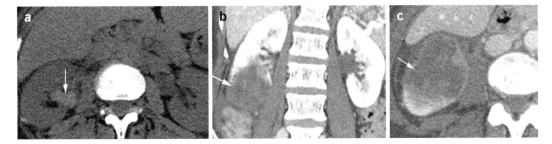

Fig. 14.48 Necrotic RCC with hemorrhage in the renal pelvis. Precontrast axial CT (**a**) shows high-density hemorrhagic fluid in the renal pelvis (*arrow*). CECT (**b**) coronal reformatted and (**c**) axial images show a large necrotic mass in the lower pole of the right kidney (*arrow*)

Diagnosis
Ureteral High-Grade TCC

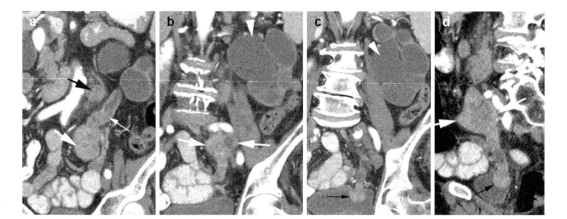

Fig. 14.49 High-grade urothelial carcinoma. CECT (**a–c**) coronal reformatted images at different levels and (**d**) sagittal reformatted images show enhancing transitional cell carcinoma at mid-ureter showing well-marginated extension beyond the ureter transversely (*thick white arrows*), proximally (*thin white arrow*), and distally to the ureterovesical junction (*thin black arrow*) resulting in hydronephrosis (*arrowhead*). Focal necrotic area is seen in the tumor. Enlarged lymph nodes are seen in the para-aortic chain (*thick black arrow*)

Diagnosis
Papillary High-Grade TCC

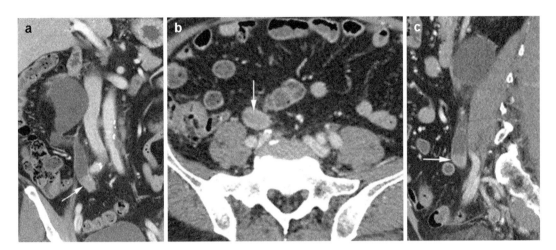

Fig. 14.50 Papillary urothelial carcinoma, high grade. CECT in the urothelial phase (**a**) coronal, (**b**) axial, and (**c**) sagittal reformatted images show focal-enhancing lesion in right mid-ureter (*arrow*) with proximal obstructive uropathy

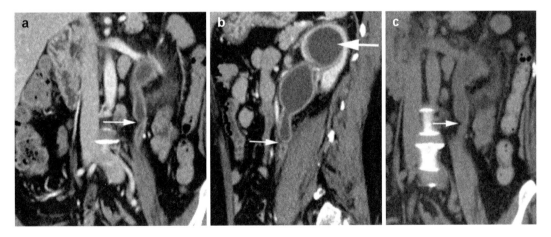

Fig. 14.51 Stricture ureter. History of ureteral stone and several catheter placement. CECT (**a**) coronal, (**b**) sagittal, and (**c**) precontrast coronal reformatted images show focal narrowing of mid-ureter (*thin arrow*) with proximal ureterectasis and hydronephrosis (*thick arrow*) with no enhancing mass

Diagnosis
Bladder Low-Grade TCC and Prostate Cancer

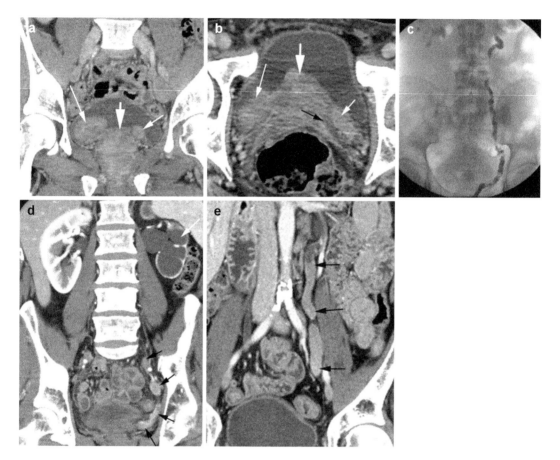

Fig. 14.52 Papillary carcinoma low grade and prostate cancer. CECT (**a**) coronal reformatted and (**b**) axial images show enlarged prostate (*thick arrow*). Two enhancing nodules on either side of the prostate at the ureteral orifices (*thin arrows*) are bladder papillary carcinomas with dilated left ureter (*black arrow*) at the UV region. (**c**) Retrograde cystogram shows irregular filling defects in mid-ureter and distal left ureter due to tumor infiltration. (**d, e**) Coronal reformatted images show the distal left ureter filled with enhancing tumor (*black arrows*) with proximal obstructive uropathy (*white arrow*)

Diagnosis

Sarcomatoid Urothelial Carcinoma

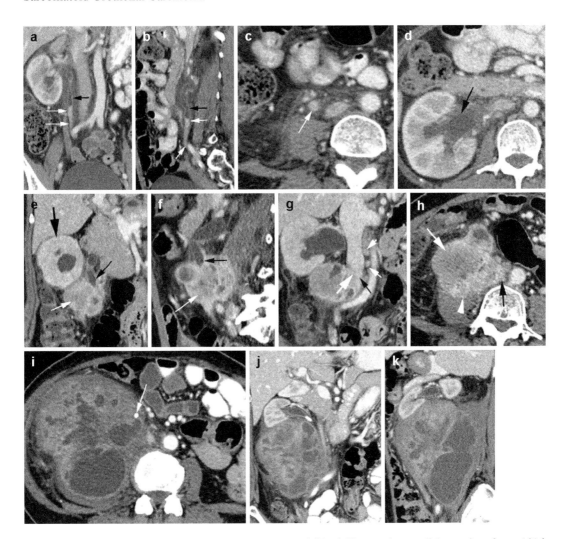

Fig. 14.53 Sarcomatoid urothelial carcinoma. CECT (**a**) coronal, (**b**) sagittal reformatted, and (**c, d**) axial images show enhancing lesion within right mid-ureter (*white arrows*) causing proximal obstructive uropathy (*black arrow*). Later date CECT, coronal (**e**), and sagittal (**f**) reformatted images show extension of the mass outside the ureter (*white arrow*) with constriction of the ureter above it (*thin black arrow*), and the right kidney remains hydronephrotic (*thick arrow*). (**g**) Coronal reformatted and (**h**) axial images show medial extension of mass (*thick white arrow*) causing extrinsic compression on IVC (*black arrow*) and posteriorly involving the psoas muscle (*arrowhead*). Enlarged lymph nodes seen in aortocaval chain (*thin white arrows*). (**i–k**) A few months later, the axial, coronal, and sagittal reformatted images show marked increase in size of the extraureteric portion of the tumor with increased necrosis. Stent is seen in the ureter (*arrow*)

Diagnosis
Bladder TCC

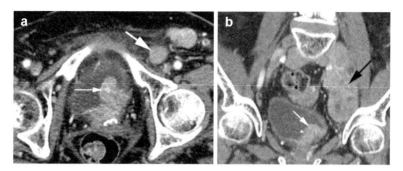

Fig. 14.54 Transitional cell carcinoma of the bladder. CECT (**a**) axial and (**b**) coronal reformatted images show enhancing mass at the base of the urinary bladder with calcification (*thin white arrow*). Enlarged lymph nodes are seen in the left inguinal region (*thick white arrow*) and in the left external iliac chain (*black arrow*)

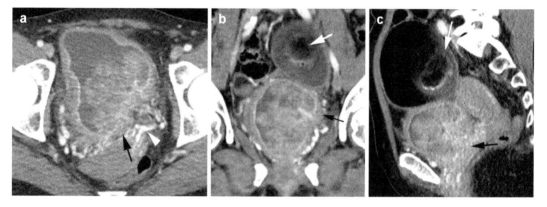

Fig. 14.55 Invasive papillary TCC. CECT (**a**) axial, (**b**) coronal, and (**c**) sagittal reformatted images show a large mass at the base of the bladder with extension outside the bladder wall (*black arrow*) showing frond-like projections within the bladder. Large vessels are seen around the bladder base supplying the mass (*arrowhead*). A dermoid is also seen in the left adnexa (*white arrow*)

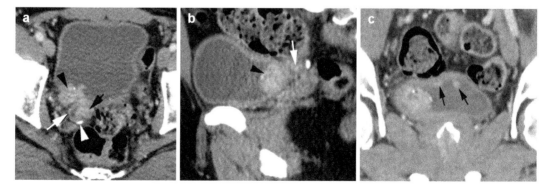

Fig. 14.56 TCC in Hutch diverticulum. (**a**) Axial CECT shows Hutch diverticulum (*white arrow*) with small fluid, stone (*white arrowhead*), and enhancing mass (*black arrow*). A second mass (*black arrowhead*) is completely filling a second diverticulum (surgically proven) and protruding into the bladder. (**b**) CECT sagittal reformatted image shows mass in Hutch diverticulum with stone (*arrow*) and portion of the second mass bulging into the bladder (*arrowhead*). (**c**) CECT coronal reformatted image shows smaller enhancing nodules at the dome of the bladder (*arrows*)

Urachus

Diagnosis
Urachal Sinus Infection

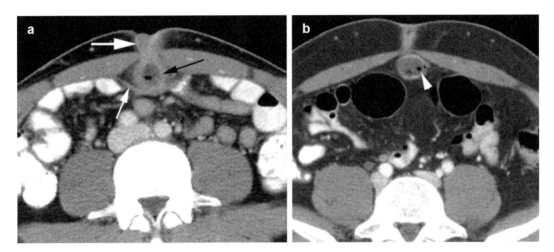

Fig. 14.57 Urachal sinus infection. Axial CECT (**a**, **b**) in two patients. Thick-walled urachal sinus (*thin black arrow*) is open at the umbilicus. The sinus tract at the umbilicus is also thick walled (*thick white arrow*). Small gas collection is seen within the urachal remnant (*arrowhead*) which is in the preperitoneal space. The peritoneum shows reactive thickening and is displaced posteriorly (*thin white arrow*)

Diagnosis
Urachal Diverticulum

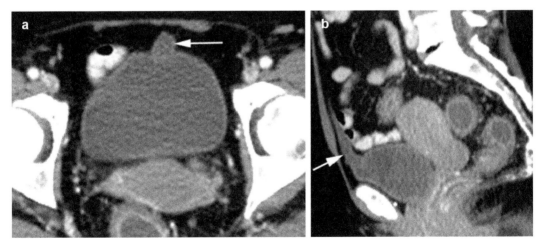

Fig. 14.58 Urachal diverticulum. CECT (**a**) axial and (**b**) sagittal reformatted images show urachus is patent at the bladder end and communicates with the bladder at the dome (*arrow*)

Diagnosis
Urachal Cyst

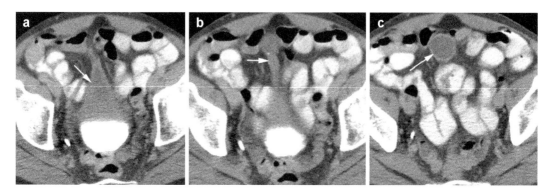

Fig. 14.59 Urachal cyst. Excretory phase CT (**a**) axial image shows the bladder end of the urachus is patent forming the bladder diverticulum (*arrow*). (**b**) Axial CT distal to the diverticulum shows the urachus to be obliter-ated (*arrow*). (**c**) Axial CT at midportion of the urachus distal to the obliterated end it is again patent and dilated forming the urachal cyst (*arrow*)

Diagnosis
Urachal Adenocarcinoma

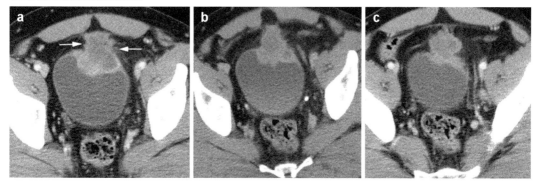

Fig. 14.60 Urachal adenocarcinoma. CECT (**a–c**) axial images show soft tissue enhancing mass at the dome of the bladder extending along the bladder end of the urachus (*arrows*)

Fig. 14.61 Urothelial carcinoma of the bladder dome. CECT (**a**, **b**) axial images show large lobulated mass at dome of the bladder extending down the bladder side walls (*arrows*)

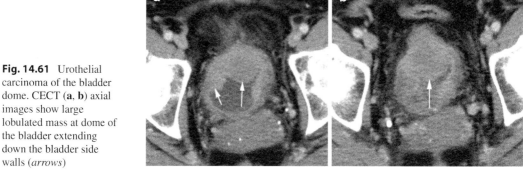

Penile Lesions

Diagnosis
Penile Condyloma

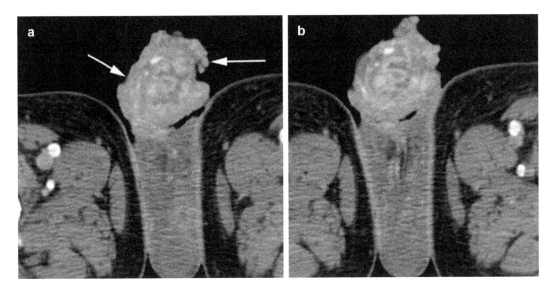

Fig. 14.62 Penile condyloma. (**a**, **b**) Postcontrast axial CT shows a lobulated heterogeneous enhancing soft tissue mass at the penile shaft (*arrows*) with areas of linear enhancement

Diagnosis
Penile Squamous Cell Carcinoma

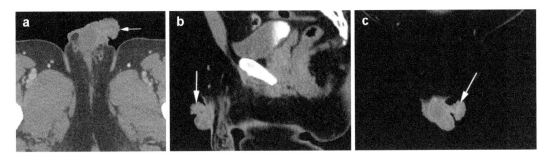

Fig. 14.63 Penile squamous cell carcinoma. CECT (**a**) axial, (**b**) sagittal, and (**c**) coronal reformatted images show a pedunculated mushroom-like mass arising from the anterior penis (*arrow*)

Diagnosis
Penile Leiomyosarcoma

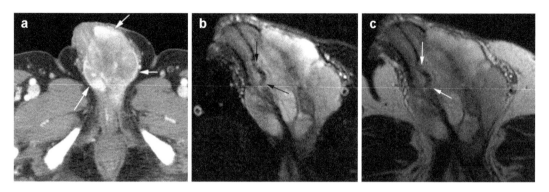

Fig. 14.64 Leiomyosarcoma of the penis. (**a**) Axial post-contrast CT shows enhancing mass at shaft of the penis, larger on the left side (*arrows*). MRI oblique axial (**b**) T2W FS and (**c**) T2W without FS images show mass at the penile shaft involving the corpus spongiosum and corpus cavernosum and extending into the urethra (*arrows*)

Diagnosis
Bladder Exstrophy

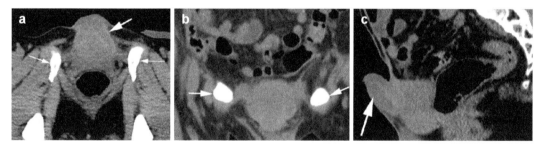

Fig. 14.65 Bladder exstrophy. Axial (**a**), coronal (**b**), and sagittal (**c**) reformatted images show widely separated pubic bones (*thin white arrows*) with absent symphysis pubis. The penis is short (*thick white arrow*) and with no identifiable bladder

Congenital Ureteral Lesions

Diagnosis
Ectopic Ureteral Insertion

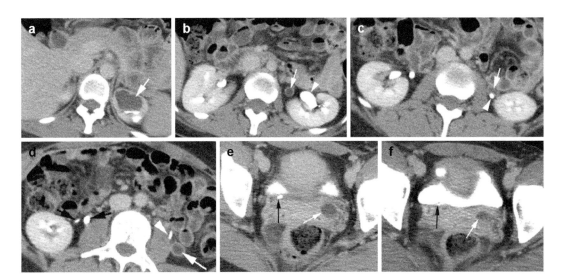

Fig. 14.66 Ectopic ureteral insertion with duplication of bilateral ureters. Axial CT (**a**) shows hydronephrosis of upper pole moiety of the left kidney (*white arrow*) and lower pole moiety (**b**) having no obstruction (*arrowhead*). The dilated upper pole ureter is seen medially (*white arrow*). (**c**) Axial CT at lower level shows the upper pole ureter crosses laterally (*white arrow*). (**d**) Duplicated right ureters travel side by side on the right side (*black arrows*) while the upper pole dilated left ureter is lateral (*white arrow*) to lower pole nondilated contrast-filled ureter (*arrowhead*). (**e**, **f**) Axial CT at bladder base show the right ureters join and enter as one ureter into the bladder (*black arrows*). The dilated left upper pole ureter inserts into the vagina below the bladder (*white arrow*)

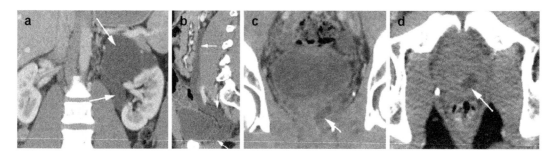

Fig. 14.67 Ectopic ureter insertion into the prostate. CECT (**a**) coronal reformatted image shows obstructed upper pole moiety with dilated upper pole ureter (*arrows*) with hydronephrosis. (**b**) Sagittal reformatted image shows insertion of the dilated upper pole ureter below the bladder (*arrows*). (**c**, **d**) Coronal reformatted and axial images show obstructed ureter ending in the prostate (*arrow*)

Diagnosis

Ureterocele

Imaging Features

1. Saccular outpouching of the ureter into the urinary bladder
2. Most often associated with duplicate ureters and involve upper pole
3. Upper pole frequently obstructs

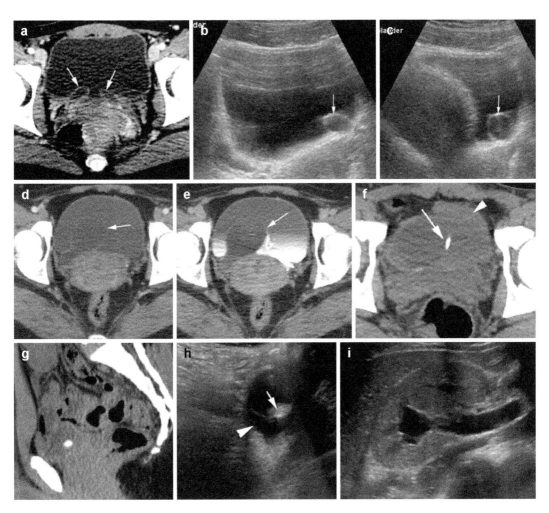

Fig. 14.68 Ureterocele in four patients. Axial CT (**a**) shows saccular outpouching of distal ureter within the bladder bilaterally (*arrows*). (**b**, **c**) Ultrasound of the bladder shows ureterocele on left side (*arrow*). (**d**, **e**) Axial postcontrast arterial and delayed-phase CT show outpouching of the right ureter into the bladder (*arrow*). (**f**) Axial and (**g**) sagittal reformatted images show stone in ureterocele (*arrow*). The bladder is partially seen (*arrowhead*). Ultrasound of the same patient (**h**) shows ureterocele with stone (*arrow*) with surrounding bladder (*arrowhead*). (**i**) Ultrasound of the right kidney shows hydronephrosis

Diseases of the Digestive Tract

15

Contents

R. Agarwala, *Atlas of Emergency Radiology:*
Vascular System, Chest, Abdomen and Pelvis, and Reproductive System,
DOI 10.1007/978-3-319-13042-2_15, © Springer International Publishing Switzerland 2015

Esophageal Lesions

Mechanical Obstruction

Diagnosis
Achalasia

Imaging Features
1. Dilated atonic esophagus filled with fluid and debris
2. Lack of normal peristalsis
3. Incomplete relaxation of the lower esophageal sphincter
4. Bird-beak sign

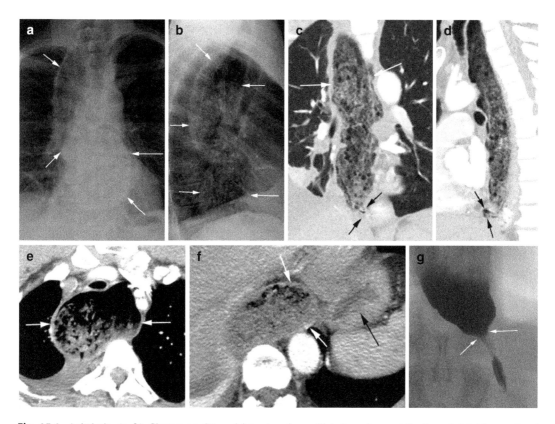

Fig. 15.1 Achalasia. (**a**, **b**) Chest x-ray PA and lateral views show debris-filled dilated esophagus (*arrows*). CT (**c**) coronal and (**d**) sagittal reformatted images show dilated debris-filled esophagus (*white arrows*) and narrowing at the GE junction (*black arrows*). Axial CT (**e**) shows dilated esophagus at the thoracic inlet (*arrows*) and (**f**) at the GE junction (*white arrows*) with collapse of the stomach (*black arrows*). (**g**) Barium swallow study shows bird-beak sign (*arrows*) with normal striation of mucosa at the gastroesophageal junction

Diagnosis
Boerhaave's Syndrome

Imaging Features

1. Periesophageal air collection in the distal esophagus from perforation
2. Gas tracking into the left subphrenic and gastrohepatic spaces

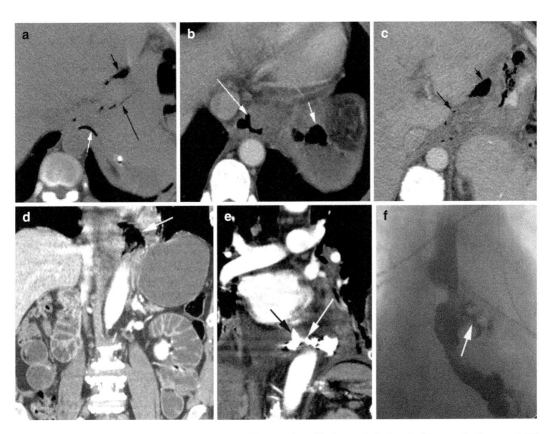

Fig. 15.2 Boerhaave's syndrome. History of vomiting and upper abdominal pain in two patients. Patient 1: CT axial (**a**) noncontrast study shows air tracking from the distal esophagus (*white arrow*), surrounding the GE junction (*long black arrow*), and in the gastrohepatic space (*short black arrow*). (**b**, **c**) Axial CECT shows extraluminal gas around the esophagus (*long white arrow*) and gas in the left subphrenic space (*short white arrow*), around the GE region (*long black arrow*) and gastrohepatic space (*short black arrow*). Patient 2: (**d**) coronal reformatted CT shows collection of gas in the left side of the distal esophagus (*arrow*). The upper abdomen shows small bowel obstruction with dilated loops. (**e**) Coronal reformatted CT shows spillage of enteric contrast in the previous region of gas collection (*arrow*). (**f**) Barium swallow study shows rupture of the esophagus with contrast spillage from the distal esophagus (*arrow*)

Candida Esophagitis

Imaging Features
1. Barium swallow study shows very irregular and shaggy appearance of the esophagus.
2. Ulcerations filled with enteric contrast.
3. CT shows diffusely thick enhancing mucosa and submucosal edema.
4. Gas tracking into the submucosa.

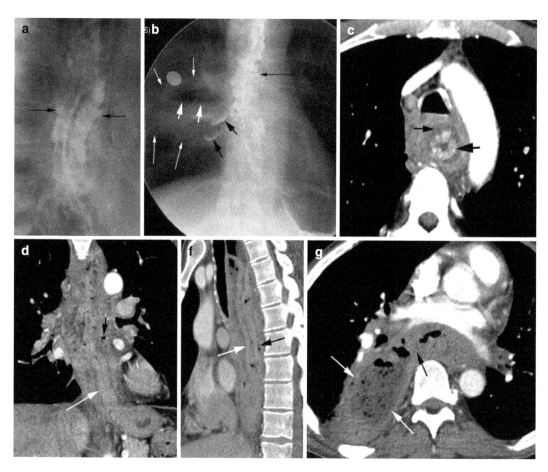

Fig. 15.3 Candida esophagitis. Esophageal swallow study (**a**) shows lobulated contour of the esophageal mucosa from ulceration filled with contrast (*black arrows*). (**b**) Large abscess (*long white arrows*) with air-fluid level (*short white arrows*) in the right perihilar region from the tracheoesophageal fistula and multiple adjacent contrast-filled bronchi (*short black arrows*). (**c**) Axial CECT shows cobblestone appearance of the mucosa (*thick black arrow*) from coalescence of plaques and submucosal edema (*thin black arrow*). (**d**, **e**) Coronal and sagittal reformatted images again show thick mucosa (*white arrow*), submucosal edema, and speckled gas in the wall (*black arrow*) from ulcerations. (**f**) Axial CT shows large abscess in the right paravertebral region (*white arrows*) tracking from the esophagus (*black arrow*)

Malignancies

Diagnosis
Squamous Cell Carcinoma

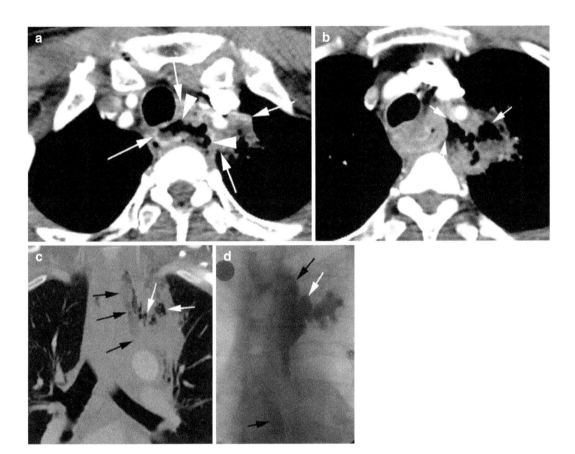

Fig. 15.4 Esophageal squamous cell carcinoma in the superior mediastinum. Axial CECT (**a**) shows a large soft tissue mass around the esophagus in the superior mediastinum extending to the left upper lobe (LUL) (*white arrows*) with irregular mucosal surface (*arrowheads*). (**b**) At a lower level, a large gas collection is seen extending from the esophagus to the mass in the LUL (*arrows*). (**c**) Coronal reformatted image again shows gas tracking from the esophagus (*black arrows*) to mass in the LUL (*white arrows*). (**d**) Esophageal swallow study shows extravasated contrast (*white arrow*) from the esophagus (*black arrow*) into the LUL

Diagnosis
Carcinoma at the Carina with Tracheoesophageal
Fistula

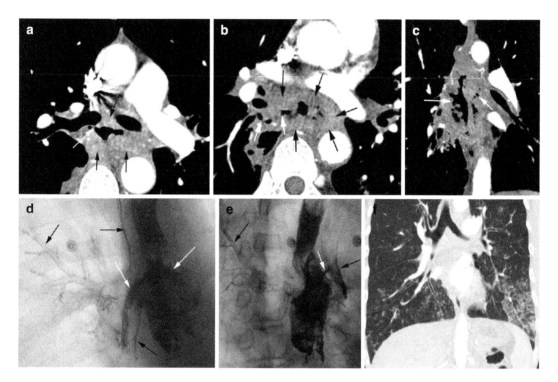

Fig. 15.5 Esophageal carcinoma at the carina with tracheoesophageal fistula. CT axial (**a**, **b**) shows a large soft tissue mass around the esophagus (*black arrows*). Fistula with gas is tracking to the right main stem and lower lobe bronchus (*white arrow*). (**c**) Coronal reformatted CT shows gas tracking on either side of the esophagus (*white arrows*). Esophageal swallow study (**d**, **e**) shows contrast spilling into main stem bronchi bilaterally (*white arrows*) with contrast lining the trachea and right middle lobe and lower lobe bronchi (*black arrows*). (**f**) Coronal reformatted CT of the chest after the swallow study shows aspiration mainly in the lung bases with bronchocentric nodules and ground-glass infiltrates

Diagnosis
Adenocarcinoma with Perforation

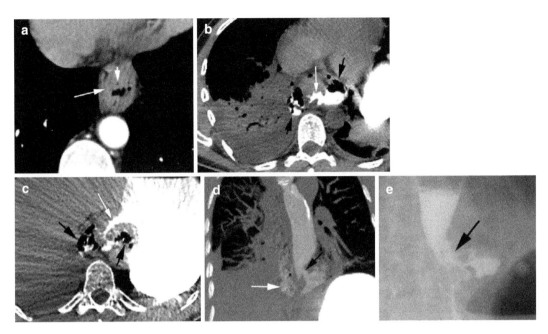

Fig. 15.6 Adenocarcinoma of the distal esophagus with perforation. (**a**) Axial CECT shows wall thickening of the esophagus (*long arrow*) with multiple small perforated gas (*short arrow*) within the tumor. (**b**, **c**) Noncontrast axial CT 1 month later shows irregular narrowing of the esophagus lumen (*white arrow*) and perforation with periesophageal gas and enteric contrast medially and laterally (*black arrows*). (**d**) Coronal reformatted image and esophageal swallow study (**e**) show contrast spillage out of the distal esophagus (*black arrow*). The CT shows gas and contrast tracking up in the mediastinum (*white arrow*)

Diagnosis
Stricture

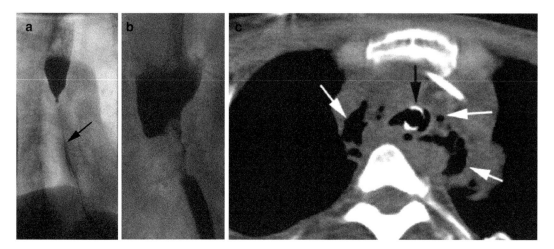

Fig. 15.7 Esophageal stricture of three patients. (**a**) Esophageal swallow study shows smooth long segment of narrowing of the esophagus (*arrow*) from the level of the arch of the aorta. History of lye ingestion. (**b**) Barium swallow study shows a short segment of irregular narrowing of the esophagus from squamous cell carcinoma.

(**c**) Axial CT shows perforation of the esophagus in the superior mediastinum with extraluminal gas (*white arrows*). Endotracheal tube in the trachea (*black arrow*). History of cocaine swallow with odynophagia. Endoscopic examination showed stricture from squamous cell carcinoma

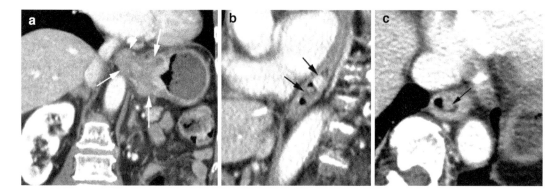

Fig. 15.8 Adenocarcinoma at the gastroesophageal junction as polypoid growth within the esophageal lumen. CECT coronal reformatted image (**a**) shows a large mass

at the GE junction (*arrows*). Sagittal reformatted (**b**) and axial images (**c**) show two small polypoid protrusions within the esophageal lumen (*arrows*)

Diagnosis
Leiomyosarcoma

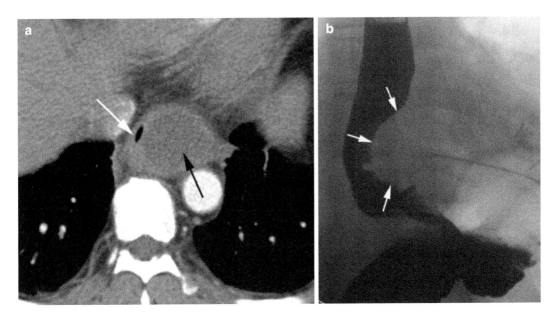

Fig. 15.9 Leiomyosarcoma of the esophagus, biopsy proven. Axial CT (**a**) image shows a large low-density intramural mass in the lower esophagus (*black arrow*) causing extrinsic compression of the esophageal lumen (*white arrow*). (**b**) Barium swallow study shows extrinsic compression of the distal esophagus by mass (*white arrows*)

Non-malignant Bowel Lesions

Mechanical Bowel Obstruction

Diagnosis
Organoaxial Gastric Volvulus

Imaging Features
1. The stomach has herniated through esophageal hiatus.
2. Twisting of the stomach along its long axis with the greater curvature superiorly positioned.

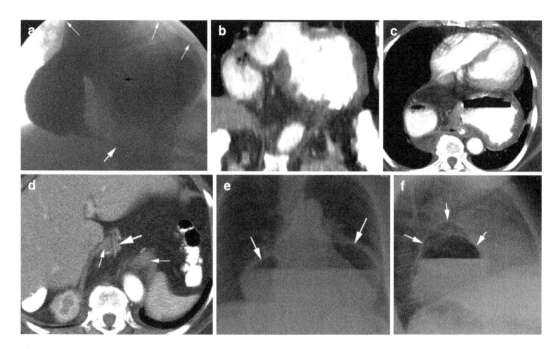

Fig. 15.10 Organoaxial volvulus. (**a**) Barium swallow study shows dilated stomach in the mediastinum with the greater curvature superiorly positioned (*thin white arrows*). Small amount of enteric contrast in the duodenum (*thick white arrow*). Nasogastric tube is seen in the distal esophagus (*black arrow*). (**b**) CT coronal reformatted image shows a similar position of the stomach as in the swallow study. (**c**) Axial CT shows nasogastric tube in the distal esophagus (*arrow*) with the twisted stomach anterior to it. (**d**) Axial CT shows the two ends of the diaphragm (*thin white arrows*) of the wide esophageal hiatus and duodenum (*thick white arrow*) entering the abdomen. (**e, f**) Chest x-ray PA and lateral views show large hiatus hernia in the posterior mediastinum (*arrows*)

Diagnosis
Mesenteroaxial Volvulus

Imaging Features
1. Transverse folding of the stomach with its distal end herniating through the hiatus into the thorax.
2. The fundus of the stomach and gastroesophageal junction is below the diaphragm.

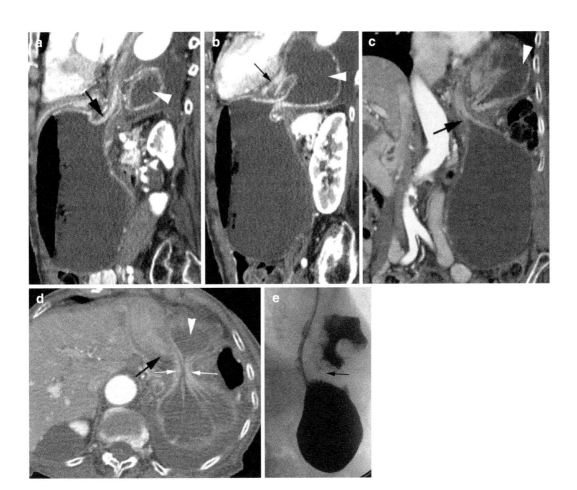

Fig. 15.11 Mesenteroaxial volvulus. CT sagittal (**a**, **b**) and coronal (**c**) reformatted images and axial (**d**) images show the fundus of the stomach with the GE junction (*thick black arrow*) below the diaphragm. The distal end of the stomach (*arrowhead*) has herniated through the narrow esophageal hiatus (*thin white arrows* in **d**) into the thorax. The duodenum is seen doubling back into the abdomen (*thin black arrow* **b**). (**e**) Barium swallow study again shows nasogastric tube entering the stomach below the diaphragm with the distal body of the stomach above the diaphragm and is constricted at the hiatus (*arrow*)

Diagnosis

Sigmoid Volvulus

Imaging Features

1. Redundant sigmoid colon
2. Coffee bean sign in supine radiograph
3. Proximal and distal ends twist in the pelvis, bird-beak sign

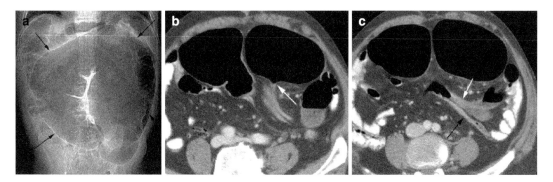

Fig. 15.12 Sigmoid volvulus. (**a**) Supine radiograph shows the coffee bean sign of the sigmoid volvulus (*arrows*). Axial CT (**b**) shows the beak of the twisted end of the sigmoid loop (*arrow*) and (**c**) shows the two collapsed ends that twist (*arrows*)

Diagnosis
Cecal Volvulus

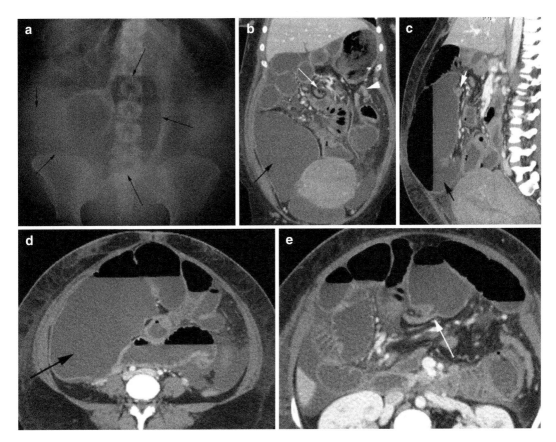

Fig. 15.13 Cecal volvulus. (**a**) Supine radiograph shows markedly a dilated cecum (*arrows*) in the lower abdomen with dilated small bowel loops. CT (**b**) coronal and (**c**) sagittal reformatted images show a markedly distended cecum (*black arrow*), ascending colon, and small bowel loops. The distal ascending colon is seen to be constricted due to twisting (*white arrow*), and the rest of the colon is collapsed (*arrowhead*). Axial CT (**d**) shows a markedly dilated right colon (*arrow*), and (**e**) shows the transition end which is collapsed with bird-beak sign (*arrow*). Patchy necrosis was seen in the cecum at surgery and the small bowel mesentery was found not to be tethered to the retroperitoneum

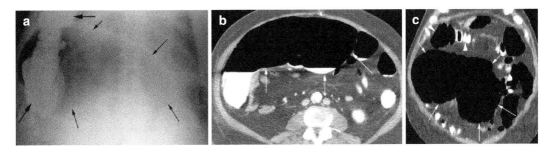

Fig. 15.14 Cecal bascule. (**a**) Supine AP radiograph of the abdomen shows dilated cecum (*thin arrows*) which is displaced medially. Barium enema contrast is seen in the distal right colon (*thick arrows*). CT (**b**) axial and (**c**) coronal reformatted images again show the dilated cecum folded and medially displaced (*white arrows*). The rest of the colon (*arrowheads*) is not dilated

Diagnosis
Transverse Colon Volvulus

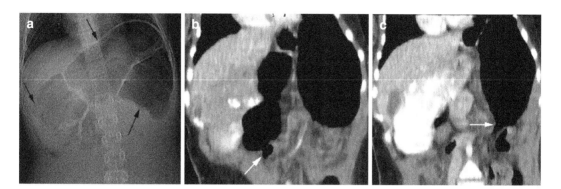

Fig. 15.15 Volvulus of the transverse colon. (**a**) Supine radiograph of the abdomen shows dilatation of the transverse colon (*arrows*). CT (**b**, **c**) coronal reformatted images show dilated transverse colon with narrowing at the hepatic and splenic flexures (*arrows*). At surgery, the transverse mesocolon was seen to be absent which was repaired. Patient had intermittent upper abdominal pain from folding of the transverse colon over the fixed points of the hepatic and splenic flexures

Diagnosis
Small Bowel Volvulus

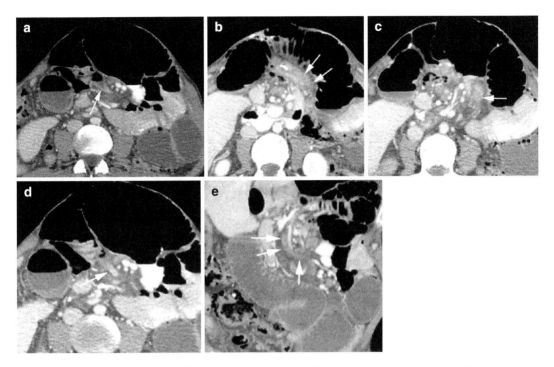

Fig. 15.16 Small bowel volvulus. CT axial (**a–d**) and coronal reformatted (**e**) shows twisting (*arrows*) of a loop of the small bowel around the superior mesenteric vessels with dilatation of the loops proximally. The twisting loop is constricted

Closed-Loop Obstruction

Diagnosis
Small Bowel Closed-Loop Obstruction

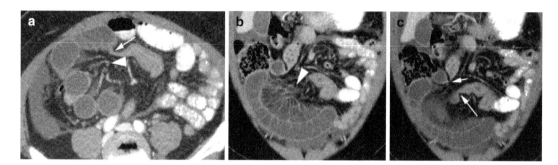

Fig. 15.17 Closed-loop small bowel obstruction from adhesion by a piece of the omentum. CT (**a**) axial and (**b**) coronal reformatted images show dilated loops of the small bowel in the right abdomen with the mesenteric blood vessels converging to a point (*arrowhead*).

A transition point is seen (*thin white arrow*). (**c**) Coronal reformatted image at a different plane shows the two constricted ends of the closed-loop small bowel obstruction (*short and long arrows*)

Diagnosis
Large Bowel Closed-Loop Obstruction

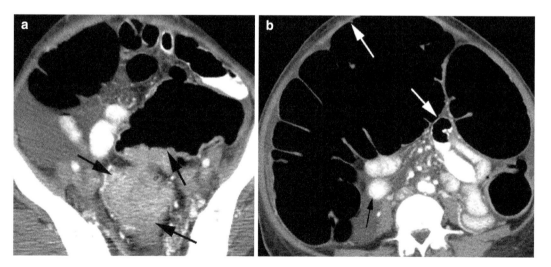

Fig. 15.18 Closed-loop obstruction of the colon by tumor and a competent ileocecal valve. Axial CT (**a**) shows a large mass obstructing the distal sigmoid colon. (**b**) The cecum which is medially deviated is dilated

(*white arrows*) more than 12 cm due to a competent ileocecal valve. The small bowel loops are of normal caliber (*black arrow*)

Diagnosis
Afferent Loop Syndrome

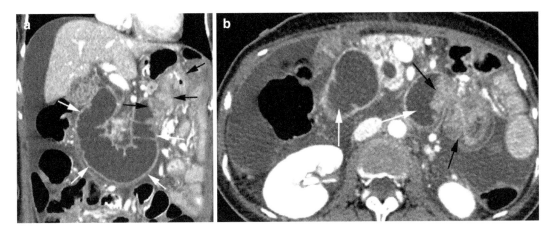

Fig. 15.19 Afferent loop syndrome. History of gastric carcinoma with Billroth II anastomosis. CT (**a**) coronal reformatted and axial (**b**) images show dilated fluid-filled duodenum (*white arrows*). The anastomosis site of the duodenojejunal junction is obstructed by enhancing soft tissue mass due to tumor recurrence (*black arrows*)

Hernia

Diagnosis
Left Paraduodenal Internal Hernia

Imaging Features
1. Encapsulated group of small bowel loops.
2. Located between the stomach and pancreas.
3. Mesenteric vessels supplying the herniated bowel loops are crowded and stretched within the hernia and constricted at the neck of the hernia.

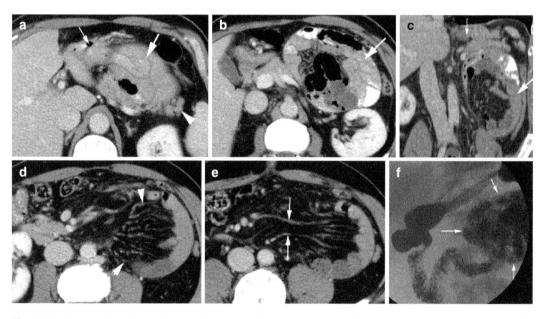

Fig. 15.20 Paraduodenal internal hernia. CT axial (**a**, **b**) and coronal reformatted images (**c**) show a cluster of the small bowel in the shape of a cocoon (*thick white arrow*) between the stomach (*thin white arrow*) and pancreas (*arrowhead*). Axial CT (**d**) shows crowding of the mesenteric vessels to the herniated loops (*arrowheads*). (**e**) The vessels at the neck of the hernia are stretched and constricted (*arrow*). (**f**) Barium swallow study shows clustered small bowel loops adjacent to the duodenojejunal junction (*arrows*)

Diagnosis
Internal Herniation into the Pelvis

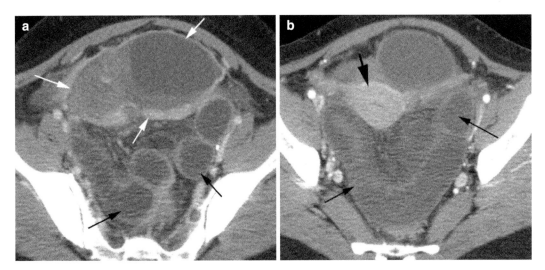

Fig. 15.21 Internal herniation into the pelvis. Axial CT (**a**, **b**) shows a large hemorrhagic ovarian cyst (*white arrows*) with dilated obstructed small bowel loops (*black arrows*) posterior to the uterus (*thick black arrow*). At surgery, the hemorrhagic cyst was adherent to the sigmoid colon and the sigmoid mesentery, and the small bowel had herniated through an opening in the adhesion

Diagnosis
Inguinoscrotal Hernia

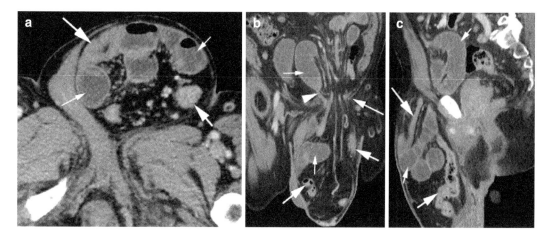

Fig. 15.22 Scrotal herniation of the small bowel with obstruction. CT axial (**a**), coronal (**b**), and sagittal (**c**) reformatted images show herniation of the small and large bowel loops through the left inguinal ring into the scrotum with obstruction of a small bowel loop (*arrowhead*) at the inguinal ring (*long thin arrow*). The herniated colon (*short thick arrow*) and some small bowel loops (*long white arrow*) are collapsed. The obstructed small bowel loops are dilated (*thin arrow*) in the hernia and in the abdomen

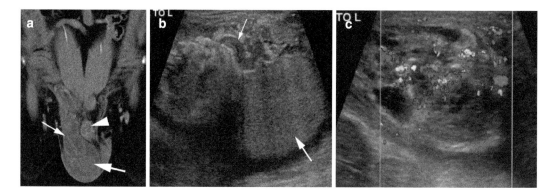

Fig. 15.23 Bowel herniation into the scrotum with no obstruction. (**a**) CT coronal reformatted image shows bowel loops in the right inguinal canal (*thin arrow*) extending to the scrotum up to the Testis (*thick arrow*) on the right side of the penis (*arrowhead*). (**b**) Grayscale ultrasound image shows fluid-filled bowel loops (*thin arrow*) anterior to the testes (*thick arrow*). (**c**) Color Doppler shows patency of the mesenteric vessels

Diagnosis
Incisional Hernia with Infarction

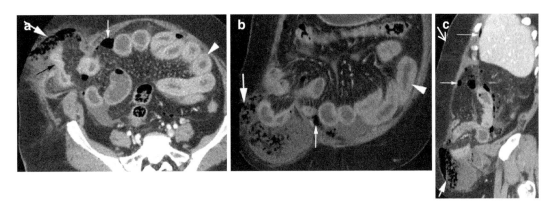

Fig. 15.24 Incisional hernia with infarction. CT axial (**a**), coronal (**b**), and sagittal (**c**) reformatted images show herniation of small bowel loops (*black arrow*) through right abdominal wall defect. The herniated loop is collapsed due to perforation but shows enhancement indicating that arterial supply is patent. Gas collection is seen in the herniated sac (*thick white arrow*) which is spilling into the peritoneal cavity (*thin white arrow*). Acute ischemic changes with wall thickening are seen in some intra-abdominal small bowel loops (*arrowhead*) and with mesenteric vascular engorgement

Diagnosis
Obstructed Abdominal Wall Hernia

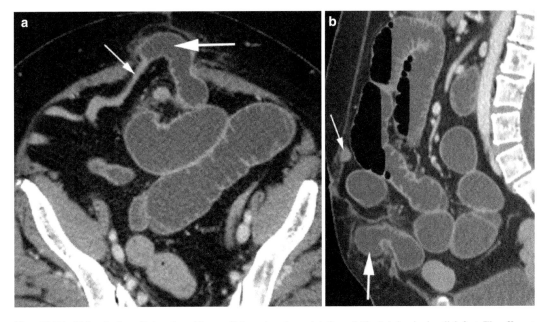

Fig. 15.25 Abdominal wall hernia with small bowel obstruction. CT axial (**a**) and sagittal reformatted (**b**) images show obstruction of herniated small bowel loop through infraumbilical abdominal wall defect. The afferent loop (*thick arrow*) is dilated with collapse of the efferent loop (*thin arrow*)

Diagnosis

Richter Hernia

Imaging Features

1. Herniation of the antimesenteric wall of a bowel loop through the anterior abdominal wall.
2. Does not cause bowel obstruction.
3. It can become necrotic and can perforate.

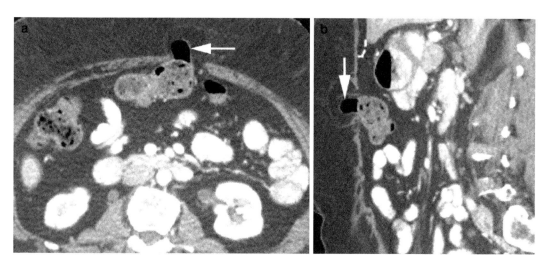

Fig. 15.26 Richter hernia. CT axial (**a**) sagittal reformatted (**b**) images show protrusion of the antimesenteric wall of the transverse colon (*arrow*) through anterior abdominal wall defect

Bowel Stricture

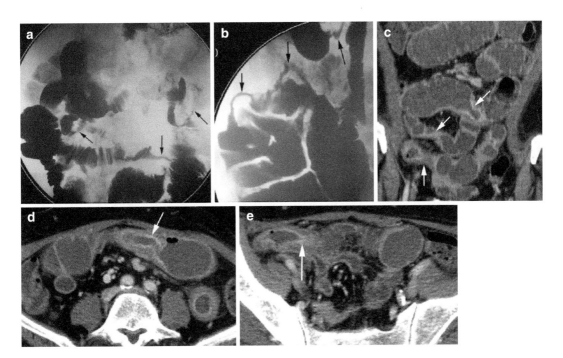

Fig. 15.27 Small bowel obstruction from multiple strictures. A patient with cytomegalovirus enteritis had balloon enteroscopy which showed multiple ulcers and strictures in the jejunum. Barium swallow study (**a**, **b**) shows multiple strictures in small bowel loops (*arrows*). CT coronal reformatted (**c**) and axial views (**d**, **e**) show small bowel obstruction with multiple focal strictures with wall thickening (*arrows*) at stricture sites

Intussusception

Diagnosis
Rectosigmoid Intussusception

Imaging Features

1. Multilayered or bowel within bowel appearance of affected bowel loop.
2. The intussusceptum with its surrounding blood vessels and mesenteric fat is surrounded by the intussuscipiens.
3. May or may not have lead points.

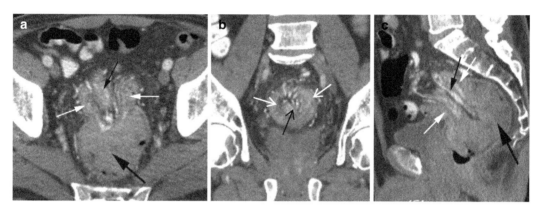

Fig. 15.28 Rectosigmoid intussusception with adenocarcinoma of the rectum as the lead point. CT axial (**a**), coronal (**b**), and sagittal (**c**) reformatted images show a large solid mass (*thick black arrow*) dragging the intussusceptum with its surrounding vessels and fatty tissue (*black arrow*) through the intussuscipiens (*white arrows*)

Diagnosis
Ileocolic Intussusception

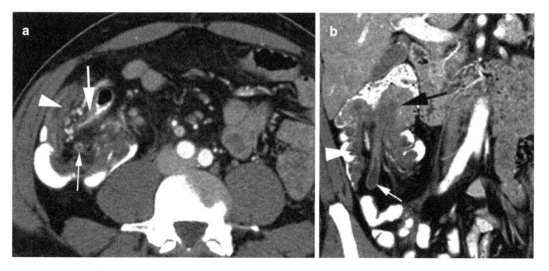

Fig. 15.29 Ileocolic intussusception with tubulovillous adenoma as lead point. CT axial (**a**) shows intussusceptum composed of the terminal ileum (*thick white arrow*), appendix (*thin white arrow*), and surrounding mesenteric vessels and adipose tissue within the cecum (*arrowhead*) which is the intussuscipiens. (**b**) Coronal reformatted image shows soft tissue mass (*black arrow*) at the tip of the intussusceptum with the appendix and mesenteric vessels and fat (*thin white arrow*) behind it and surrounded by the ascending colon as intussuscipiens (*arrowhead*)

Diagnosis
Colocolic Intussusception

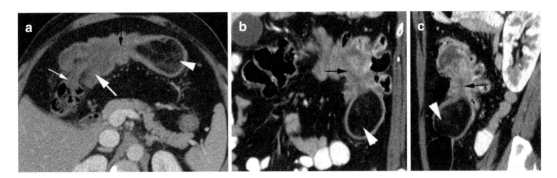

Fig. 15.30 Colocolic intussusception with lipoma as lead point in two patients. CT axial (**a**) view shows the proximal transverse colon as intussusceptum (*thin white arrow*) surrounded by mid-transverse colon as intussuscipiens (*thick white arrow*). The lipoma (*arrowhead*) at the distal end has a long thin pedicle (*black arrow*) traversing the intussuscipiens. CT coronal (**b**) and sagittal (**c**) reformatted views in the second patient show lipoma (*arrowhead*) as the lead point of the intussusceptum with long pedicle (*black arrow*) in the splenic flexure

Diagnosis
Jejunal Intussusception

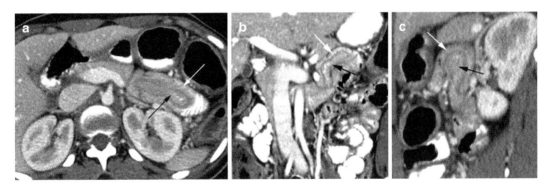

Fig. 15.31 Intussusception of the proximal jejunum with no lead point. CT axial (**a**), coronal (**b**), and sagittal (**c**) reformatted images show the intussusceptum (*black arrow*) surrounded by a halo of adipose tissue within the intussuscipiens (*white arrow*)

Gastric Outlet Obstruction

Imaging Features
1. Distended stomach
2. Collapsed small and large bowel loops

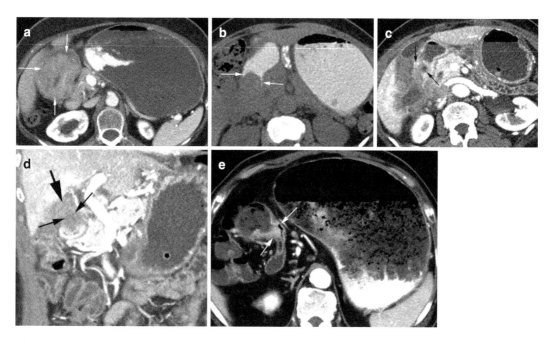

Fig. 15.32 Gastric outlet obstruction in three patients with different causes. Patient 1: (**a**) axial CT shows large enhancing adenocarcinoma at the gastric antrum causing obstruction (*arrows*). Patient 2: (**b**) axial CT with enteric contrast and no IV contrast shows a large filling defect in the proximal duodenum (*arrows*). CECT axial (**c**) and coronal reformatted (**d**) images show enhancing mass obstructing the second part of the duodenal sweep (*thin arrows*) adjacent to liver metastasis (*thick arrow*). Both lesions metastasized from squamous cell cervical cancer. Patient 3: axial CT (**e**) shows sclerosing constriction (*arrows*) of the duodenum from chronic ulcer resulting in gastric outlet obstruction

Small Bowel Feces Sign

Imaging Features

1. Low-grade or subacute small bowel obstruction.

2. Obstructed dilated end shows bubbles of gas within the lumen.
3. Bowel loops collapse beyond this end.

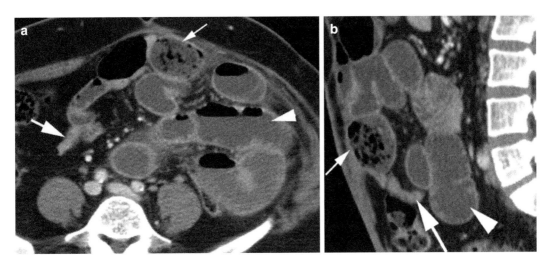

Fig. 15.33 Small bowel obstruction with feces sign. CT axial (**a**) and coronal reformatted (**b**) images show an obstructed loop of the small bowel with a cluster of gas bubbles (*thin arrow*) adherent to the anterior abdominal wall from adhesion. SB loops proximal to this site are dilated (*arrowhead*) and distal loops are collapsed (*thick arrow*)

Diagnosis
Small Bowel Bezoar

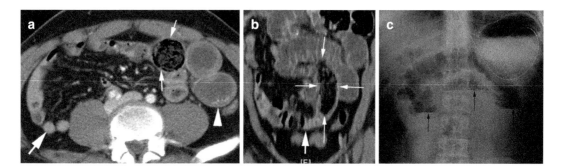

Fig. 15.34 Bezoar with small bowel obstruction. CT axial (**a**) and coronal reformatted (**b**) images show round luminal filling of a mid-small bowel loop with gas collections (*thin arrows*) causing proximal dilated loops (*arrowhead*) and distal collapsed loops (*thick arrow*). (**c**) Upright radiograph shows mid-small bowel obstruction with multiple dilated small bowel loops with air-fluid levels (*arrows*)

Diagnosis
Duodenal Bezoar

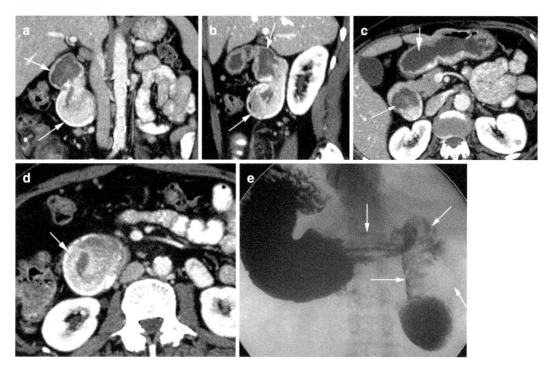

Fig. 15.35 Bezoar duodenum. History of Crohn's disease with stricture at the distal second part of the duodenal sweep and upper abdominal pain. CT (**a**) coronal and (**b**) sagittal reformatted images show dilated first and second parts of the duodenal sweep with intraluminal high- and low-density mass (*arrows*). Axial CT (**c**, **d**) at lower level shows mild gastric outlet obstruction (*thick arrow*) by the mass (*thin arrow*). (**e**) Upper GI study shows irregular filling defect of the antrum to the second part of the duodenal sweep (*arrows*)

Diagnosis
Gastric Bezoar

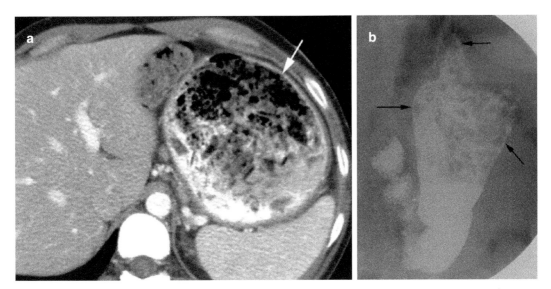

Fig. 15.36 Gastric bezoar. History of peptic ulcers with multiple previous surgeries presents with gastric outlet obstruction. (**a**) Axial CT shows diffuse filling defects within the distended stomach (*arrow*). (**b**) Barium swallow study again shows distended proximal stomach with multiple filling defects (*arrows*). Endoscopic examination showed filling defects to be bezoar

Bowel Ischemia

Diagnosis
Acute Bowel Ischemia

Diagnosis
Pneumatosis Intestinalis

Imaging Features: Depending on Cause
1. Homogeneous or heterogeneous and hypoattenuating or hyperattenuating wall thickening.
2. Bowel dilatation.
3. Bowel wall can be thinned.
4. Mesenteric edema and engorgement of mesenteric veins.
5. Pneumatosis intestinalis.
6. Pneumatosis portalis—gas in mesenteric and portal veins.
7. Pneumoperitoneum and variable free fluid.

Imaging Features
1. Gas in the bowel wall
2. Gas in mesenteric and portal veins

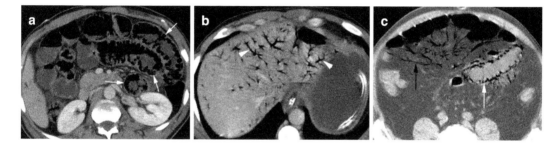

Fig. 15.37 Pneumatosis intestinalis in two patients. Patient 1 with bowel adhesion: (**a**, **b**) axial CT shows diffuse small bowel dilatation with air in the wall of some bowel loops (*white arrows*) and extensive portal gas (*arrowhead*). Patient 2 with atrial fibrillation: (**c**) axial CT shows dilated small bowel loop with air in the wall (*white arrow*) and extensive gas in mesenteric veins (*black arrow*)

Diagnosis
Emphysematous Gastritis

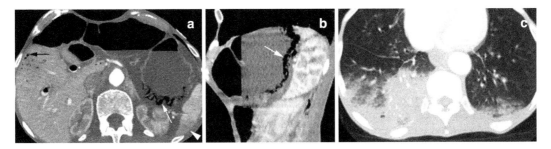

Fig. 15.38 Emphysematous gastritis in a cachectic patient with hypotension, sepsis, and ischemic hepatitis. CT (**a**) axial and (**b**) sagittal reformatted images show gas in the stomach wall (*white arrow*) and gas in the portal veins (*black arrow*). Focal ischemic changes are seen in the spleen (*arrowhead*) and the kidneys show poor perfusion. (**c**) Axial CT of the lung bases shows pneumonia more in the right base

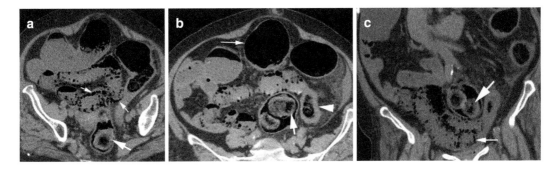

Fig. 15.39 Diffuse bowel ischemia in Alzheimer patient with bloody diarrhea. Noncontrast CT (**a**, **b**) axial and coronal reformatted images show diffuse pneumatosis of distal small bowel loops (*short thin arrows*), dilated ascending and transverse colon (*long thin arrow*), and wall thickening of the left colon (*arrowhead*) with large retained stool (*short thick arrow*) in the distal colon causing obstruction

Diagnosis
SLE Vasculitis

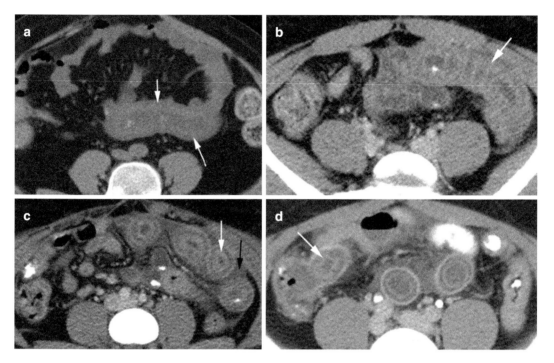

Fig. 15.40 Systemic lupus erythematosus causing bowel ischemia of multiple small bowel loops. Axial CTs (**a**) pre- and (**b**) postcontrast study show wall thickening of mid-small bowel with faint enhancement (*arrows*). (**c, d**) Axial CT shows target sign in the proximal and distal small bowel (*white arrow*) with mesenteric edema (*black arrow*)

Diagnosis
Radiation Enteritis

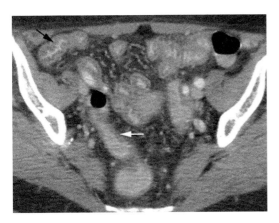

Fig. 15.41 Radiation enteritis in a patient with rectal cancer. Axial CT shows diffuse wall thickening of the distal small bowel (*black arrow*) and rectosigmoid colon (*white arrow*). The mesentery shows vascular congestion

Diagnosis
Shock Bowel

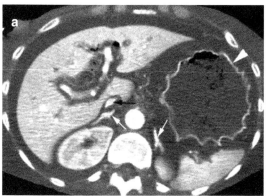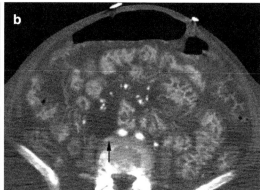

Fig. 15.42 Shock bowel in a patient with septic shock. Postcontrast axial CT (**a**) shows intense mucosal enhancement of the stomach (*arrowhead*), extensive periportal edema, increased enhancement of bilateral adrenal glands (*thin white arrows*), and small IVC (*thin black arrow*). Gas in porta hepatis is in the dilated bile ducts from recent cholecystectomy. (**b**) Lower abdominal axial CT shows diffuse mucosal enhancement of small and large bowel loops, very small slit-like IVC (*black arrow*), and ascites

Diagnosis

Acute Colonic Ischemia

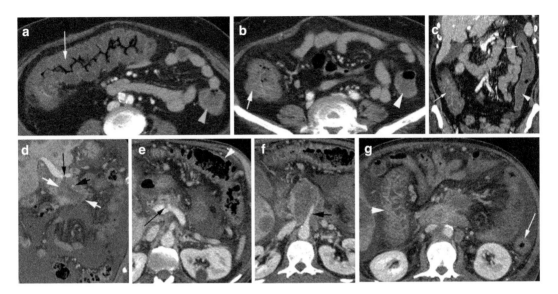

Fig. 15.43 Ischemic colon in two patients. Patient 1: patient had sick sinus syndrome with paroxysmal tachycardia with arterial ischemia in SMA distribution. Axial CECT (**a**, **b**) and coronal reformatted (**c**) images show ischemia of the right and transverse colon up to the splenic flexure (*thin arrows*) with marked wall thickening confirmed at surgery. The transverse colon (*arrow* in **a**) shows increased haustral thickening with poor enhancement. The ascending colon (*thin arrow* in **b**) shows a thick colon with lack of haustra and decreased enhancement. The descending colon is dilated due to ileus (*arrowhead*) but shows no wall thickening and was not ischemic at surgery. Patient 2: pancreatic cancer with SMV thrombus. CECT (**d**) coronal reformatted (**e**) axial images show bland and tumor thrombus (*black arrows*) in the SMV at the confluence above the necrotic pancreatic mass (*white arrow*). The SMA (*short black arrow* in **d**, **f**) is encased by tumor but patent. (**f**, **g**) Axial CT shows wall thickening and enhancement of the ascending and transverse colon up to the splenic flexure (*arrowhead*). The descending colon (*thin white arrow* in **g**) shows no wall thickening

Diagnosis
Cecal Infarction

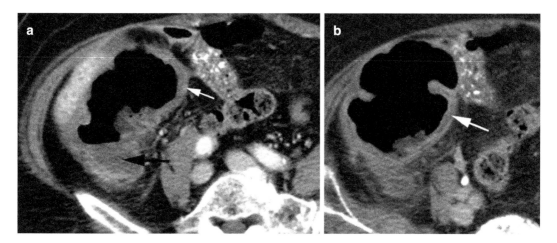

Fig. 15.44 Cecal infarction. History of diabetes, NSAID use, and non-ST segment myocardial infarction. Axial postcontrast CT (**a**, **b**) shows dilatation of the cecal lumen (*black arrow*) with wall thickening (*white arrow*) and no wall enhancement. The cecum was resected

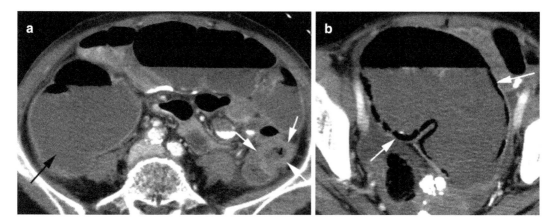

Fig. 15.45 Cecal infarction due to closed-loop obstruction from adenocarcinoma of the left colon and competent ileocecal valve. Axial CT (**a**) shows a constricting mass at the mid-left colon (*white arrows*) and dilatation of the colon proximal to it (*black arrow*). Small bowel loops show no obstruction due to a competent ileocecal valve. (**b**) Axial CT shows the cecum to be markedly dilated with pneumatosis (*white arrows*). The cecum was perforated at surgery

Infection and Inflammation

Diagnosis
Pseudomembranous Colitis

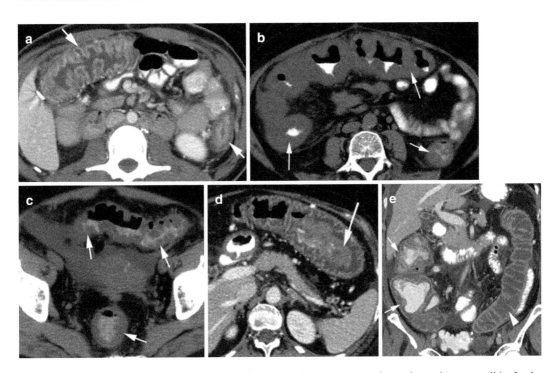

Fig. 15.46 Pseudomembranous colitis in three patients. Axial CT (**a**) shows marked diffuse thickening of the colonic wall. The mucosa shows enhancement and shows pronounced undulation giving the typical accordion appearance (*arrow*). (**b**, **c**) Noncontrast axial CT in a patient with watery diarrhea shows pancolitis with marked wall thickening (*arrows*) and thick haustral folds. Colonoscopy proved pseudomembranous colitis. In the third patient, CECT (**d**) axial image shows target sign at the distal transverse colon. (**e**) Coronal reformatted image shows marked colonic wall thickening (*arrows*) of the ascending colon (*arrows*). The descending colon (*arrowhead*) is very dilated with no wall thickening but with prominent haustra

Diagnosis

Typhlitis or Neutropenic Colitis

Imaging Features

1. Circumferential wall thickening and distension mainly of the cecum with diffuse hyperemia, edema, superficial ulcers, pericolonic stranding, and fluid
2. Can involve the ascending colon and terminal ileum
3. Can have pneumatosis and pneumoperitoneum

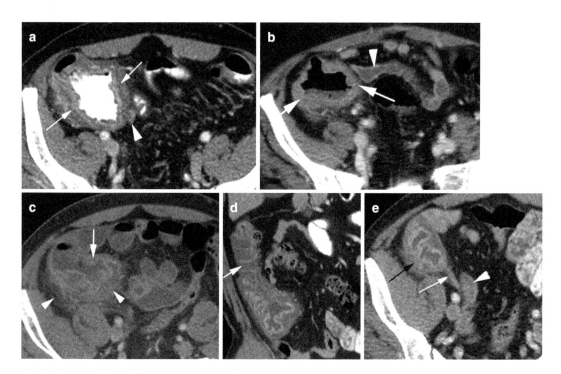

Fig. 15.47 Typhlitis in different patients. Axial CT (**a**) in a patient with acute myeloid leukemia having pancytopenia shows diffuse wall thickening of the cecum (*arrow*). The appendix (*arrowhead*) is of normal size. (**b**) Axial CT in a neutropenic patient with leukemia shows distended thick-walled cecum (*arrows*) and also involvement of the terminal ileum which is mildly dilated (*arrowhead*). (**c**) Axial CT in a neutropenic patient with lower abdominal pain and fever shows dilated thick-walled cecum (*arrow*), surrounding pericolonic edema (*arrowheads*), and dilated surrounding distal small bowel loops. (**d**) Coronal reformatted CT at a later date shows involvement of the ascending colon showing thick wall (*arrow*). (**e**) Axial CT at the same time shows normal appendix (*white arrow*), dilated terminal ileum (*arrowhead*), and thick-walled cecum (*black arrow*) unchanged as seen in other planes

Diagnosis
Diverticulitis of the Cecum

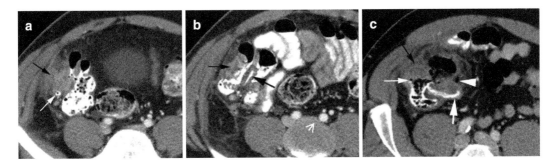

Fig. 15.48 Diverticulitis of the cecum in two patients. Patient 1: axial CT (**a**, **b**) images show diffuse edema around the cecum (*thin black arrow*) and terminal ileum (*thick black arrow*) causing compression of the lumen of both the cecum and terminal ileum. Contrast-filled diverticulum is seen (*white arrow*). (**c**) Patient 2: axial CT shows a deformed cecum from compression by surrounding inflammatory edema. A small diverticulum (*white arrow*) is within the edema. A small extraluminal gas bubble from perforation is seen medially (*white arrowhead*). Reactive edema is seen in the terminal ileum (*thick arrow*)

Diagnosis
Appendicitis

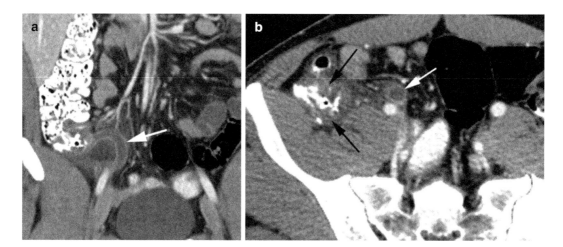

Fig. 15.49 Appendicitis. CT coronal reformatted (**a**) and axial images show dilated appendix with enhancing thick wall (*white arrow also in b*) and surrounding edema. (**b**) Cecal wall is thick (*black arrows*)

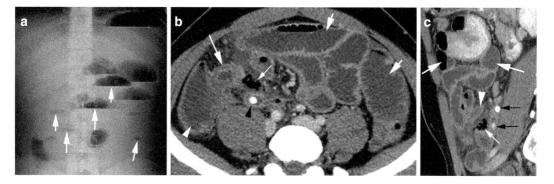

Fig. 15.50 Appendicitis with small bowel obstruction. (**a**) Upright radiograph of the abdomen shows multiple dilated partially fluid-filled small bowel loops with air-fluid levels and string-of-pearl sign (*arrows*). (**b**) Axial CT shows thick appendicitis with stone in it (*black arrowhead*) and adjacent extraluminal air from perforation of the appendix (*thin white arrow*). The terminal ileum shows edematous wall thickening (*long thick white arrow*). The cecum (*arrowhead*) and the small bowel loops are dilated (*thick short arrows*). (**c**) Sagittal reformatted CT shows diffuse dilated small bowels, some with air-fluid levels (*thick arrows*). Also seen are two stones in the appendix (*black arrows*) and perforated gas (*thin white arrow*) and wall edema of the narrow terminal ileum (*arrowhead*)

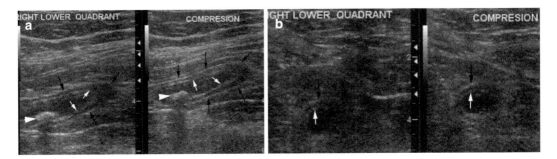

Fig. 15.51 Appendicitis by ultrasound. (**a**) Longitudinal and (**b**) transverse views. The appendix is seen as a long tube with wall edema and with fluid between the two echogenic walls (*black-white arrows*) and echogenic stone (*arrowhead*) with echo shadowing and lack of compression

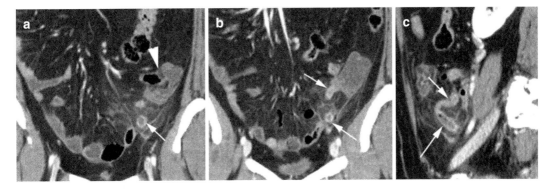

Fig. 15.52 Bowel malrotation with appendicitis. CT (**a**, **b**) coronal and (**c**) sagittal reformatted images show the cecum and terminal ileum (*arrowhead*) in the left lower quadrant of the abdomen with the inflamed appendix originating from the tip of the cecum (*arrows*) surrounded by edema

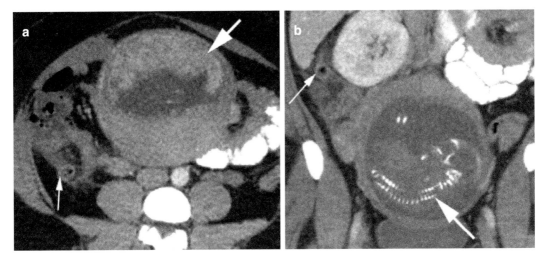

Fig. 15.53 Appendicitis with pregnancy. (**a**) Axial CT shows inflamed appendix with surrounding edema (*thin arrow*) and enlarged uterus with placenta (*thick arrow*). (**b**) Coronal reformatted image shows inflamed appendix in the subhepatic space with surrounding edema (*thin arrow*) and intrauterine gestation (*thick arrow*)

Diagnosis
Ileocecal TB

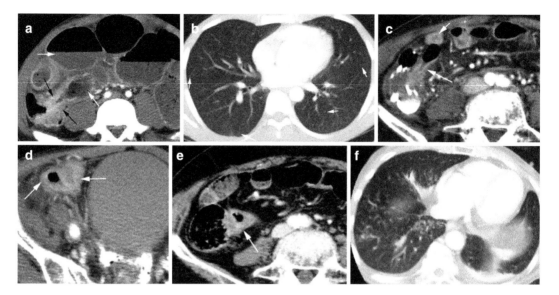

Fig. 15.54 Tuberculosis ileocecal region in two patients. Patient 1: axial CT (**a**, **b**) images show marked stenosis of the ileocecal region, thick enhancing walls (*black arrows*), and with prestenotic dilatation (*white arrows*) of the SB. The lung bases show bilateral miliary TB nodules. Patient 2: axial CT (**c**, **d**) shows wall thickening with hyperemia of the terminal ileum to the ileocecal region (*arrows*) with no bowel obstruction. (**e**) Axial CT a few months later shows that the TI and ileocecal valve show increased wall thickening (*arrow*) and increased hyperemia. (**f**) Axial CT of the lung bases shows TB with centrilobular nodules

Diagnosis
Crohn's Ileitis

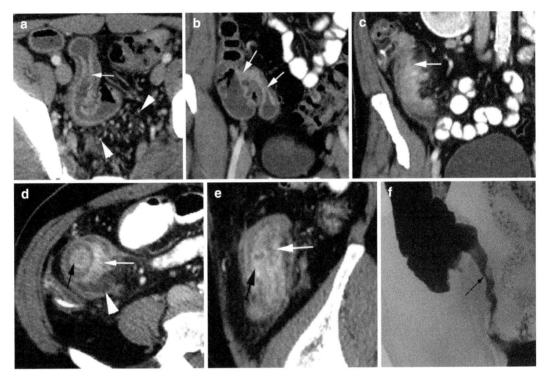

Fig. 15.55 Crohn's disease at the terminal ileum in two patients. Patient 1: CT (**a**) axial and (**b**) coronal reformatted images show stratified thickening of the terminal ileum wall with prominent mucosal thickening (*white arrows*) and prominent vasa recta (*arrowhead*). Patient 2: CT coronal (**c**), axial (**d**), and sagittal (**e**) images show mucosal thickening (*black arrow*), diffuse thickening of the muscularis layer (*white arrow*), and edema of the submucosa between the two layers and with inflammatory changes extending to the surrounding mesentery of the terminal ileum (*arrowhead*) and with no obstructive signs. (**f**) Barium swallow study shows irregular narrowing of the terminal ileum (*black arrow*)

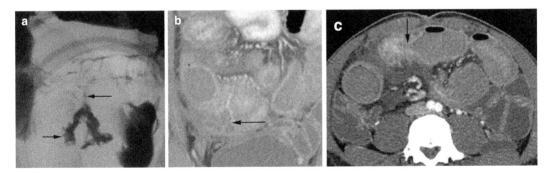

Fig. 15.56 Crohn's terminal ileum with sinus tract. (**a**) The small bowel follow-through study shows a blind sinus tract from the terminal ileum (*arrows*). (**b**) Coronal reformatted CT also shows the same sinus tract (*arrow*). (**c**) Axial CT shows narrowing of the thick-walled terminal ileum and prestenotic obstruction (*arrow*)

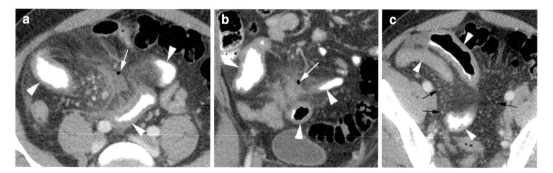

Fig. 15.57 Crohn's distal small bowel with perforation. CT (**a**) axial and (**b**) coronal reformatted images show small gas collection and edema in the distal small bowel mesentery (*thin arrow*) surrounded by thick-walled stiff loops of the small bowel (*arrowheads*). (**c**) Axial CT at the lower level shows very rigid thick-walled small bowel loops (*arrowheads*) with dilated vasa recta (*black arrows*)

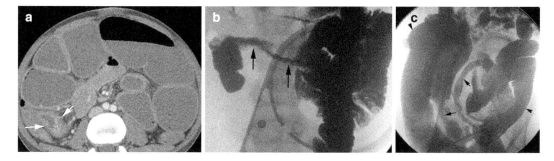

Fig. 15.58 Crohn's stricture with obstruction. (**a**) Axial CT shows wall thickening and narrowing of the terminal ileum (*arrows*). (**b**) Barium swallow study shows long segment of narrowing of the terminal ileum, the string sign (*arrows*). (**c**) Barium swallow study shows two strictures of the distal small bowel (*black arrows*) with dilatation of the obstructed small bowel between the strictures (*arrowheads*)

Diagnosis
Crohn's Colitis

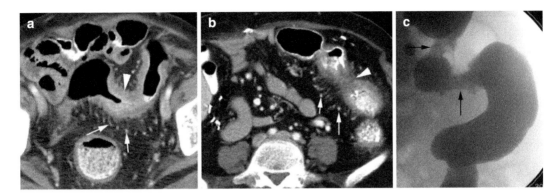

Fig. 15.59 Crohn's colitis. CT axial (**a**, **b**) shows multiple focal thick-walled strictures in the descending and sigmoid colon (*arrowheads*) and dilated vasa recta (*arrows*). (**c**) Barium enema study on a different patient shows two areas of stricture in the distal descending colon (*arrows*)

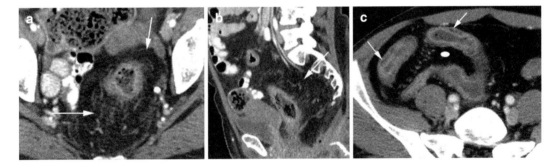

Fig. 15.60 Crohn's disease with fibrofatty proliferation and fat halo sign. (**a**, **b**) Axial and sagittal reformatted CTs show a thick-walled sigmoid colon surrounded by fatty tissue which is slightly heterogeneous in attenuation (*arrow*). (**c**) Axial CT shows chronic Crohn's disease with thick-walled distal small bowel loops with fat halo sign with fatty tissue in the submucosa (*arrows*). The stiff loops are also separated by fatty tissue (*ellipse*)

Diagnosis
Ulcerative Colitis

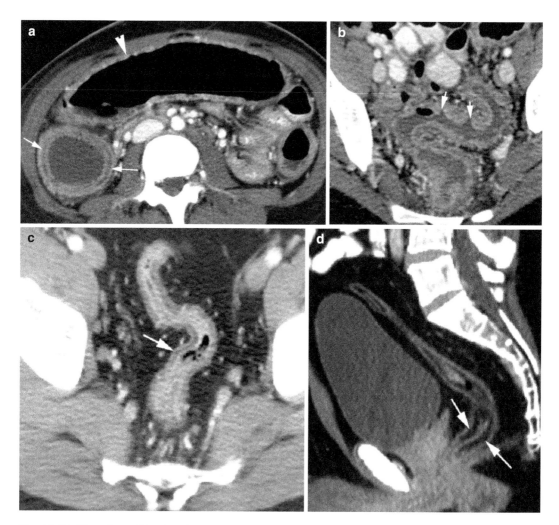

Fig. 15.61 Ulcerative colitis. CT of different patients with pancolitis. (**a**) Axial CT image shows wall thickening with mural stratification (*arrow*) of the right colon with fluid in the submucosa. The transverse and left colon is dilated and with lack of haustra (*arrowhead*). (**b**) Axial CT image shows mucosal thickening of the fluid-filled sigmoid and rectum with ulcerations (*arrows*). (**c**, **d**) Axial and sagittal reformatted images in two patients show low-density mural stratification with fatty tissue, the fat halo sign (*arrows*)

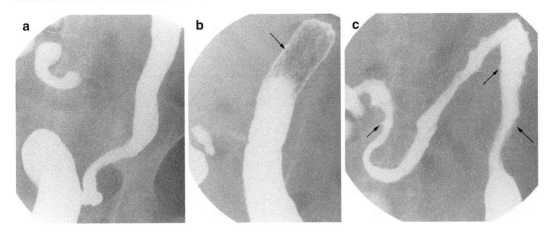

Fig. 15.62 Ulcerative colitis by barium enema study. (**a**) Ahaustral shortening of the left colon. (**b**) Granular mucosa (*arrow*). (**c**) Multiple ulcers mostly in the splenic flexure (*arrows*)

Diagnosis

Perforated Small Bowel Diverticulitis

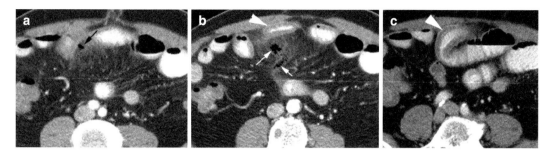

Fig. 15.63 Small bowel diverticulitis with perforation. Axial CT (**a–c**) shows focal diverticulum with gas (*black arrow*) in the wall of a small bowel loop and edema in the adjacent mesentery. Perforation of the diverticulum with spillage of gas into the adjacent edematous mesentery (*white arrows*) is seen adjacent to the diverticulum. Edema of the small bowel wall is seen surrounding the perforation (*arrowheads*)

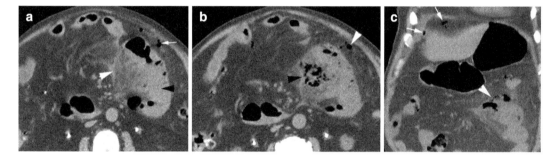

Fig. 15.64 Small bowel diverticulitis rupture. CT axial (**a**) shows marked thickening of a jejunal loop (*black arrowhead*) with edema of the adjacent mesentery (*white arrowhead*) and extraluminal gas pockets laterally (*arrow*). (**b**) Axial CT at the lower level shows spillage of gas into the mesentery (*black arrowhead*) and also laterally (*white arrowhead*). (**c**) Coronal reformatted image shows the site of perforation (*arrowhead*) from the jejunum and free gas in the peritoneal cavity (*arrows*)

Fig. 15.66 Diverticulitis of the left colon with abscess. CT axial (**a**) shows abscess in the sigmoid mesocolon with enhancing margins and gas pockets. The sigmoid colon is edematous and extrinsically compressed by the abscess. In a different patient, (**b**) axial, (**c**) coronal, (**d, e**) and sagittal reformatted images show thick-walled left colon (*black arrows*) with abscess (*white arrows*) extending from the wall into the adipose tissue medially. Secondary epiploic appendagitis is also seen (*arrowheads*)

Diagnosis
Perforated Sigmoid Diverticulitis

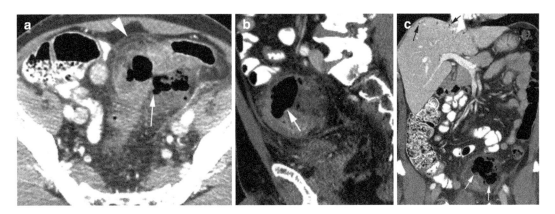

Fig. 15.65 Sigmoid diverticulitis perforation with portal gas. CT axial (**a**), sagittal (**b**), and coronal reformatted images show rupture of sigmoid diverticula into the sig-moid mesocolon (*thin white arrow*) with surrounding edema (*arrowhead*) and portal gas (*thin black arrows*)

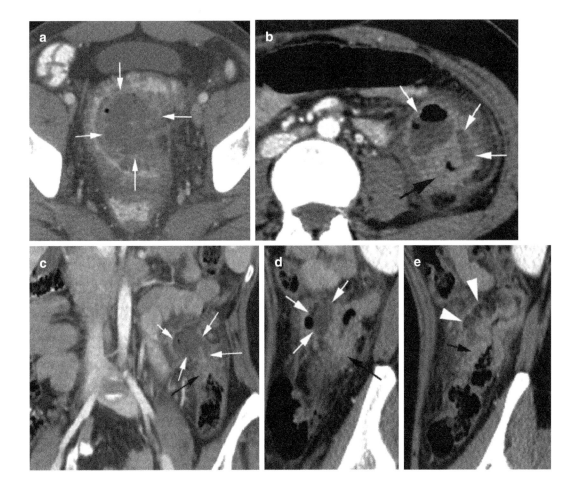

Diagnosis
Diverticulitis of the Ascending Colon

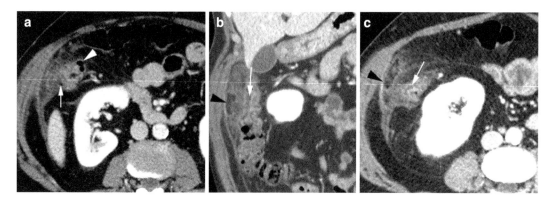

Fig. 15.67 Diverticulitis of the ascending colon and omental infarction. Axial CT (**a**) shows wall thickening at the distal right colon with fat stranding involving the lateral border surrounding an inflamed diverticulum (*arrow*). Diverticula without inflammation are seen medially (*arrowhead*). (**b**) Coronal reformatted image and (**c**) axial CT at the lower level show omental infarction (*arrowhead*) as elliptical low-density focus with central high-density and peripheral high-attenuating halo which is discontinuous with the colon. Edema of the omentum is causing extrinsic compression of the colon which also shows wall edema as submucosal low attenuation (*white arrow*)

Fistula

Diagnosis
Colovesical Fistula

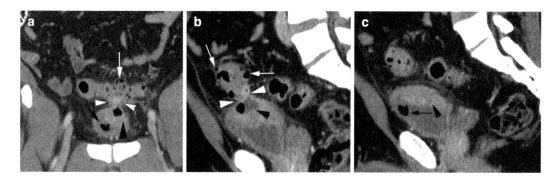

Fig. 15.68 Chronic diverticulitis with colovesical fistula. CT coronal (**a**) and sagittal (**b**, **c**) reformatted images show multiple diverticula in the sigmoid colon (*white arrow*). A thick fistulous tract (*white arrowheads*) is extending from the colon to the thick-walled bladder (*black arrowhead*) with gas in the lumen of the bladder (*black arrow*)

Diagnosis
Colouterine Fistula

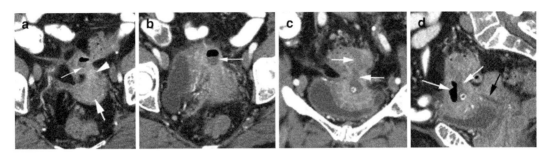

Fig. 15.69 Chronic diverticulitis with colouterine fistula. CT axial (**a**) shows chronic diverticulitis of the sigmoid colon with a pocket of gas and fluid collection (*thin arrow*) tethered to the fundus of the uterus (*thick arrow*) by thick tissue (*arrowhead*). (**b**) At the lower level, it shows the same fluid and gas within the fundus of the uterus (*arrow*). (**c**) Coronal and (**d**) sagittal reformatted images show fluid and gas tracking within the fundus of the anteverted uterus (*arrows*). Small fluid is also seen in the endometrial canal (*black arrow*)

Diagnosis
Cervical Cancer with Colonic Fistula

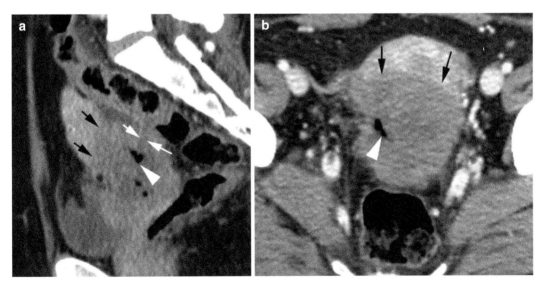

Fig. 15.70 Cervical cancer with colonic fistula. History of vaginal bleeding and lower abdominal pain in a 38-year-old patient. CT (**a**) sagittal reformatted and (**b**) axial images show a low-density mass in the cervix with extrinsic pressure to the rest of the uterus (*black arrows*). Fistulous connection is seen between the sigmoid colon and the mass (*white arrows*) with gas pockets in the mass (*arrowhead*)

Diagnosis
Coloenteric Fistula

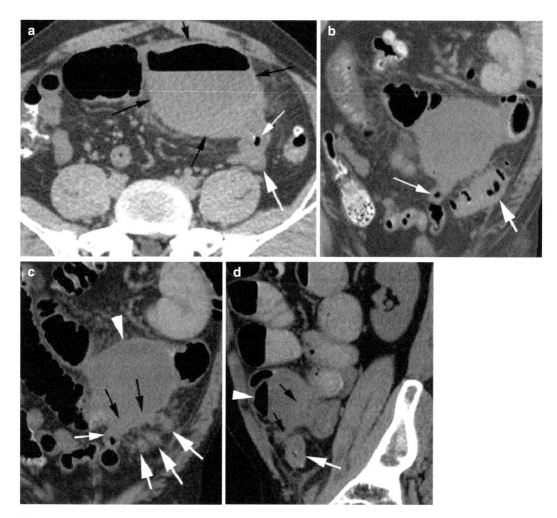

Fig. 15.71 Diverticulitis with coloenteric fistula. Noncontrast CT (**a**) axial image shows the sigmoid colon (*thick arrow*) adherent to the small bowel (*thin arrow*) with a large abscess (*thin black arrows*) in the small bowel mesentery. (**b**) Coronal reformatted image shows multiple diverticula in the sigmoid colon (*thick arrow*) lateral to the small bowel loop (*thin arrow*). (**c**) Coronal reformatted image at anterior plane to (**b**) and (**d**) sagittal reformatted images show a minimally higher attenuated tract (*black arrows*) connecting the sigmoid colon (*thick arrows*) to the small bowel (*thin arrow*) with anterior abscess (*white arrowhead*). At surgery, the small bowel was seen to be jejunum

Diagnosis
Colourachal Fistula

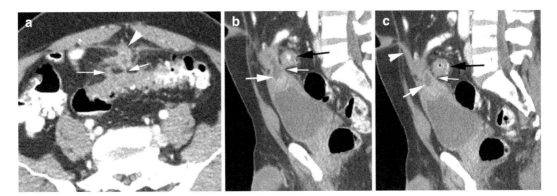

Fig. 15.72 Diverticulitis with colourachal fistula. CT (**a**) axial and (**b**, **c**) sagittal reformatted images at different levels show multiple diverticula in the sigmoid colon (*black arrow*) with two fistula tracts (*thin white arrows*) extending into the urachus (*arrowhead*). Small abscess (*thick white arrow*) is seen within the urachus which is continuous with the urinary bladder and communicating with the umbilicus (*arrowhead*)

Peptic Ulcer

Diagnosis
Gastric Ulcer

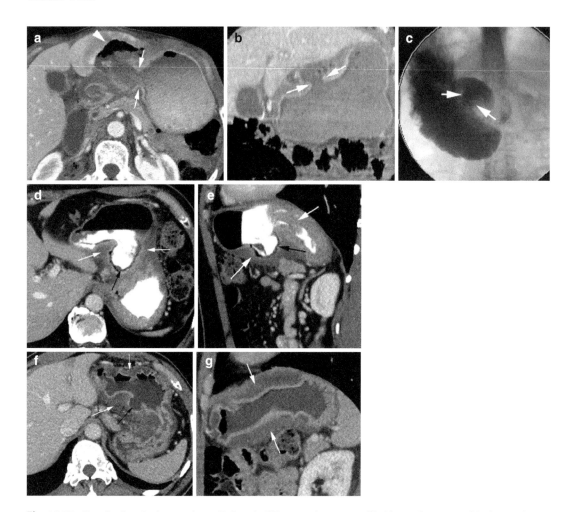

Fig. 15.73 Gastric ulcer in three patients. Patient 1: CT axial (**a**) and coronal reformatted (**b**) images and barium swallow (**c**) show a benign gastric ulcer at the lesser curvature of the stomach with ulcer collar (*white arrows*) abutting the left liver lobe (*arrowhead*). Patient 2: CT axial (**d**) and sagittal reformatted (**e**) images show positive enteric contrast-filled large ulcer crater (*black arrow*) projecting posteriorly with the surrounding gastric wall edema (*white arrows*). Patient 3: CT axial (**f**) and sagittal reformatted (**g**) images show diffuse edema of the stomach (*white arrows*) with fluid-filled ulcer crater (*black arrow*) at the lesser curvature

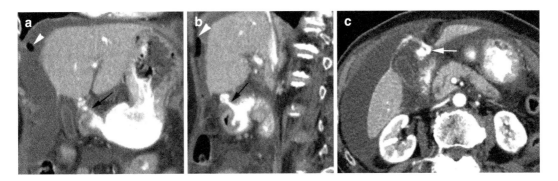

Fig. 15.74 Perforated gastric ulcer. CT coronal (**a**) and sagittal (**b**) reformatted and axial (**c**) images show contrast leaking out from a perforated gastric ulcer at the antrum (*arrow*) with pneumoperitoneum (*arrowhead*) and ascites

Diagnosis
Duodenal Ulcer

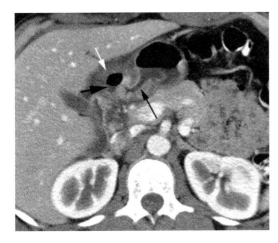

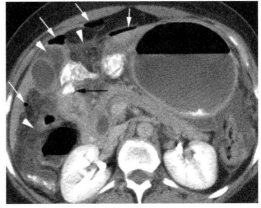

Fig. 15.75 Duodenal ulcer. Axial CT shows fluid and gas within the ulcer crater (*thick black arrow*) at the duodenal bulb and with surrounding edematous soft tissue (*white arrow*). The gastric antrum shows reactive wall thickening and narrow lumen (*thin black arrow*)

Fig. 15.76 Duodenal ulcer perforation. Axial CT shows large contrast-filled duodenal ulcer at the posterior wall of the first part of the duodenum (*black arrow*) with pneumoperitoneum (*white arrow*) and edema surrounding the duodenum, gallbladder, and right and left colon (*arrowheads*)

Neoplasm

Gastric Malignancy

Diagnosis
Malignant Gastric Ulcer

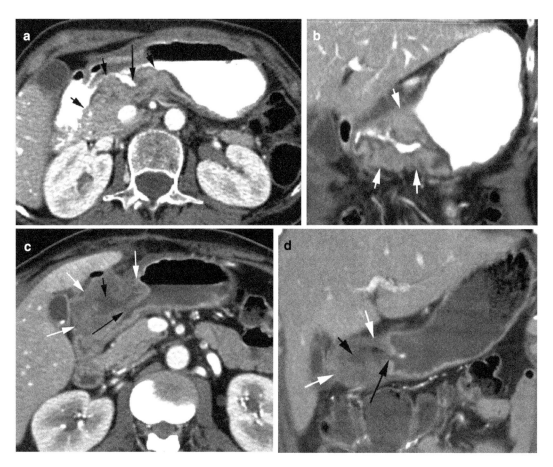

Fig. 15.77 Malignant gastric ulcer in two patients. CT in patient 1: axial (**a**) and coronal reformatted images (**b**) show contrast-filled ulcer crater (*long arrow*) surrounded by enhancing thick soft tissue mass (*short arrows*) causing extrinsic compression of the gastric lumen. Patient 2: axial (**c**) and coronal reformatted (**d**) images show thick soft tissue-enhancing mass (*short white arrows*) with central ulcer crater (*short black arrow*) communicating with the lumen of the stomach (*long black arrow*)

Diagnosis

Adenocarcinoma

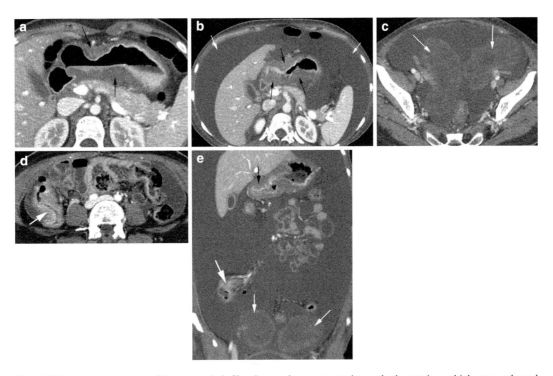

Fig. 15.78 Adenocarcinoma of the stomach, infiltrative, with drop metastasis. CT (**a**) axial image shows diffuse infiltrative mildly enhancing mass narrowing the gastric lumen (*arrows*). Axial CT (**b**) at a later date shows diffuse ascites (*white arrows*). The stomach again shows the infiltrating mildly enhancing mass narrowing of the lumen (*black arrows*). Axial CT through (**c**) the pelvis shows drop metastasis to both ovaries which are enlarged (*arrow*). (**d**) CT through the lower abdomen shows metastasis to the colon (*arrow*) showing a thick enhancing wall and lumen narrowing. (**e**) Coronal reformatted image shows metastasis to the colon (*thick arrow*) and ovaries (*thin white arrow*) and the gastric mass (*black arrow*) and large ascites

Diagnosis

Adenocarcinoma of the Stomach and Duodenum

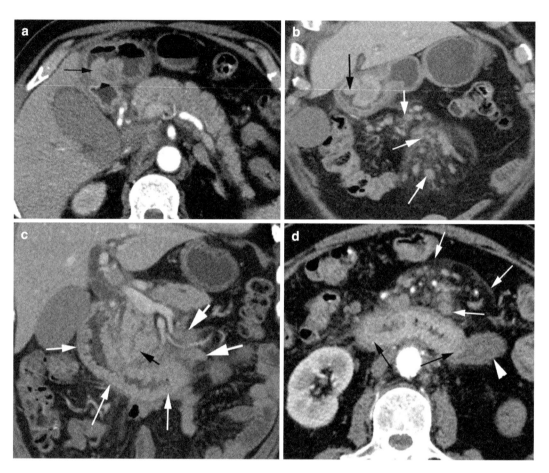

Fig. 15.79 Adenocarcinoma of the stomach and duodenum, polypoid and infiltrative. CT (**a**) axial and coronal reformatted (**b**) images show polypoid growth within the antrum of the stomach (*black arrow*). Small bowel mesentery shows edema and enlarged lymph nodes (*white arrows*). (**c**) Coronal reformatted image shows diffuse wall thickening and enhancement of the duodenal sweep up to the third part (*white arrows*). The small bowel mesentery with lymphadenopathy (*thick white arrows*) is lateral to the head of the pancreas (*black arrow*). (**d**) Axial image shows infiltrating mass of the duodenum (*black arrows*) with normal mucosa of the fourth part of the duodenum (*arrowhead*). The mesentery again shows edema with lymphadenopathy (*white arrows*)

Periampullary Mass

Diagnosis
Adenocarcinoma of the Head of the Pancreas

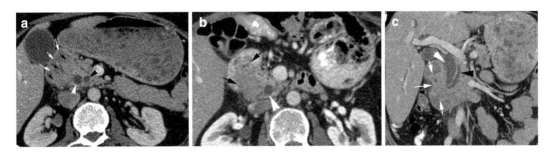

Fig. 15.80 Periampullary mass, adenocarcinoma of the head of the pancreas. CT axial (**a**) and (**b**) post-Whipple procedure show a low-density mass (*black arrows*) at the second part of the duodenal sweep surrounded by fluid in the obstructed duodenum (*white arrows*). The obstructed CBD (*white arrowhead*) and pancreatic duct (*black arrowhead*) are dilated. (**c**) Coronal reformatted image again shows pancreatic mass completely filling the second part of the duodenum (*thin white arrows*). The CBD (*white arrowhead*) and pancreatic ducts (*black arrowhead*) are dilated

Diagnosis
Carcinoid Duodenum

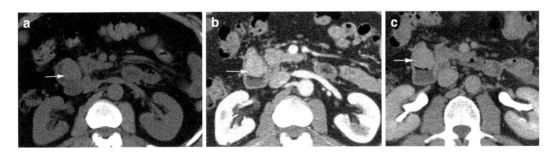

Fig. 15.81 Periampullary mass, carcinoid duodenum. CT axial (**a**) noncontrast study shows high-density polypoid mass in the second part of the duodenal sweep (*arrow*). (**b**) Portal venous phase shows good enhancement and (**c**) delayed phase shows decrease in enhancement of the mass

Diagnosis

Colon Cancer Metastasis to the Duodenum

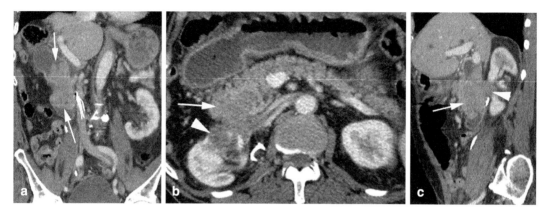

Fig. 15.82 Periampullary metastatic mass from right colon cancer. Coronal reformatted CECT (**a**) Large mass in the second part of the duodenal sweep (*arrows*). (**b**) Axial and (**c**) coronal reformatted CTs show the mass (*arrow*) to extend posteriorly to involve the right kidney (*arrowhead*)

Linitis Plastica

Fig. 15.83 Linitis plastica. Axial CT abdomen shows diffuse infiltrative adenocarcinoma of the stomach at stage T4N1 with diffuse wall thickening (*thick arrows*) of a rigid stomach. Gastric mucosa shows good enhancement (*thin arrow*). The mass is infiltrating posteriorly with lymphadenopathy around the aorta

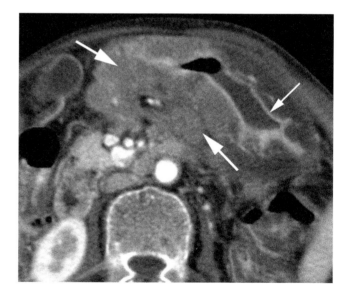

GI Lymphoma

Diagnosis
Gastric Lymphoma

Imaging Features
1. Marked gastric wall thickening with submucosal spread
2. Uncommon to cause gastric outlet obstruction or infiltrate perigastric fat
3. Usually homogeneous but may have areas of necrosis
4. Regional or retroperitoneal lymphadenopathy

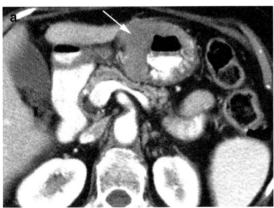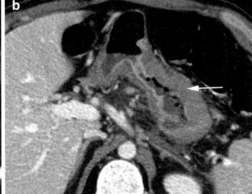

Fig. 15.84 Gastric lymphoma in two patients. Patient 1: (**a**) axial CT shows segmental involvement of the stomach with homogenous tumor mass (*arrow*). Patient 2: (**b**) axial CT shows diffuse involvement with diffuse homogeneous wall thickening (*arrow*) and narrowing of the lumen with linitis plastica appearance

Diagnosis

Small Bowel Lymphoma

Imaging Features

1. Circumferential bulky mass in the intestinal wall, extending to the mesentery and regional lymph nodes.
2. Can show aneurysmal dilatation of the bowel lumen.
3. Involve long segments, may ulcerate and perforate or be focal polypoid mass.
4. Obstruction is uncommon.

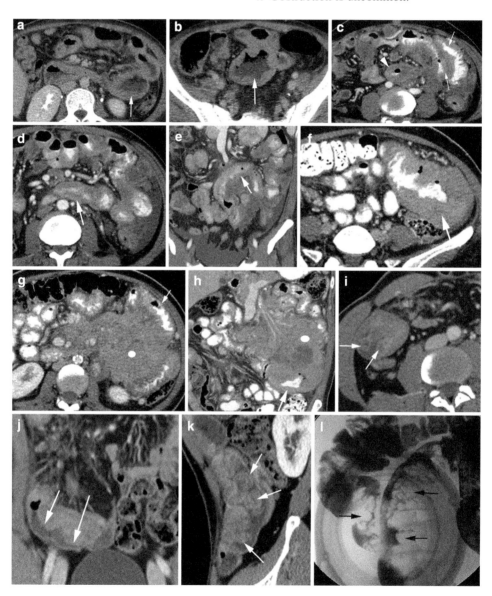

Fig. 15.85 Small bowel lymphoma in four patients. Patient 1: axial CT (**a**, **b**) shows aneurysmal dilatation of some small bowel loops with diffuse wall thickening (*arrow*). Patient 2: CT (**c**, **d**) axial and (**e**) coronal reformatted images show wall thickening of some small bowel loops in the left abdomen; some show symmetrical thickening (*thick arrows*), while some are asymmetrically thickened (*thin arrow*). Patient 3: axial CT (**f**, **g**) and coronal reformatted (**h**) images show large soft tissue mass with necrotic areas in small bowel mesentery (*ellipse*) causing displacement of some small bowel loops (*thin arrow*) and encasing some loops (*thick arrow*). Patient 4: CT axial (**i**), coronal (**j**), and sagittal (**k**) reformatted images and (**l**) barium small bowel study show multiple polypoid nodules in a segment of dilated small bowel (*arrows*)

Diagnosis
Follicular Lymphoma Causing Bowel Obstruction

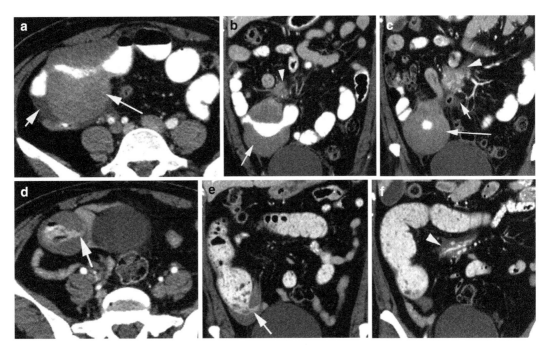

Fig. 15.86 Follicular lymphoma causing bowel obstruction. (**a**) Axial CECT shows a large circumferential low-density mass around a distal small bowel loop (*long arrow*) with small surrounding fluid (*short arrow*). (**b, c**) Coronal reformatted images show infiltration into the small bowel mesentery with lymph node enlargement (*arrowhead*). (**d–f**) CT done 1 year later for abdominal pain shows marked constriction of the SB within the mass (*arrow*), which is smaller in size and with prestenotic dilatation. The mesenteric panniculitis has also decreased (*arrowhead*)

Diagnosis
Large Bowel Lymphoma

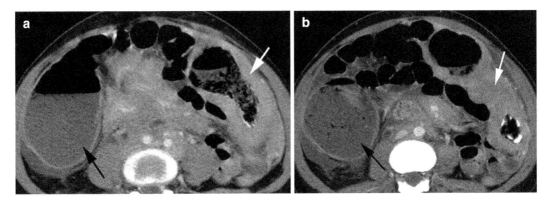

Fig. 15.87 Large bowel lymphoma. Axial CT (**a, b**) shows diffuse circumferential wall thickening of the left colon (*white arrow*) with some obstructive pattern with the dilated right colon (*black arrow*). The mass remained within the confines of the bowel wall

Adenocarcinoma of the Colon

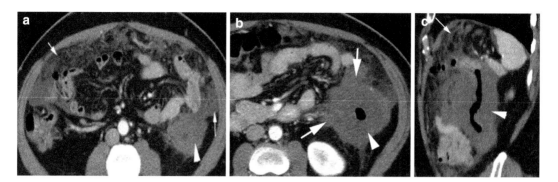

Fig. 15.88 Adenocarcinoma of the descending colon. CT (**a**, **b**) axial images at different levels and (**c**) sagittal reformatted images show marked wall thickening of the left colon (*arrowhead*) with narrowing of the lumen, with focal lobulated extension outside the wall (*thick arrows*), and with omental metastasis (*thin arrows*)

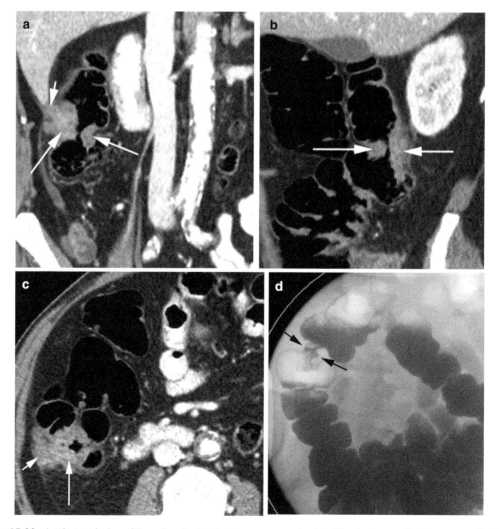

Fig. 15.89 Apple core lesion of the colon. Lesion in the right colon was a tubulovillous adenoma with no carcinomatous change. CT (**a**) coronal and (**b**) sagittal reformatted and (**c**) axial images show circumferential soft tissue mass causing focal luminal narrowing (*long arrows*) of the right colon and extension laterally outside the colon (*short arrow*). (**d**) Barium enema of a different patient shows constriction lesion of the sigmoid by adenocarcinoma

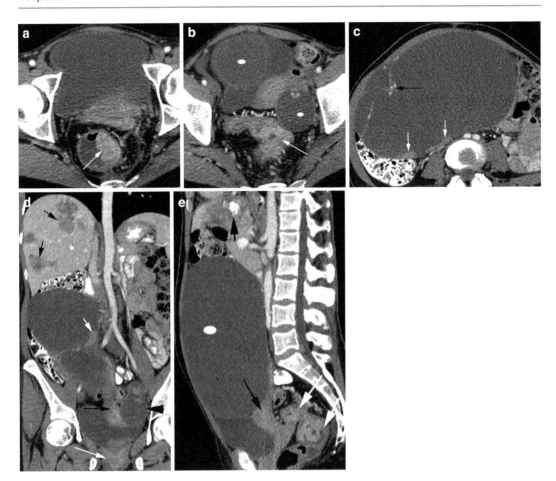

Fig. 15.90 Rectal adenocarcinoma with ovarian and hepatic metastasis. CT (**a**, **b**) axial shows enhancing thick-walled mass of the rectosigmoid colon with polypoid protrusion into the lumen inferiorly (*arrow*). Large cystic masses are seen in both ovaries (*ellipse*). (**c**) Axial CT of mid-abdomen shows the upper extent of large complex cyst in the right ovary with calcification in septations (*black arrow*) and mural nodules (*short white arrows*). (**d**) Coronal and (**e**) sagittal reformatted images show the rectal mass (*white arrows*), uterus (*long black arrow*) and large cyst at the right ovary (*ellipse*), complex cyst at the left ovary (*black arrowhead*) with mural nodules (*short white arrow*), and liver metastasis (*short thin black arrow*) some with calcifications (*thick black arrow*)

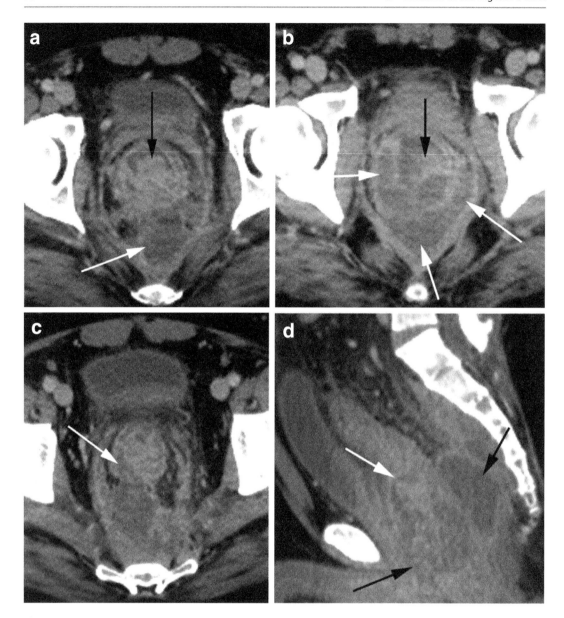

Fig. 15.91 Rectal adenocarcinoma with perirectal abscess. CT axial (**a**, **b**) shows a solid enhancing polypoid mass projecting into the lumen of the rectum (*black arrow*) and perirectal abscess within the puborectal sling (*white arrows*). (**c**) Axial CT shows continuation of abscess within the rectal mass (*white arrow*). (**d**) Sagittal reformatted image shows extension of the abscess from the rectal mass (*white arrow*) collecting around the anus (*black arrows*)

Carcinoid

Diagnosis
Carcinoid Appendix

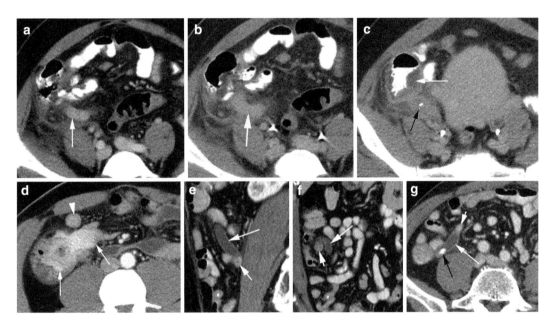

Fig. 15.92 Carcinoid appendix in three patients. Patient 1: (**a**, **b**) axial CT shows uniformly enhancing solid mass filling a long segment of the mid- and distal appendix (*white arrow*) with surrounding edema. (**c**) Axial CT at lower level shows acute appendicitis proximal to the mass with stone, wall thickening (*black arrow*), and edema of the cecum (*white arrow*). Patient 2: axial CT (**d**) shows markedly thickened appendix with avid enhancing mass extending into the cecum (*white arrows*) and metastasis to a lymph node (*arrowhead*). This was stage IV carcinoid. Patient 3: CT (**e**) sagittal and (**f**) coronal reformatted (**g**) axial images show a dilated fluid-filled appendix (*long white arrow*) with proximal stone (*black arrow*). The tip of the appendix shows a small enhancing mass (*short white arrow*)

Diagnosis
Gastric Carcinoid

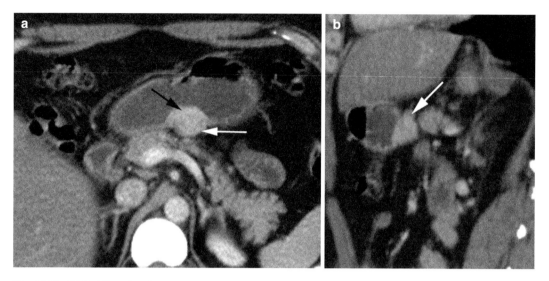

Fig. 15.93   Well-differentiated type 3 gastric neuroendo-crine tumor. Axial CT (**a**) and (**b**) sagittal reformatted images show a focal solid well-defined enhancing mass at the body of the stomach (*black arrow*) with extension pos-teriorly outside the stomach (*white arrow*)

Diagnosis
Carcinoid Duodenum

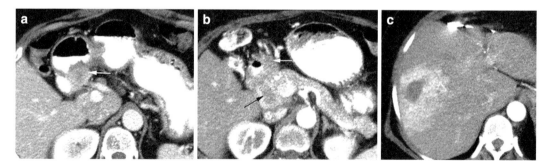

Fig. 15.94   Carcinoid duodenum. Axial CT (**a**) shows an enhancing mass in the medial wall of the duodenal bulb (*white arrow*). (**b**, **c**) A few months later, the mass has extended to the second part of the duodenum (*black arrow*) with metastasis to the liver

Diagnosis

Neuroendocrine Carcinoma of the Cecum

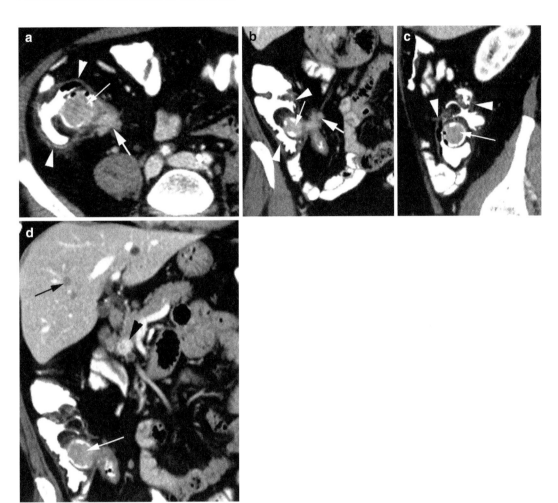

Fig. 15.95 Neuroendocrine carcinoma of the cecum, well differentiated. CT (**a**) axial, (**b**) coronal, and (**c**) sagittal reformatted images show enhancing mass causing filling defect in the contrast-filled cecum and ileocecal valve (*thin arrow also in d*) . Extension of the lesion is seen to the adjacent lymph nodes (*thick arrow*) and the serosal surface of the cecum (*arrowheads*), confirmed at surgery. (**d**) Coronal reformatted image shows distant metastases to the liver (*black arrow*) and mesenteric lymph node (*black arrowhead*)

Appendix Lesions

Diagnosis
Adenocarcinoma

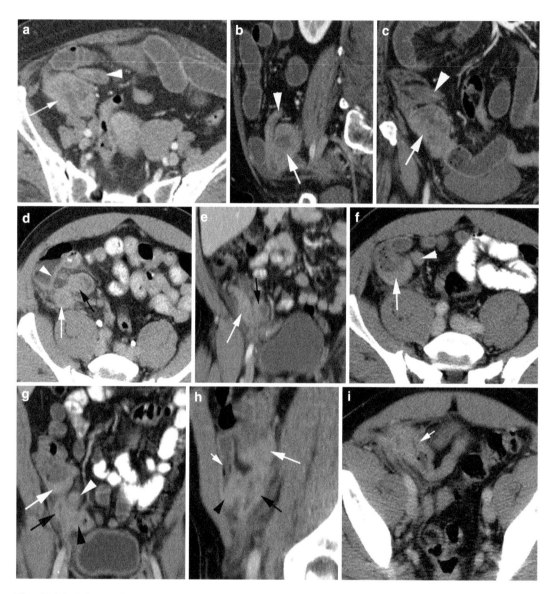

Fig. 15.96 Adenocarcinoma of the appendix in two patients. Patient 1: CT axial (**a**), sagittal (**b**), and coronal (**c**) reformatted images show heterogeneous enhancing mass in the appendix (*thin arrow*). The TI shows tumor infiltration with enhancing wall thickening (*arrowhead*) causing low-grade obstruction with proximal bowel dilatation. Patient 2: axial (**d**) and coronal reformatted CTs (**e**) show enhancing mass in the appendix (*white arrow*) extending to the adjacent ileum (*black arrow*) and thickening of the adjacent cecum (*arrowhead*). (**f**) Axial, (**g**) coronal, and (**h**) sagittal reformatted CTs a few months later show increased thickening of the cecum (*long white arrow*), enlarged lymph nodes (*white arrowhead*), and diffuse thickening of the appendix (*black arrow*) and the ileum adjacent to the appendix (*black arrowhead*). The ileum distal to the lesion shows normal wall thickness (*short white arrow*). (**i**) Axial CT shows focal thick-walled terminal ileum (*short white arrow*). Focal involvement of the ileum was also seen at surgery

Diagnosis
Mucocele

Fig. 15.97 Mucocele of the appendix. CT axial (**a**) and coronal reformatted (**b**) images show markedly dilated fluid-filled appendix (*arrow*) with thin walls and no periappendiceal edema

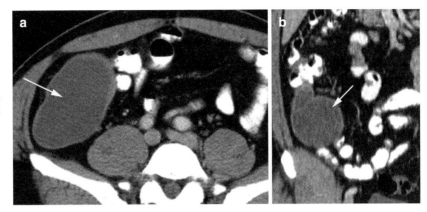

Diagnosis
Mucinous Cystadenoma

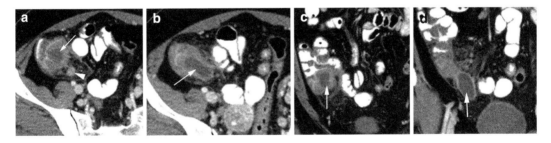

Fig. 15.98 Mucinous cystadenoma of the appendix with superimposed appendicitis. CT axial (**a**, **b**) and coronal (**c**, **d**) reformatted images show a dilated appendix (*long arrow*) with wall thickening proximally, periappendiceal inflammation, and reactive lymph nodes (*arrowhead*). The thick wall has heterogeneous density with areas of poor enhancement. Ulcerations of the appendix were seen at pathology

GIST

Diagnosis
GIST of the Stomach

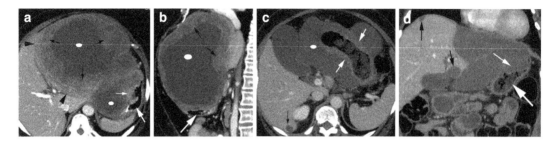

Fig. 15.99 Gastrointestinal stromal tumor of the stomach. CT (**a**) axial and (**b**) sagittal reformatted images show a large mass with central necrosis (*ellipse also in c*) and peripheral enhancing soft tissue (*thin black arrows*) with the large extragastric component in the gastrohepatic space causing extrinsic pressure on the liver with edema of the compressed liver surface (*black arrowheads*). The gas-filled stomach (*thick white arrow*) is also compressed with small intramural component of the tumor at the lesser curvature (*thin white arrow*). (**c**, **d**) CT done at a later date during treatment shows absence of the soft tissue component of the tumor and liver metastasis (*black arrows*). Intramural component (*thin white arrow*) of the stomach (*thick white arrow*) with wall thickening is still seen

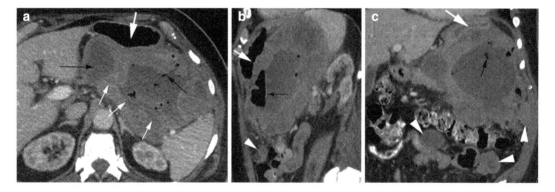

Fig. 15.100 Gastric stromal tumor with fistulization and metastasis. CT axial image shows a large necrotic mass with gas collections (*black arrows*) arising from the stomach and growing posteriorly into the lesser sac between the gas-filled stomach (*thick arrow*) and the pancreas posteriorly (*thin arrows*). Gas was from a fistula within the stomach lumen. Sagittal (**b**) and coronal (**c**) reformatted images show omental metastasis (*arrowheads*)

Diagnosis
GIST of the Duodenum

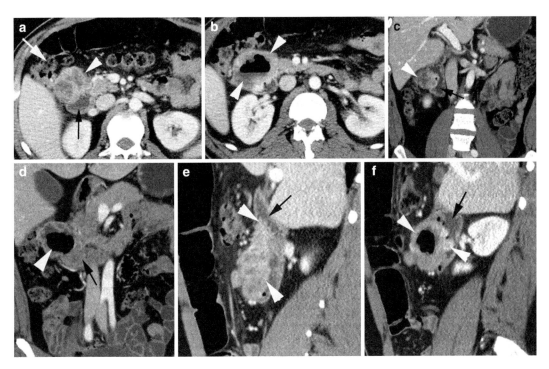

Fig. 15.101 GIST of the duodenum. CECT axial images (**a**, **b**) at different planes show an enhancing mass with central necrosis (*arrowheads*) arising from the second part of the duodenal sweep (*black arrow*) with central gas from fistulization with the duodenal lumen and abutting the hepatic flexure (*white arrow*). (**c**, **d**) Coronal reformatted images at different planes show the necrotic mass (*arrowhead*) with the intramural portion indenting the duodenal lumen (*black arrow*). (**e**, **f**) Sagittal reformatted images at different planes show the solid portion of the mass (*arrowheads*) originating from the duodenum and narrowing the lumen (*black arrow*). The large necrotic central portion shows gas due to fistula formation. The duodenum and hepatic flexure were surgically removed since the mass was adherent to the colon

Diagnosis
GIST of the Small Bowel

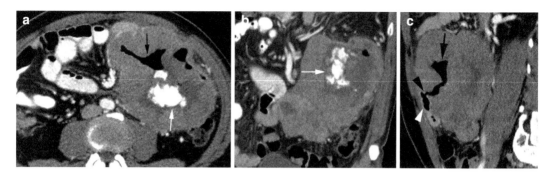

Fig. 15.102 Small bowel stromal tumor. Axial (**a**) and coronal (**b**) and sagittal reformatted (**c**) CTs show sharply demarcated exophytic mass of the small bowel (*white arrowhead* in **c**) with coarse calcification (*white arrow*). Gas in the necrotic center (*black arrow*) is due to fistulization (*black arrowhead*) with the small bowel lumen from which it is arising (best seen in **c**)

Diagnosis
Perirectal GIST

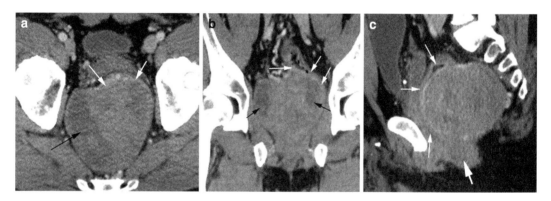

Fig. 15.103 Perirectal stromal tumor. CT (**a**) axial and (**b**) coronal reformatted images show a sharply demarcated solid mass arising from the posterior wall of the rectum (*thin white arrows*) showing peripheral necrosis (*black arrows*). (**c**) Sagittal reformatted image shows the rectum to be displaced anteriorly (*thin white arrows*) but not the anus (*thick white arrow*)

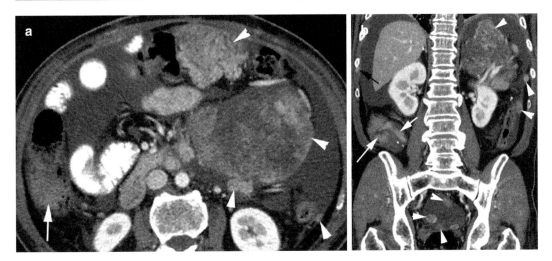

Fig. 15.104 GIST with diffuse metastasis. History of past gastric GIST with resection and chemotherapy. CT (**a**) axial and (**b**) coronal reformatted images show multiple enhancing nodular metastasis to the peritoneum (*arrowheads*), cecum, terminal ileum and ascending colon (*thick arrow*), and right intercostal muscle (*black arrow*)

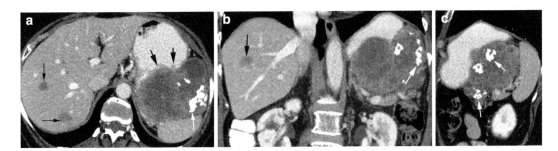

Fig. 15.105 Stromal tumor with calcification. Axial (**a**), coronal (**b**), and (**c**) sagittal reformatted images show a large low-density GIST arising from the stomach (*thick black arrows*), growing into the gastrosplenic ligament, with calcifications (*white arrow*) and liver metastasis (*thin black arrows*)

Peritoneal and Retroperitoneal Diseases

16

Contents

R. Agarwala, *Atlas of Emergency Radiology:*
Vascular System, Chest, Abdomen and Pelvis, and Reproductive System,
DOI 10.1007/978-3-319-13042-2_16, © Springer International Publishing Switzerland 2015

Peritonitis

Diagnosis
Bacterial Peritonitis

Imaging Features
1. Peritoneal fluid collection
2. Enhancement of peritoneum

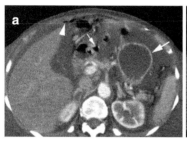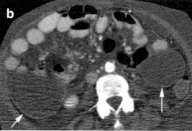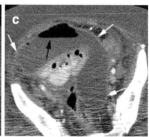

Fig. 16.1 Bacterial peritonitis from ruptured duodenal ulcer. CT axial (**a**) shows small pneumoperitoneum (*arrowhead*) with perforation of the first part of duodenal sweep (*thin white arrow*). The stomach shows ischemic changes with only the mucosa enhancing (*thick arrow*). Fluid is seen in the peritoneal cavity with mild peritoneal enhancement. (**b**, **c**) Later date axial CT shows peritonitis of the mid-abdominal and pelvic peritoneum which now shows increased enhancement and thickening (*white arrows*) with increased intraperitoneal gas collection (*black arrow*)

Diagnosis
Bile Peritonitis

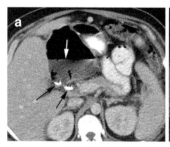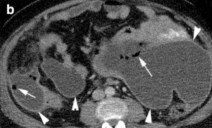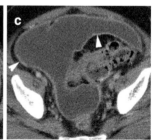

Fig. 16.2 Bile peritonitis with superimposed infection from recent cholecystectomy. Axial CT (**a–c**) images show large amount of ascites with thick enhancing peritoneum (*arrowheads*) and with gas collection (*white arrows*). The gas is predominant in the gastrohepatic space adjacent to the cholecystectomy clips (*black arrows*)

Pneumoperitoneum

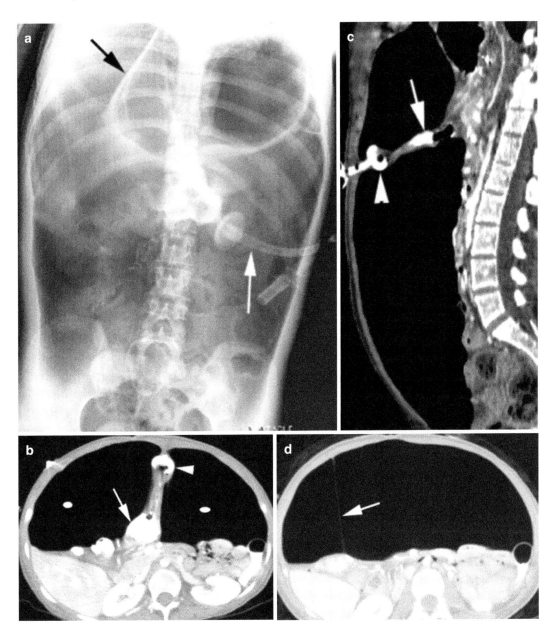

Fig. 16.3 Pneumoperitoneum from gastrocolocutaneous fistula and peritoneal leak from malposition of gastrostomy tube. (**a**) Flat plate of abdomen shows large pneumoperitoneum surrounding the falciform ligament (*black arrow*) and the gastrostomy tube (*white arrow*). CT axial (**b**) and sagittal (**c**) reformatted images show gastrostomy tube (*arrowhead*) connected to the colon (*arrow*). The large peritoneal gas (*ellipse*) is displacing and compressing the bowel loops. (**d**) Axial CT showing falciform ligament (*arrow*) with surrounding pneumoperitoneum

Hemoperitoneum

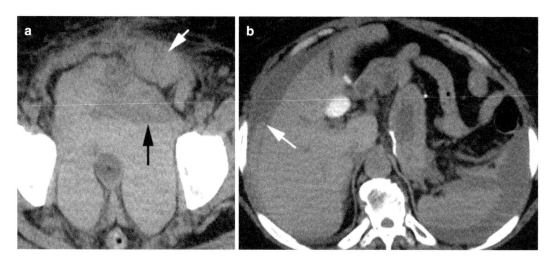

Fig. 16.4 Hemoperitoneum. Patient on Coumadin for PE and high INR had trauma. CT axial (**a**) image shows large hemoperitoneum in posterior cul-de-sac with hematocrit level (*black arrow*). Large hematoma in left rectus abdominis muscle (*white arrow*). Axial CT of upper abdomen (**b**) shows hemoperitoneum with hematocrit level in right subphrenic space (*white arrow*)

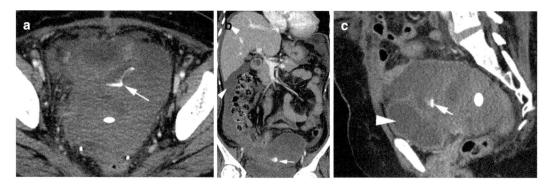

Fig. 16.5 Active arterial bleeding. CT axial (**a**), coronal (**b**), and sagittal (**c**) reformatted images show active extravasation of contrast (*arrow*) from a branch of the internal iliac artery surrounded by high-density lobulated sentinel clot (*ellipse*). The rest of the peritoneal cavity is filled with lower density hemorrhagic fluid (*thin arrowheads*) but of higher attenuation than urine in the bladder (*thick arrowhead*)

Chylous Ascites

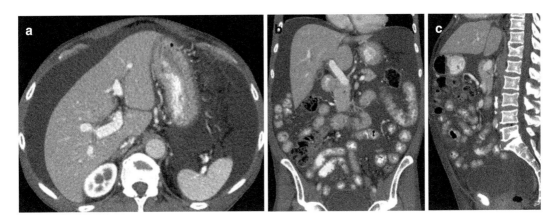

Fig. 16.6 Chylous ascites: CT axial (**a**), coronal (**b**), and sagittal (**c**) reformatted images show low-density ascites distending the peritoneal cavity with no lymphadenopathy. Milky fluid was tapped. Cause not known

TB Peritonitis

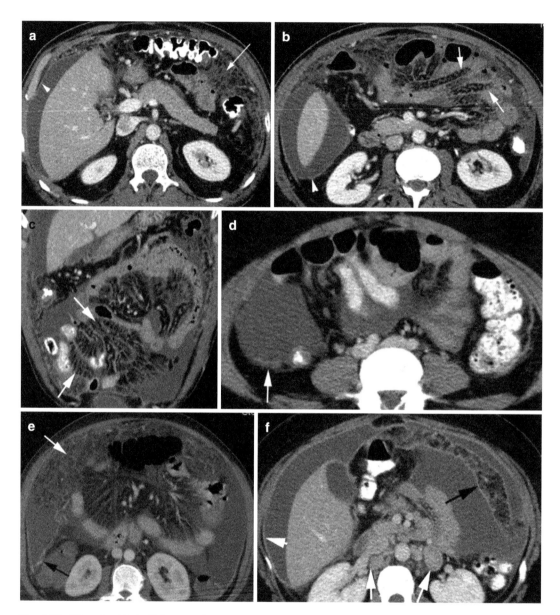

Fig. 16.7 TB peritonitis in different patients. Patient 1: CT axial (**a**, **b**) and coronal reformatted (**c**) images show thickening of the omentum (*long white arrow*) and small bowel mesentery (*short white arrows*) with vascular congestion. Peritoneal fluid is surrounded by enhancing peritoneum (*arrowhead*). Patient 2: Axial CT (**d**) shows nodular thickening of peritoneum (*arrow*). Patient 3: Axial CT (**e**) shows very thickened omentum with prominent vessels (*white arrow*) which are also seen on the peritoneal surface (*black arrow*). Patient 4: Axial CT (**f**) shows enlarged lymph nodes in the retroperitoneum (*white arrows*), thick peritoneum (*arrowhead*), and thick omentum (*black arrow*)

Peritoneal Lymphomatosis

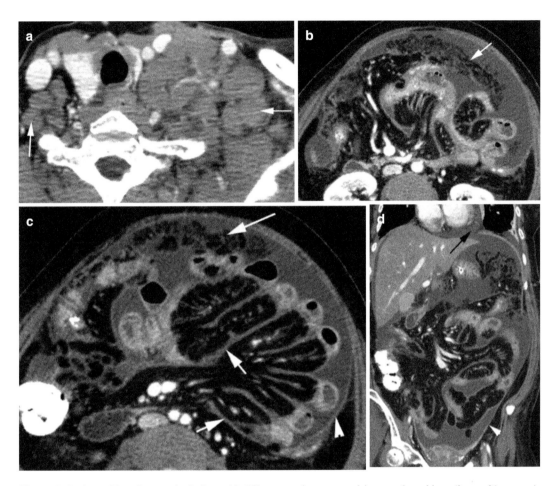

Fig. 16.8 Peritoneal lymphomatosis. Patient with diffuse large B-cell lymphoma. CT (**a**) axial image of the neck shows large lymph nodes in the supraclavicular region more on the left side (*arrow*). CECT of the abdomen, axial (**b**, **c**) and coronal reformatted (**d**) images show moderate ascites, omental increased markings (*long white arrow*), and diffuse thickening of leaves of the mesentery (*short arrows*) displacing small bowel loops. Peritoneum shows enhancement (*arrowhead*); small pericardial fluid (*black arrow*) is seen. No abdominal lymphadenopathy

Mucinous Ascites

Diagnosis
Perforated Mucocele Appendix

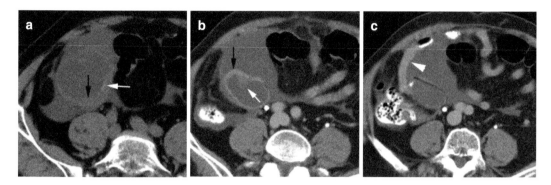

Fig. 16.9 Perforated mucocele appendix. Axial CT (**a**) noncontrast image shows dilated mucus-filled thick-walled (*black arrow*) appendix with a faint curvilinear calcification (*white arrow*) surrounded by extruded mucus. Delayed phase axial CECT (**b**, **c**) shows mild enhancement of the irregular thick wall (*black arrow*) and soft tissue mural nodule (*white arrow*). The extruded mucus is causing extrinsic pressure on the adjacent small bowel (*arrowhead*)

Diagnosis
Pseudomyxoma Peritonei

Imaging Features
1. Diffuse low-density peritoneal mucinous ascites with soft tissue strands
2. Scalloping surface of liver, spleen, and mesentery
3. Rim-like or punctate calcifications

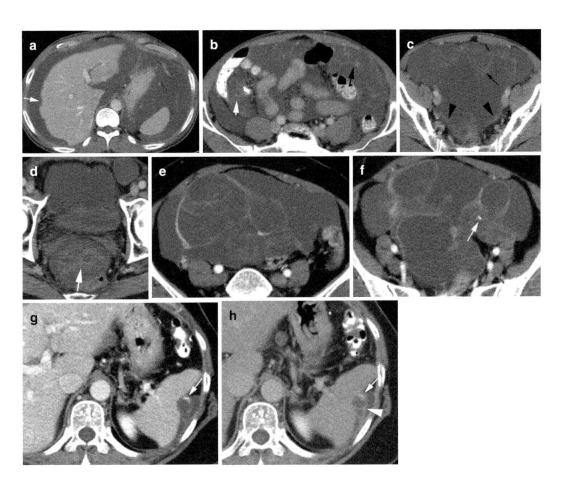

Fig. 16.10 Pseudomyxoma peritonei in two patients. Patient 1: Axial CT (**a–d**) shows the peritoneal cavity is distended with low-density fluid. Stranding (*thin black arrows*) in the fluid is mostly in the ileocecal region (*short white arrows*) and pelvis (*thick white arrow*) with thick peritoneum in the posterior cul-de-sac (*arrowheads*) and scalloping liver surface (*thin white arrow*). Patient 2 with perforated mucinous cystadenoma of the appendix: Axial CT (**e, f**) show thick septation in the mucinous ascites and a focal calcification (*arrow*). (**g, h**) Axial CT of the same patient with recurrence after 2 years shows septated mucinous tumor (*arrowhead*) with rim-like calcification (*white arrow*) in left subphrenic space scalloping on the spleen surface

CSF Pseudocyst

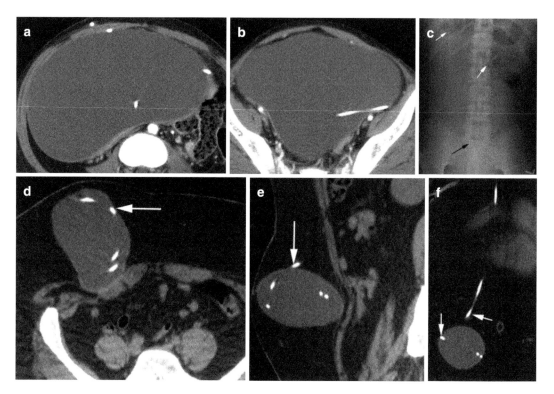

Fig. 16.11   CSF pseudocyst. Patient 1: Axial CT (**a**, **b**) show a large thin-walled cystic mass around the ventriculoperitoneal shunt catheter. (**c**) Flat plate of the abdomen shows large fluid collection around the VP shunt displacing bowel loops (*white arrows*), with the tip of the catheter at the level of the right SI joint (*black arrow*). Patient 2: CT (**d**) axial, (**e**) sagittal, and (**f**) coronal reformatted images show the shunt catheter is coiling in the subcutaneous tissue in the right lower abdominal wall (*arrow*) surrounded by well-marginated fluid collection

Mesenteric Lesions

Sclerosing Mesenteritis

Diagnosis
Retractile Mesenteritis

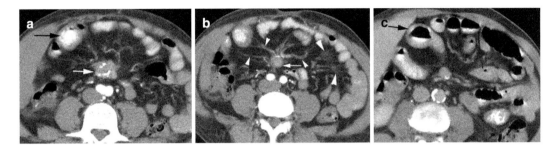

Fig. 16.12 Retractile mesenteritis. Axial CT (**a**, **b**) shows a soft tissue mass at the root of mesentery with coarse calcification (*white arrow*) and radiating desmoplastic reaction (*small arrowheads*). Patchy areas of mesenteric edema (*thick arrowhead*) also seen. (**c**) Low-grade obstruction from kinking is seen in a loop of the small bowel which is a little dilated (*black arrow*)

Diagnosis
Mesenteric Panniculitis

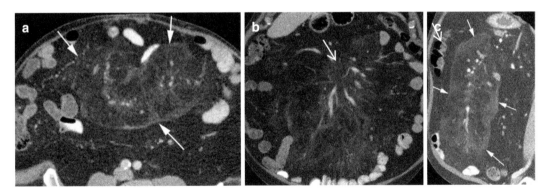

Fig. 16.13 Mesenteric panniculitis. CT axial (**a**), coronal (**b**), and (**c**) sagittal reformatted images show a well-demarcated area of ground-glass density of the small bowel mesentery (*arrows*), which is aligned with the root of the jejunal mesentery, has a mass effect on the jejunal loops, and envelopes the vessels

Mass in Mesentery

Diagnosis
Carcinoid Metastasis to Root of Mesentery

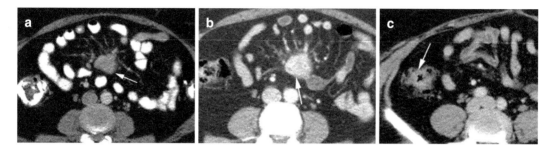

Fig. 16.14 Carcinoid metastasis to mesentery with adenocarcinoid tumor of the right colon. Axial CT (**a**) in early arterial and (**b**) delayed phases show enhancing solid mass in the root of mesentery with radiating tentacles (*arrow*). Axial CT (**c**) shows focal small solid enhancing mass right colon (*arrow*)

Diagnosis
Carcinoid Terminal Ileum

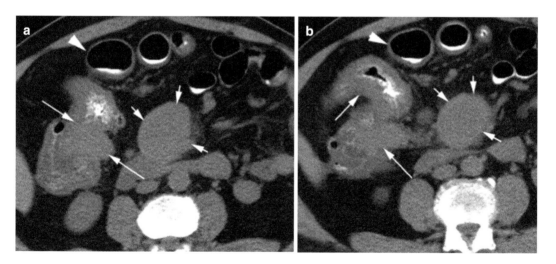

Fig. 16.15 Carcinoid at terminal ileum with metastasis to mesentery. Noncontrast axial CT (**a**, **b**) shows a large soft tissue mass causing wall thickening of terminal ileum (*long arrow*) with mild adjacent small bowel obstruction (*arrowhead*). Large smooth soft tissue mass is seen at root of mesentery (*short arrow*). Both lesions are proven to be carcinoids

Diagnosis
Aggressive Fibromatosis

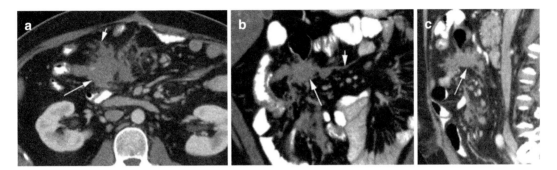

Fig. 16.16 Aggressive fibromatosis with history of colon surgery. CT (**a**) axial, (**b**) coronal, and (**c**) sagittal reformatted images show a large irregular soft tissue mass in the mesentery (*long arrow*) with strands extending into the mesenteric fat (*short arrow*). No bowel obstruction or vascular compromise

Diagnosis
Desmoid Tumor

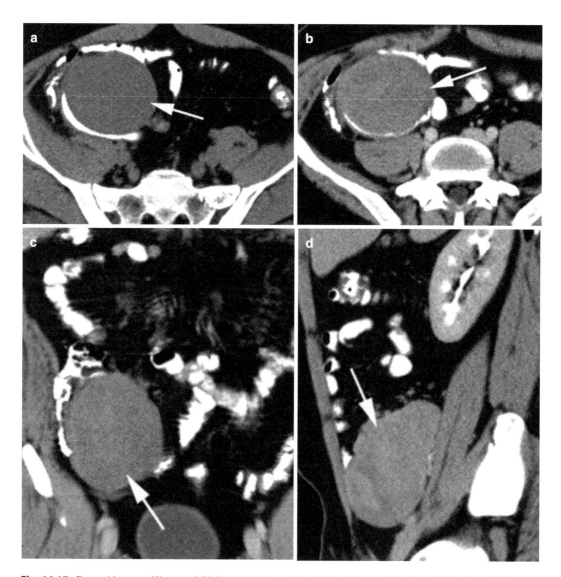

Fig. 16.17 Desmoid tumor. History of RLQ mass with pain in a 29-year-old man. (**a**) Noncontrast CT shows a well-marginated mass (*arrow*) in the mesentery of TI causing extrinsic compression on the bowel loops. CECT (**b**) axial, (**c**, **d**) coronal and sagittal reformatted images show faint enhancement of the mass (*arrow*). Histologically proven

Diagnosis
Granulocytic Sarcoma

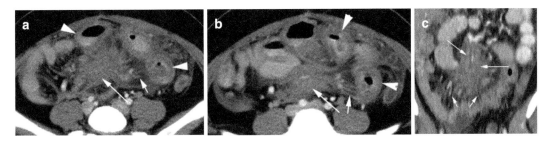

Fig. 16.18 Granulocytic sarcoma at mesenteric root. CT axial (**a**, **b**) and coronal reformatted (**c**) images show a large irregular soft tissue mass at root of mesentery (*long white arrow*) with linear extensions (*short white arrows*) to the adjacent small bowel causing obstruction and ischemic changes with wall thickening (*arrowheads*). The affected small bowel with the mass was surgically removed

Diagnosis
Dermoid Mesentery

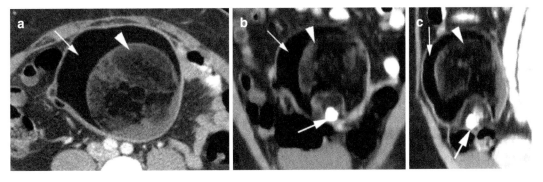

Fig. 16.19 Dermoid mesentery. CT axial (**a**), coronal (**b**), and sagittal (**c**) reformatted images show a large dermoid with fat (*thin arrow*), soft tissue (*white arrowhead*), and calcification (*thick arrow*) within the mesentery and displacing bowel loops

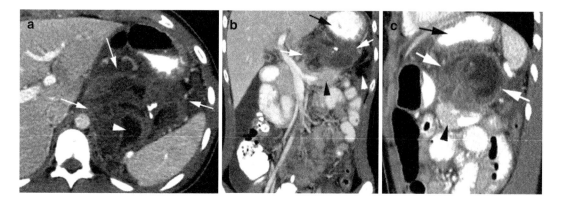

Fig. 16.20 Ruptured dermoid in lesser sac. History of left upper abdominal pain in a 15-year-old female. CT axial (**a**), coronal (**b**), and sagittal (**c**) reformatted images show a large heterogeneous mass (*white arrows*) in the lesser sac, between the stomach anteriorly (*black arrow*), pancreas inferiorly (*black arrowhead*), and spleen with gastrosplenic ligament posteriorly and in superior location. The mass has soft tissues, calcification, and fatty tissue (*white arrowhead* in **a**). Small amount of fatty tissue seen outside the mass (*arrowhead* in **b**) in the left paracolic gutter due to rupture and with ascites in the right paracolic gutter

Fig. 16.21 Retroperitoneal dermoid. Axial CT shows mass with rim calcification, linear fat, and soft tissues in anterior pararenal space (*arrow*) displacing mesenteric vessels anteriorly (*arrowhead*)

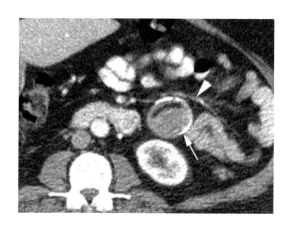

Diagnosis
Gossypiboma

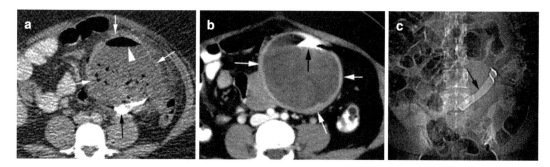

Fig. 16.22 Gossypiboma in two patients. Retained opaque surgical material (*black arrow*) in small bowel mesentery in both patients. Patient 1: Axial CT (**a**) shows a radio-opaque foreign body (*black arrow*) with soft tissue encapsulation (*white arrows*). The encapsulation has gas collections and gas fluid level (*arrowhead*) from superimposed infection. Patient 2: Axial CT shows (**b**) thick-walled encapsulation (*white arrows*) of the foreign body (*black arrow*). (**c**) Scanogram showing the soft tissue mass with radio-opaque foreign body (*black arrow*) displacing the bowel loops

Peritoneal Tumors

Diagnosis
Desmoplastic Peritoneal Tumor

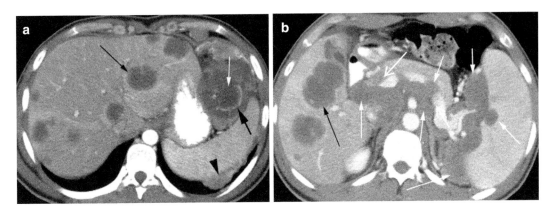

Fig. 16.23 Desmoplastic peritoneal tumor. CT axial (**a**, **b**) show low-density soft tissue mass (*white arrow*) in the gastrophrenic ligament with calcification (*thick black arrow*). Diffuse soft tissue mass at the splenic hilum and surrounding the aortocaval region with no vascular obstruction (*white arrows*). Diffuse metastasis is seen in the liver (*thin black arrows*) and left subphrenic region (*arrowhead*)

Diagnosis
Metastasis from Desmoplastic Ovarian Tumor

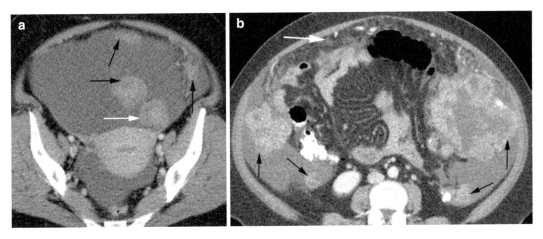

Fig. 16.24 Desmoplastic ovarian tumor with peritoneal metastasis. Axial CT (**a**, **b**) show small enhancing mass in the left ovary (*white arrow*). Diffuse metastases are seen in the peritoneum (*black arrows*) and omentum (*thick white arrow*), some of which are necrotic.

Diagnosis

Leiomyomatosis Peritonealis Disseminata

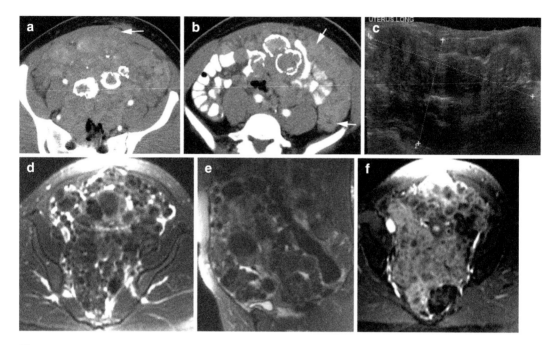

Fig. 16.25 Leiomyomatosis peritonealis disseminata. Patient with history of uterine fibroids. Axial CT (**a**, **b**) show multiple uterine fibroids; some calcified also involving the peritoneal surface of the lower abdomen and pelvis more on the left side (*arrows*). The uterus cannot be differentiated. (**c**) Longitudinal ultrasound of the pelvis shows diffuse heteroechogenicity in the region of the uterus (*cursors*). MRI study (**d**) axial T2 fat-sat and (**e**) sagittal T2 fat-sat show diffuse nodules in the region of the uterus and lower abdominal peritoneal surface with the same signal as skeletal muscles. Post-gad T1 fat-sat (**f**) shows mild enhancement of the nodules

Diagnosis

Calcified Peritoneal Metastasis from Ovarian Carcinoma

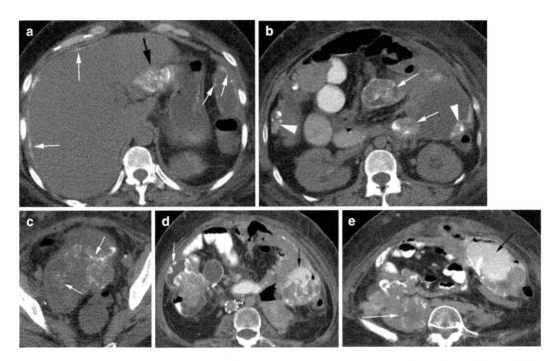

Fig. 16.26 Calcified peritoneal metastasis from papillary carcinoma of the ovary. Axial CT (**a**) shows diffuse calcification of the peritoneum over the liver (*long white arrows*), lesser omentum (*black arrow*), and left subphrenic region (*short white arrows*). (**b**, **c**) Peritoneal calcification in paracolic gutters (*arrowheads*), over retroperitoneal vessels, and in the mesentery and posterior cul-de-sac (*white arrows*). (**d**, **e**) Axial CT at later date shows peritoneal hemorrhage from catheter placement (*black arrow*) and increased peritoneal calcification which is extending to the right psoas muscle (*white arrows*)

Omental Torsion

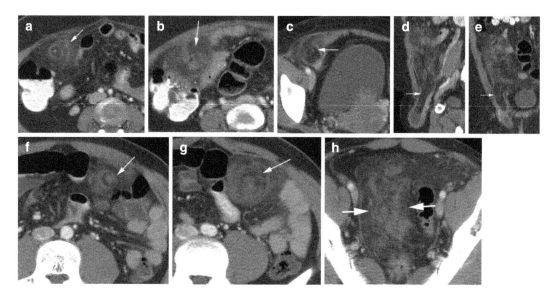

Fig. 16.27 Omental torsion with infarction. Patient 1: CT axial (**a**, **b**) shows the whorling (*arrow*) of torsed segment of omentum with layers of linear high and low density of ischemia and edema. CT axial (**c**), sagittal (**d**), and coronal (**e**) reformatted images show herniation of the omentum into the right inguinal canal (*arrow*). Patient 2: Axial CT (**f–h**) showing torsion of omentum on the left side (*thin arrow*) with high-density infarcted omentum in the pelvis (*thick arrows*)

Omental Infarction

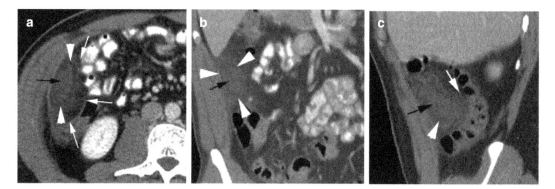

Fig. 16.28 Omental infarction. CT axial (**a**), coronal (**b**), and sagittal (**c**) reformatted images show a large nonenhancing omental mass in subhepatic space. It has a central higher attenuation (*black arrow*) with thin lucent rim (*arrowhead*). A halo of edema surrounding the affected omentum is causing extrinsic pressure on the bowel loops medially (*white arrow*)

Epiploic Appendagitis

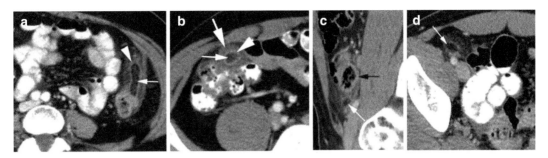

Fig. 16.29 Epiploic appendagitis. CT of different patients. Axial image (**a**) in descending and (**b**) in ascending colon shows thin high-density ring (*arrowhead*) surrounding focal fat (*thin arrow*) adjacent to the colon with surrounding edema (*thick arrow*). (**c**, **d**) Sagittal and axial images of epiploic appendagitis (*white arrow*) at tip of cecum (*black arrow*)

Retroperitoneal Lesions

Retroperitoneal Air

Diagnosis
Mediastinal Extension

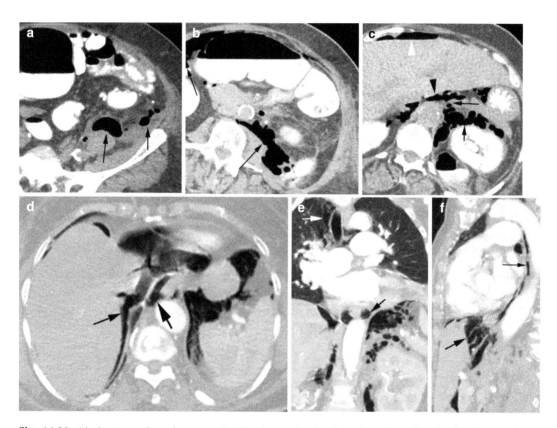

Fig. 16.30 Air in retroperitoneal space extending to mediastinum from leaking anastomosis. Axial CT (**a**) shows gas in the inferior cone of perirenal space over left iliopsoas muscle (*arrow*). (**b**) Gas tracking over the left psoas muscle in perirenal space (*arrow*). (**c**) Perirenal gas (*short black arrow*) extending into pararenal space (*black arrowhead*) beside the aorta (*long black arrow*) and also extending into the peritoneal cavity (*white arrowhead*). Axial (**d**), coronal (**e**), and sagittal (**f**) reformatted images show gas extending to bare area of the liver around the IVC (*thin arrow*) and extending to the mediastinum (*thin black arrow* in **f** and *white arrow* in **e**) through the esophageal hiatus (*thick arrow*)

Diagnosis
Ruptured Sigmoid Diverticulitis

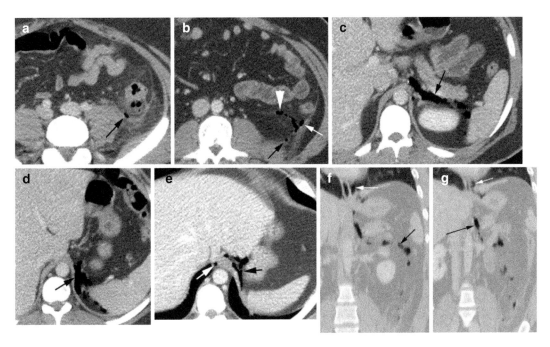

Fig. 16.31 Ruptured diverticulitis with air along the interfascial space. Axial CT (**a**) shows extraluminal air next to diverticulitis of the left colon (*arrow*). (**b**) Air in the anterior (*arrowhead*), posterior (*black arrow*), and lateroconal (*white arrow*) interfascial space. (**c–e**) Air in the anterior interfascial space (*black arrow* **c–g**) between perirenal and pararenal spaces entering the mediastinum around the aortic and esophageal hiatus (*white arrow*). Coronal reformatted images (**f, g**) show air tracking up to the mediastinum through the anterior interfascial space around the aorta and esophagus into the mediastinum (*white arrows*)

Diagnosis
Post ERCP

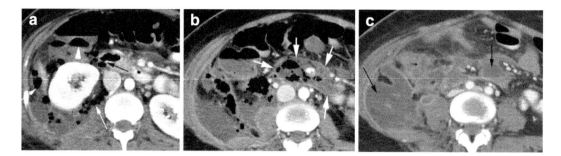

Fig. 16.32 Perforation of the duodenum in the perirenal space post ERCP examination. CT axial (**a**) shows perforation of the third part of the duodenum with leaking air (*black arrow*) surrounding the kidney (*white arrow*) and air-fluid collections (*arrowhead*). (**b**) Axial CT at a lower plane shows that air and fluid are tracking across the midline to the left side through space anterior to the aorta and root of mesenteric vessels (*arrows*). (**c**) Axial CT at a later date shows decrease of air but increase in fluid collections forming abscess (*arrows*) with enhancing walls around the fluid collections

Retroperitoneal Hemorrhage

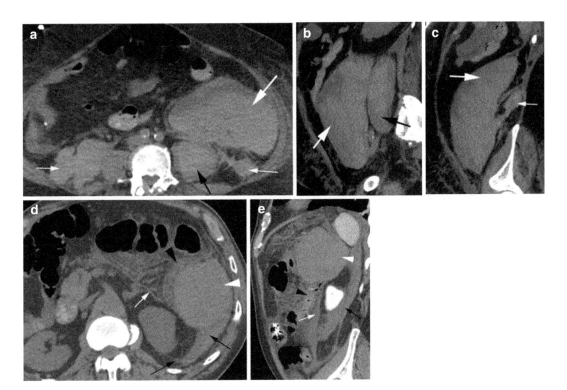

Fig. 16.33 Retroperitoneal hemorrhage. Patient 1 with thrombocytopenia: Axial (**a**) and sagittal reformatted (**b**, **c**) images show a large hematoma with hematocrit level in the left anterior pararenal space (*thick arrow*). Smaller hemorrhage is also seen in the posterior pararenal spaces bilaterally (*thin white arrows*) and hemorrhage in left psoas muscle (*black arrow*). Patient 2 with postcolonos-copy hemorrhage: Axial and sagittal reformatted images (**d**, **e**) show a large hematoma (*white arrowhead*) in latero-conal space displacing the descending colon (*black arrowhead*) medially. Anterior (*white arrow*) and poste-rior (*black arrow*) renal fascia are thickened from hemor-rhage. Stranding in anterior pararenal space from edema or hemorrhage

Retroperitoneal Abscess

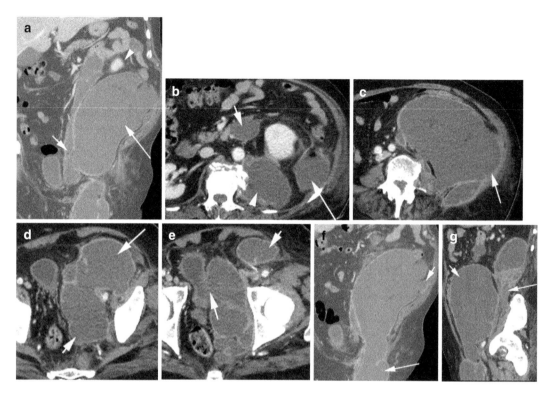

Fig. 16.34 Abscess in anterior pararenal space. Patient with diabetes. (**a**) Coronal reformatted image shows large thick rimmed abscess distending the inferior APS (*long arrow*) laterally. This large abscess has ruptured medially into the PPS between psoas and quadratus lumborum fascia (*short arrow*) and reaches cranially towards the inferior phrenic fascia. The kidney with the perirenal space is compressed but not involved (*arrowhead*). (**b**) Axial CT shows abscess in the lateral portion of APS (*long arrow*), PPS between the psoas and quadratus lumborum muscles (*arrowhead*), and small collection at the medial part of APS superiorly (*short arrow*). (**c**) Axial CT shows abscess involving the strap muscles (*arrow*) through the PPS. (**d**)

Axial CT shows APS abscess dividing around the common iliac artery and extending medially to the pelvis (*short arrow*) and laterally to the inguinal canal (*long arrow*). (**e**) Axial CT shows the abscess extending to the right side of APS in the lower pelvis (*long arrow*) and portion into the inguinal canal (*short arrow*). (**f**) Coronal reformatted CT shows abscess extending into the inguinal canal (*long arrow*) and focal rupture in PPS to strap muscles (*short arrow*). (**g**) Sagittal reformatted CT shows abscess between the psoas and quadratus lumborum fascia posteriorly (*long arrow*) and larger abscess (*short arrow*) in the APS. The abscess grew *Streptococcus anginosus*

Necrotic Lymphadenopathy

Diagnosis
TB Infection

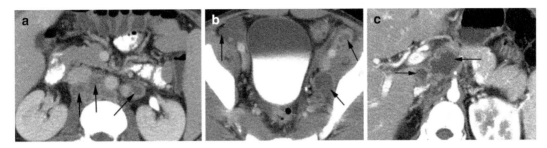

Fig. 16.35 Necrotic lymph nodes from TB infection in the retroperitoneum. Axial CT (**a**) shows enlarged, necrotic lymph nodes in the para-aortic, aortocaval, and retrocaval regions (*arrows*). (**b**) Necrotic nodes in the external iliac and obturator chains (*arrows*). (**c**) Necrotic nodes in the celiac axis (*arrow*)

Diagnosis
Metastasis

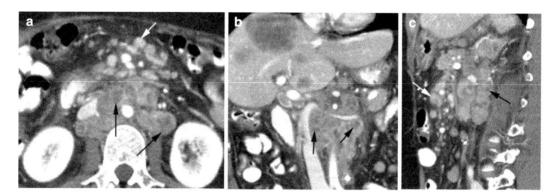

Fig. 16.36 Necrotic lymph nodes from colon cancer. CT axial (**a**), coronal (**b**), and sagittal (**c**) reformatted images show retroperitoneal necrotic lymph nodes (*black arrow*). Enlarged mesenteric lymph nodes are also seen (*white arrow*)

Diagnosis
Lymphoma

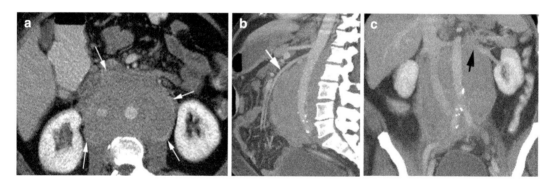

Fig. 16.37 Lymphoma mantle cell. CT axial (**a**), sagittal (**b**), and coronal (**c**) reformatted images show a large low-density homogeneous soft tissue mass (*short arrows*) surrounding the aorta and IVC and causing mass effect on the SMA (*thick white arrow*) and renal vessels (*black arrow*)

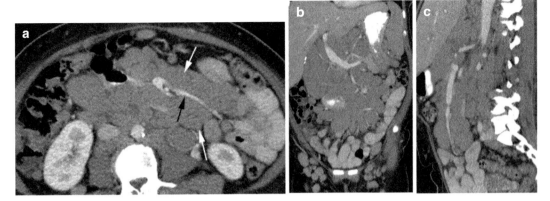

Fig. 16.38 Sandwich sign of lymphadenopathy. History of CLL. CT axial (**a**) shows enlarged lymph nodes in the mesentery (*white arrows*) with contrast-enhanced vessels (*black arrow*) traversing in the middle giving the sandwich appearance. CT coronal (**b**) and sagittal (**c**) reformatted images show large lymph nodes in the mesentery, retroperitoneum, and inguinal region

Retroperitoneal Lipoma

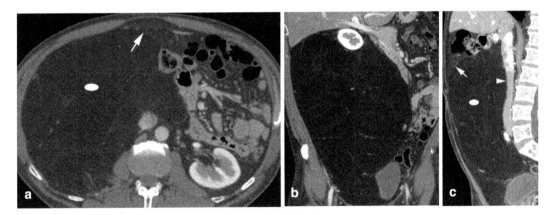

Fig. 16.39 Retroperitoneal benign lipoma. CT axial (**a**), coronal (**b**), and sagittal (**c**) reformatted images show a large low-density fatty mass with small internal vessels (*ellipse*) causing displacement of the adjacent organs with compression on IVC (*arrowhead*). It has a lower density than the omentum (*arrow*)

Retroperitoneal Liposarcoma

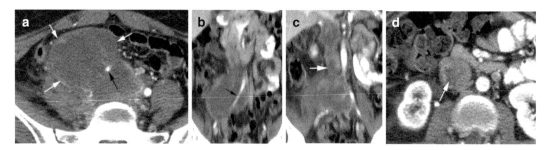

Fig. 16.40 Retroperitoneal leiomyosarcoma. CT (**a**) axial and (**b**) coronal reformatted images show a large necrotic mass (*white arrows*) encasing the right common iliac artery (*black arrow*). Coronal reformatted image (**c**) and axial CT (**d**) show tumor invasion into IVC (*arrow*)

The Spleen and Adrenal Glands

17

Contents

R. Agarwala, *Atlas of Emergency Radiology:*
Vascular System, Chest, Abdomen and Pelvis, and Reproductive System,
DOI 10.1007/978-3-319-13042-2_17, © Springer International Publishing Switzerland 2015

Splenic Lesions

Extramedullary Hematopoiesis

Diagnosis
Thalassemia with Extramedullary Hematopoiesis

Imaging Features
1. Intramedullary widening of bones with coarse trabeculation
2. Extramedullary hematopoiesis
3. Hepatosplenomegaly

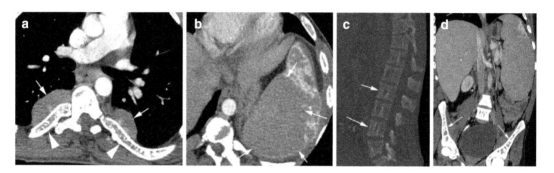

Fig. 17.1 Thalassemia with extramedullary hematopoiesis. CT axial image (**a**) shows extramedullary hematopoiesis as paraspinal soft tissues (*white arrows*) and undertubulation of the posterior ribs with coarse trabeculation of the ribs (*arrowheads*). (**b**) Axial CT shows a large extramedullary hematopoiesis as a nonenhancing mass in the spleen (*arrows*) compressing the normal splenic parenchyma. (**c, d**) Sagittal and coronal reformatted images show increased trabeculation of the lumbar vertebrae and iliac bones (*arrows*). The liver and spleen are enlarged

Diagnosis
Myelofibrosis with Extramedullary Hematopoiesis

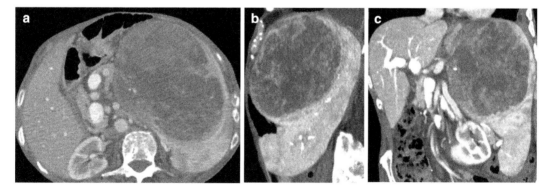

Fig. 17.2 Splenic extramedullary hematopoiesis in myelofibrosis. CT axial (**a**), sagittal (**b**), and coronal (**c**) reformatted images show extramedullary hematopoiesis as a large well-marginated low-density heterogeneous mass in the upper pole of the spleen having mass effect

Lymphoma

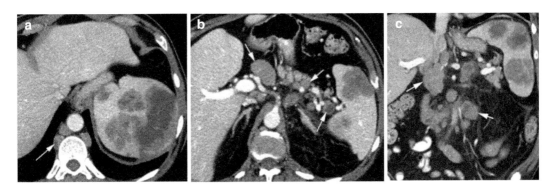

Fig. 17.3 Lymphoma of the spleen. History of diffuse B-cell lymphoma. CT axial (**a**, **b**) and coronal (**c**) reformatted images show multifocal low-density nodular involvement of the spleen with enlarged lymph nodes in the retrocrural region, mesenteric region, and portacaval region (*arrows*)

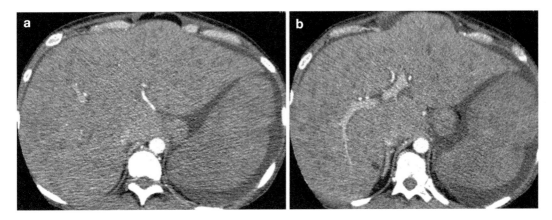

Fig. 17.4 Hepatosplenomegaly from non-Hodgkin's lymphoma. Axial CT (**a**, **b**) shows hepatosplenomegaly with diffuse low-density nodular involvement of the liver and spleen

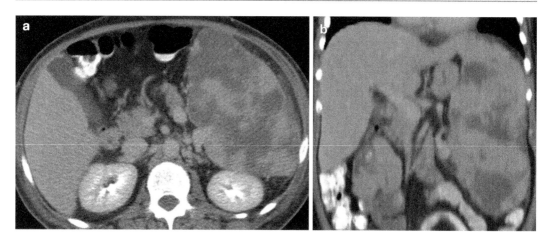

Fig. 17.5 Lymphoma of the spleen. History of T-cell lymphoma. Axial CT (**a**, **b**) shows enlarged spleen with multiple irregular confluent low-density lesions

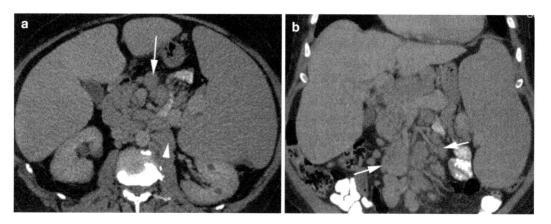

Fig. 17.6 Hepatosplenomegaly from chronic lymphoid leukemia. Axial CT (**a**) and coronal reformatted (**b**) images show diffusely enlarged liver and spleen, focal low-density lesions of the left kidney, and lymphadenopathy in the small bowel mesentery (*arrow*) and para-aortic region (*arrowhead*)

Coccidioidomycosis

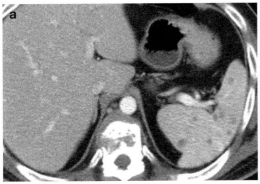

Fig. 17.7 Coccidioidomycosis of the spleen and vertebra. Axial CT (**a**) shows multiple small low-density lesions in the spleen. (**b**) Bone windowing shows destructive changes of the T12 vertebral body (*arrowheads*) with increased paravertebral soft tissue (*arrow*) which was biopsy proven as coccidioidomycosis infection

Sarcoid

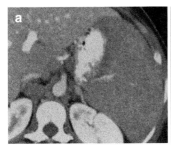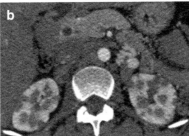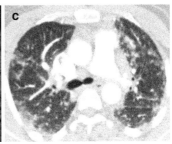

Fig. 17.8 Sarcoidosis. Axial CT (**a**) shows a large spleen with diffuse low-density lesions. (**b**) Axial CT a few years later after splenectomy, developed renal sarcoidosis with multiple low-density nodules. (**c**) Axial CT of the chest shows multiple centrilobular nodules in lymphatic distribution

Infarction

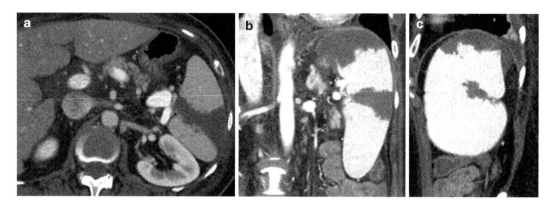

Fig. 17.9 Splenic infarction in a patient with atrial fibrillation and hypotension. CT axial (**a**), coronal (**b**), and sagittal (**c**) reformatted images show well-defined low-attenuating infarctions in the upper pole and midpoles

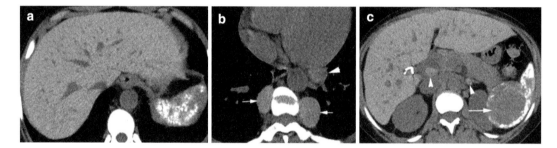

Fig. 17.10 Splenic calcification and extramedullary hematopoiesis in a sickle cell anemia patient. Noncontrast axial CT (**a–c**) shows hemochromatosis of the liver with increased attenuation. Multiple high-density lymph nodes are seen in the abdomen, paraspinal region of the lower thorax (*arrows*), and left hilum (*arrowhead*) from hemochromatosis (hemosiderosis). Low-density areas in a calcified spleen are from extramedullary hematopoiesis (*long arrow*)

Adrenal Lesions

Pheochromocytoma

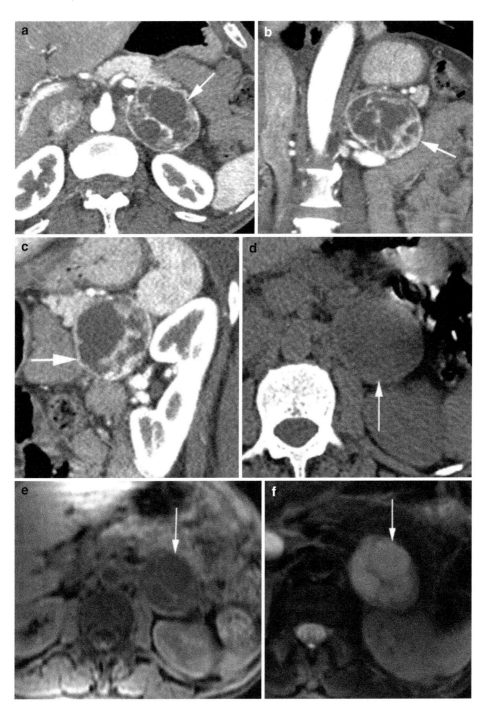

Fig. 17.11 Pheochromocytoma with neurofibromatosis type 1. CT postcontrast axial (**a**), coronal (**b**), and sagittal (**c**) reformatted images and unenhanced axial image (**d**) show a large left adrenal enhancing mass with low-density cystic areas (*arrow*). Axial MRI in T1W (**e**) and T2W fat-sat (**f**) images again shows a large adrenal mass (*arrow*) with cystic areas with low signal in T1W image and high signal in T2W images

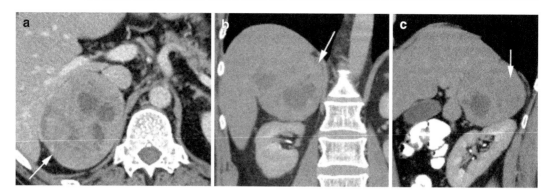

Fig. 17.12 Pheochromocytoma of the right adrenal gland. CT axial (**a**), coronal (**b**), and sagittal (**c**) reformatted images show a large adrenal mass (*arrows*) causing extrinsic compression on the liver. The tumor shows poor enhancement with multiple cystic areas

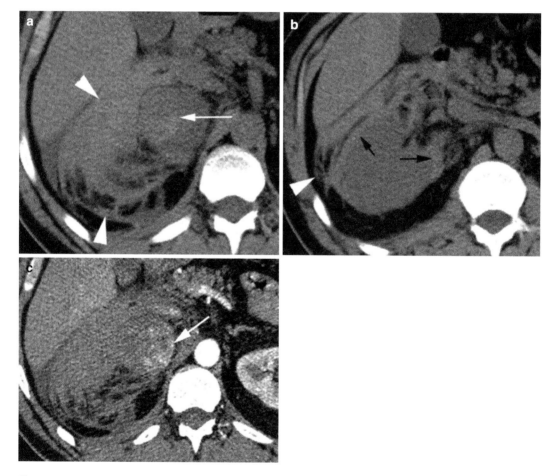

Fig. 17.13 Pheochromocytoma with spontaneous hemorrhage. Axial unenhanced CT (**a**, **b**) shows a large right adrenal gland mass with high-density hemorrhage from the mass (*white arrow*) extending into the perirenal space (*arrowheads*) and causing subcapsular hemorrhage in the right kidney (*black arrows*). Postcontrast image (**c**) shows enhancement of the nonhemorrhagic portion of the tumor (*arrow*)

Retroperitoneal Paraganglioma

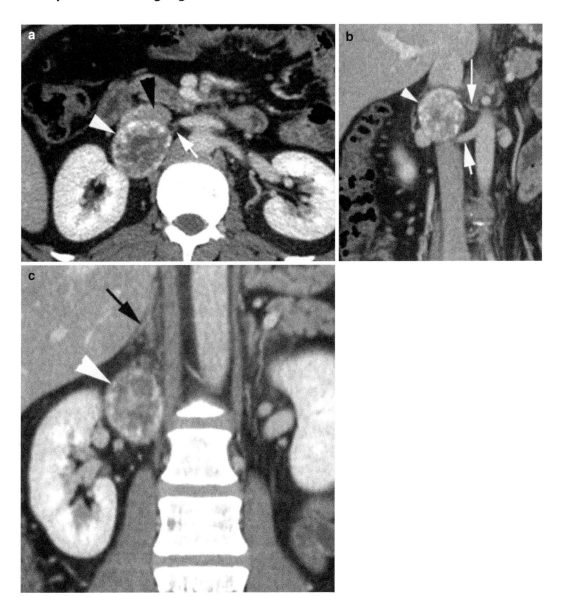

Fig. 17.14 Retroperitoneal paraganglioma. Incidental finding for appendicitis CT. CECT (**a**) shows a solid mass mostly with peripheral enhancement and central low density (*white arrowhead*) behind the IVC (*black arrowhead*) with a small renal artery (*white arrow*) supplying the mass (surgically proven). Coronal reformatted image (**b**) shows the mass (*arrowhead* also in **c**) supplied by the small renal artery (*long arrow*) with the large main renal artery coursing inferior to the mass (*thick arrow*). (**c**) Shows the adrenal gland (*black arrow*) to be separate (*black arrow*)

Adrenocortical Carcinoma

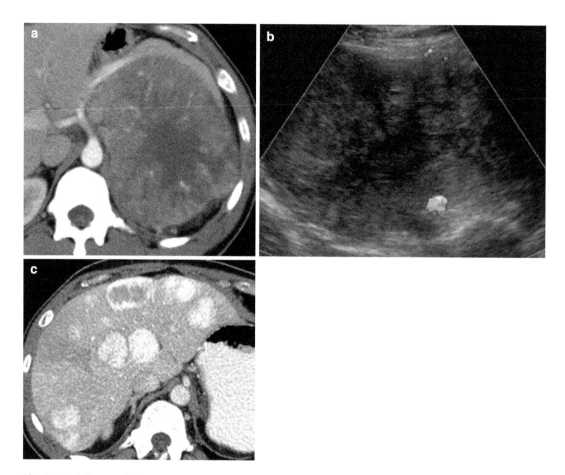

Fig. 17.15 Adrenocortical carcinoma. Axial CT (**a**) shows a large solid mass with linear vasculature within the solid portion and with central necrosis. (**b**) Ultrasound shows heteroechoic mass with central low echogenicity. (**c**) Later CT done after adrenalectomy shows enhancing hepatic metastasis

Adrenal Cyst

Diagnosis
Adrenal Pseudocyst

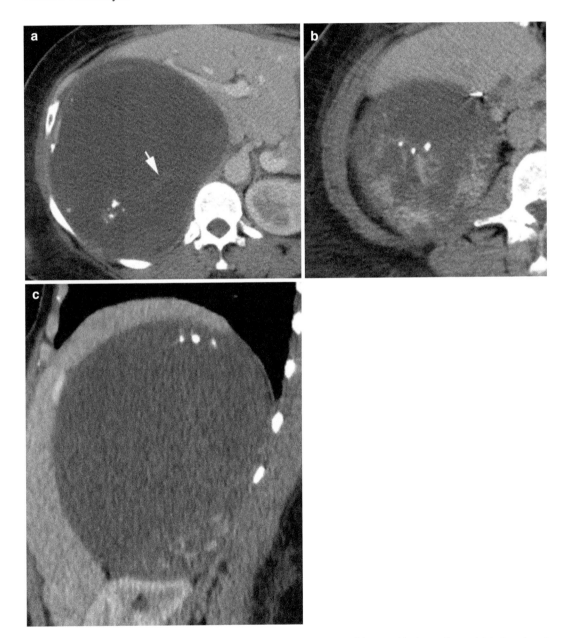

Fig. 17.16 Adrenal pseudocyst. Axial CT (**a**, **b**) and sagittal reformatted images (**c**) show a large right adrenal cyst with septation (*arrow*) and coarse calcification and enhancing soft tissues inferiorly

Diagnosis

Complex Adrenal Cyst with Adenoma

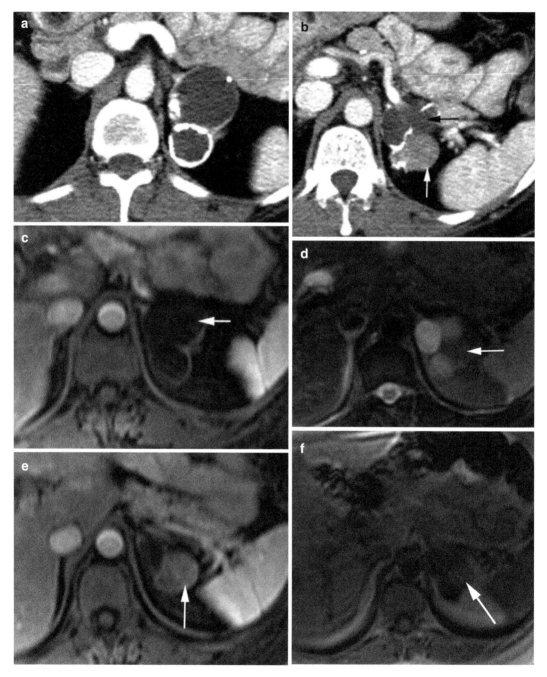

Fig. 17.17 Left adrenal complex cyst with calcification and adenoma. Axial CT (**a**, **b**) shows lobulated cyst of the left adrenal gland with rim calcification (*black arrow*). Soft tissue enhancing nodule had features of adenoma (*white arrow*). Axial MRI (**c**) T1W shows no signal in the cysts (*arrow*) and high signal in T2W image with low signal in the adenoma (*arrow*) (**d**). Postcontrast study (**e**) shows enhancement of the adenoma (*arrow*) and no enhancement of the cyst. (**f**, **g**) In- and out-phase images show signal drop-off in the opposed phase (*arrow*)

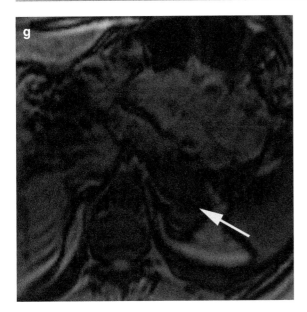

Fig. 17.17 (continued)

Diagnosis
Adrenal Simple Cyst

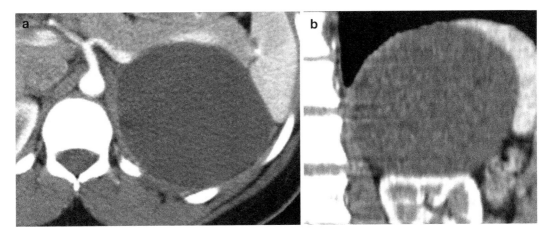

Fig. 17.18 Simple cyst of the adrenal gland. CT axial (**a**) and coronal (**b**) reformatted images show a simple cyst in the left adrenal gland as an incidental finding

Metastasis

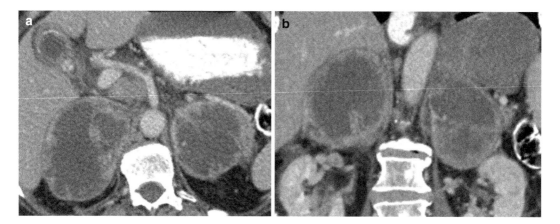

Fig. 17.19 Adrenal metastasis from Merkel cell cancer. Axial (**a**) and coronal (**b**) reformatted CT images show a large necrotic mass in each adrenal gland with peripheral enhancement

Myelolipoma

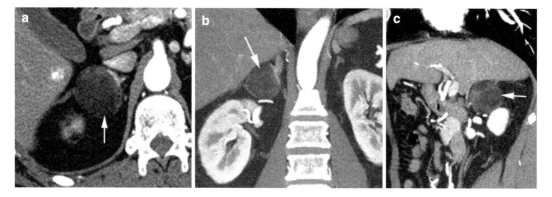

Fig. 17.20 Myelolipoma of the right adrenal gland. CT axial (**a**), coronal (**b**), and sagittal (**c**) reformatted images show a well-defined mass in the right adrenal gland (*arrow*), predominantly fatty tissue

Adrenal Hemorrhage

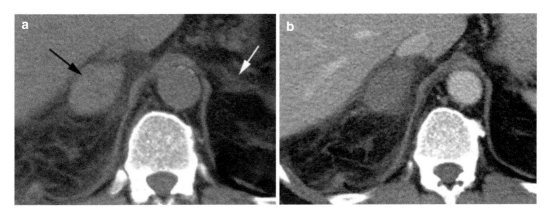

Fig. 17.21 Adrenal hemorrhage with insufficiency. Axial non-enhanced CT (**a**) shows a well-defined right adrenal mass (*black arrow*) with high density from hemorrhage and edema of surrounding perinephric space and normal left adrenal gland (*white arrow*). (**b**) Postcontrast study shows no enhancement of any part of the adrenal hemorrhage

Bibliography

1. Akbar SA, Jafri SZH, Amendola M, et al. Renal infections: an update. Appl Radiol. 2009;25–38.
2. Alsaif HS, Venkatesh SK, Chan DSG, et al. CT appearance of pyogenic liver abscesses caused by klebsiella pneumonia. Radiology. 2011;260(1):129–38.
3. Anderson SW, Kruskal JB, Kane RA. Benign hepatic tumors and iatrogenic pseudotumors. Radiographics. 2009;29:211–29.
4. Antila KM, Makisalo H, Arola J, et al. Biliary papillomatosis. Radiographics. 2008;28:2059–63.
5. Avery LL, Scheinfeld MH. Imaging of penile and scrotal emergencies. Radiographics. 2013;33:721–40.
6. Balthazar EJ, Yen BC, Gordon RB. Ischemic colitis: CT evaluation of 54 cases. Radiology. 1999;211:381–8.
7. Ba-Ssalamah A, Prokop M, Uffmann M, et al. Dedicated multidetector CT of the stomach? Spectrum of diseases. Radiographics. 2003;23:625–44.
8. Bechtold RE, Dyer RB, Zagoria RJ, et al. The perirenal space: relationship of the pathologic processes to normal retroperitoneal anatomy. Radiographics. 1996;16:841–54.
9. Boscak AR, Al-Hawary M, Ramsburgh SR. Adenomyomatosis of the gallbladder. Radiographics. 2006;26:941–6.
10. Boudiaf M, Sayer P, Terem C, et al. CT evaluation of small bowel obstruction. Radiographics. 2001;21:613–24.
11. Brody MJ, Leighton DB, Murphy BL, et al. CT of blunt bowel and mesenteric injury: typical findings and pitfalls in diagnosis. Radiographics. 2000;20:1525–36.
12. Brofiman N, Atri M, Epid D, et al. Evaluation of bowel and mesenteric blunt trauma with multidetector CT. Radiographics. 2006;26:1119–31.
13. Browne RFJ, Meehan CP, Colville J, et al. Transitional cell carcinoma of the upper urinary tract: spectrum of imaging findings. Radiographics. 2005;25:1609–27.
14. Buckley JA, Fishman EK. CT evaluation of small bowel neoplasms: spectrum of disease. Radiographics. 1998;18:379–92.
15. Catalano OA, Sahani DV, Forcione DG, et al. Biliary infections: spectrum of imaging findings and management. Radiographics. 2009;29:2059–80.
16. Chang S, Choi D, Lee SJ, et al. Neuroendocrine neoplasms of the gastrointestinal tract: classicification, pathologic basis, and imaging features. Radiographics. 2007;27:1667–79.
17. Chung YE, Kim MJ, Park YN, et al. Varying appearances of cholangiocarcinoma: radiologic-pathologic correlation. Radiographics. 2009;29:683–700.
18. Craig WD, Wagner BJ, Travis MD. Pyelonephritis: radiologic-pathologic review. Radiographics. 2008;28:255–76.
19. Elsayes KM, Narra VR, Mukundan G, et al. MR imaging of the spleen: spectrum of abnormalities. Radiographics. 2005;25:967–82.
20. Fasel JH, Selle D, Evertsz CJ, et al. Segmental anatomy of the liver: poor correlation with CT. Radiology. 1998;206:151–6.
21. Federie MP, Courcoulas AP, Powell M, et al. Blunt splenic injury in adults: clinical and CT criteria for management, with emphasis on active extravasation. Radiology. 1998;206:137–42.
22. Feldman D. The coffee bean sign. Radiology. 2000;216:178–9.
23. Fernback SK, Feinstein KA, Spencer K, et al. Ureteral duplication and its complications. Radiographics. 1997;17:109–27.
24. Fielding JR, Practical MR. Imaging of the female pelvic floor weakness. Radiographics. 2002;22:295–304.
25. Fishman EK, Urban BA, Hruban RH. CT of the stomach: spectrum of disease. Radiographics. 1996;16:1035–54.
26. Fuchsjager MH. The small-bowel feces sign. Radiology. 2002;225:378–9.
27. Furukawa A, Saotome T, Yamasaki M, et al. Cross-sectional imaging in Crohn disease. Radiographics. 2004;24:689–702.
28. Ghai S, Pattison J, Ghai S, et al. Primary gastrointestinal lymphoma: spectrum of imaging findings with pathologic correlation. Radiographics. 2007;27:1371–88.
29. Guermazi A, Brice P, Kerviler ED, et al. Extranodal Hodgkin disease: spectrum of disease. Radiographics. 2001;21:161–79.
30. Gupta A, Stuhlfaut JW, Flemming KW, et al. Blunt trauma of the pancreas and biliary tract: a multimodality imaging approach to diagnosis. Radiographics. 2004;24:1381–95.
31. Han JK, Choi BI, Kim TK, et al. Hilar cholangiocarcinoma: thin-section spiral CT findings with cholangiographic correlation. Radiographics. 1997;17:1475–85.
32. Han JK, Choi BI, Kim AY, et al. Cholangiocarcinoma: pictorial essay of CT and cholangiographic findings. Radiographics. 2002;22:173–87.
33. Hanbidge AE, Buckler PM, O'Malley ME, et al. Imaging evaluation for acute pain in the right upper quadrant. Radiographics. 2004;24:1117–35.
34. Hanna RF, Aguirre DA, Kased N, et al. Cirrhosis-associated hepatocellular nodules: correlation of histopathologic and MR imaging features. Radiographics. 2008;28:747–69.
35. Harris AC, Zwirewich CV, Lyburn ID, et al. CT findings in blunt renal trauma. Radiographics. 2001;21:S201–14.
36. Helenon O, Merran S, Paraf F, et al. Unusual fat-containing tumors of the kidney: a diagnostic dilemma. Radiographics. 1997;17:129–44.
37. Ho VB, Allen SF, Hood MN, et al. Renal masses: quantitative assessment of enhancement with dynamic MR imaging. Radiology. 2002;224:695–700.
38. Hoeffel C, Crema MD, Belkacem A, et al. Multidetector row CT: spectrum of diseases involving the ileocecal area. Radiographics. 2006;26:1373–90.
39. Hong X, Choi H, Loyer EM, et al. Gastrointestinal stromal tumor: role of CT in diagnosis and in

response evaluation and surveillance after treatment with imatinib. Radiographics. 2006;26:481–95.

40. Hopkins JK, Giles HW, Wyatt-Ashmead J, et al. Cystic nephroma. Radiographics. 2004;24:589–93.

41. Horton KM, Lawler LP, Fishman EK. CT findings in sclerosing mesenteritis (panniculitis): spectrum of disease. Radiographics. 2003;23:1561–7.

42. Horwitz BM, Zamora GE, Marcela G. Gastrointestinal stromal tumor of the small bowel. Radiographics. 2011;31:429–34.

43. Hotron KM, Corl FM, Fishman EK. CT evaluation of the colon: inflammatory disease. Radiographics. 2000;20:399–418.

44. Israel GM, Bosniak MA. How I do it: evaluating renal masses. Radiology. 2005;236:441–50.

45. Israel GM, Bosniak MA. Pitfalls in renal mass evaluation and how to avoid them. Radiographics. 2008; 28:1325–38.

46. Johnson PT, Horton KM, Fishman EK. Nonvascular mesenteric disease: utility of multidetector CT with 3D volume rendering. Radiographics. 2009;29: 721–40.

47. Kang Y, Lee JM, Kim SH, et al. Intrahepatic mass-forming cholangiocarcinoma: enhancement pattern on gadoxetic acid-enhanced MR images. Radiology. 2012;264(3):751–60.

48. Kanne JP, Mankoff DA, Baird GS, et al. Gastric linitis plastica from metastatic breast carcinoma: FDG and FES PET appearances. AJR Am J Roentgenol. 2007;188:W503–5.

49. Katabathina VS, Vikram R, Nagar AM, et al. Mesenchymal neoplasms of the kidney in adults: imaging spectrum with radiologic-pathologic correlation. Radiographics. 2010;30:1525–40.

50. Kawamoto S, Horton KM, Lawler LP, et al. Intraductal papillary mucinous neoplasm of the pancreas: can benign lesions be differentiated from malignant lesions with multidetector CT? Radiographics. 2005; 25:1451–70.

51. Kawamoto S, Horton KM, Fishman EK. Pseudomembranous colitis: spectrum of imaging findings with clinical and pathologic correlation. Radiographics. 1999;19:887–97.

52. Kawashima A, Sandler CM, Fishman EK, et al. Spectrum of CT findings in nonmalignant disease of the adrenal gland. Radiographics. 1998;18: 393–412.

53. Kim YH, Blake MA, Harisinghani MG, et al. Adult intestinal intussusception: CT appearances and identification of a causative lead point. Radiographics. 2006;26:733–44.

54. Kim TK, Choi BI, Han JK, et al. Peripheral cholangiocarcinoma of the liver: two-phase spiral CT findings. Radiology. 1997;204:539–43.

55. Kim OH, Chung HJ, Choi BG. Imaging of the choledochal cyst. Radiographics. 1995;15:69–88.

56. Kim JU, Lee JM, Kim SH, et al. Differentiation of intraductal growing-type cholangiocarcinomas from nodular-type cholangiocarcinomas at biliary MR imaging with MR cholangiography. Radiology. 2010;257(2):364–72.

57. Kim YH, Saini S, Sahani D, et al. Imaging diagnosis of cystic pancreatic lesions: pseudocyst versus nonpseudocyst. Radiographics. 2005;25:671–85.

58. Krebs TL, Wagner BJ. MR imaging of the adrenal gland: radiologic-pathologic correlation. Radiographics. 1998;15:1425–40.

59. Lane MJ, Liu DM, Huynh MD, et al. Suspected acute appendicitis: nonenhanced helical CT in 300 consecutive patients. Radiology. 1999;213:341–6.

60. Lee HY, Kim SH, Lee JM, et al. Preoperative assessment of resectability of hepatic hilar cholangiocarcinoma: combined CT and cholangiography with revised criteria. Radiology. 2006;239(1): 113–21.

61. Lee WJ, Lim HK, Jang KM, et al. Radiologic spectrum of cholangiocarcinoma: emphasis on unusual manifestation and differential diagnosis. Radiographics. 2001; 21:S97–116.

62. Leite NP, Kased N, Hanna RF, et al. Cross-sectional imaging of extranodal involvement in abdominopelvic lymphoproliferative malignancies. Radiographics. 2007;27:1613–34.

63. Levine MS, Pantongrag-Brown L, Aguilera NS, et al. Non-Hodgkin lymphoma of the stomach: a cause of linitis plastica. Radiology. 1996;201:375–8.

64. Levine MS, Rubesin SE. Diseases of the esophagus: diagnosis by esophagography. Radiology. 2005;237: 414–27.

65. Levy AD, Murakata LA, Abbott RM, et al. Benign tumors and tumorlike lesions of the gallbladder and extrahepatic bile ducts: radiologic-pathologic correlation. Radiographics. 2002;22:387–413.

66. Levy AD, Murkata LA, Rohrmann CA. Gallbladder carcinoma: radiologic-pathologic correlation. Radiographics. 2001;21:295–314.

67. Levy AD, Patel N, Dow N, et al. Abdominal neoplasms in patients with neurofibromatosis type 1: radiologic-pathologic correlation. Radiographics. 2005;25:455–80.

68. Levy AD, Remotti HE, Thompson WM, et al. Gastrointestinal stromal tumors: radiologic features and pathologic correlation. Radiographics. 2003;23: 283–304.

69. Levy AD, Rimola J, Mehrotra AK, et al. Benign fibrous tumors and tumorlike lesions of the mesentery: radiologic-pathologic correlation. Radiographics. 2006;26:245–64.

70. Levy AD, Sobin LH. Gastrointestinal carcinoids: imaging features with clinicopathologic comparison. Radiographics. 2007;27:237–57.

71. Lim JH, Kim MH, Kim TK, et al. Papillary neoplasms of the bile duct that mimic biliary stone disease. Radiographics. 2003;23:447–55.

72. Lim JH, Lee G, Lyun Y. Radiologic spectrum of intraductal papillary mucinous tumor of the pancreas. Radiographics. 2001;21:323–40.

73. Lubner M, Menias C, Rucker C, et al. Blood in the belly: CT findings of hemoperitoneum. Radiographics. 2007;27:109–25.

74. Lucey BC, Stuhlfaut JW, Soto JA. Mesenteric lymph nodes seen at imaging: causes and significance. Radiographics. 2005;25:351–65.

75. Lvoff N, Breiman RS, Coakley FV, et al. Distinguishing features of self-limiting adult small-bowel intussusception identified at CT. Radiology. 2003;227:68–72.

76. Madureira AJ. The comb sign. Radiology. 2004;230: 783–4.

77. Menias CO, Surabhi VR, Prasad SR, et al. Mimics of cholangiocarcinoma: spectrum of disease. Radiographics. 2008;28:1115–29.

78. Mergo PJ, Helmberger TK, Buetow PC, et al. Pancreatic neoplasms: MR imaging and pathologic correlation. Radiographics. 1997;17:281–301.

79. Metser U, Goldstein MA, Chawla TP, et al. Detection of urothelial tumors: comparison of urothelial phase with excretory phase CT urography—a prospective study. Radiology. 2012;264:110–8.

80. Mindell HJ, Mastromatteo JF, Dickey KW. Anatomic communications between the three retroperitoneal spaces: determination by CT-guided injections of contrast material in cadavers. AJR Am J Roentgenol. 1995;164:1173–8.

81. Molmenti EP, Balfe DM, Kanterman RY, et al. Anatomy of the retroperitoneum: observation of the distribution of pathologic fluid collections. Radiology. 1996;200:95–103.

82. Morgan DE, Lockhart ME, Canon CL, et al. Polycystic liver disease: multimodality imaging for complications and transplant evaluation. Radiographics. 2006;26: 1655–68.

83. Mortele KF, Segatto E, Ros PR. The infected liver: radiologic-pathologic correlation. Radiographics. 2004;24:937–55.

84. Nicolau C, Torra R, Badenas C, et al. Autosomal dominant polycystic kidney disease types 1 and 2: assessment of US sensitivity for diagnosis. Radiology. 1999;213:273–6.

85. O'Sullivan SG. Accordion sign. Radiology. 1998;206: 177–8.

86. Oliva MR, Mortele KJ, Erturk SM, et al. Magnetic resonance imaging of the pancreas. Appl Radiol 2006:7–21.

87. Pear BL. Pneumatosis intestinalis: a review. Radiology. 1998;207:13–9.

88. Pedrosa I, Saiz A, Arrazola J, et al. Hydatid disease: radiologic and pathologic features and complications. Radiographics. 2000;20:795–817.

89. Pernas JC, Catala J. Pseudocyst around ventriculo-peritoneal shunt. Radiology. 2004;232:239–43.

90. Persaud T, Swan N, Torreggiani WC. Giant mucinous cystadenoma of the appendix. Radiographics. 2007;27:553–7.

91. Peterson CM, Anderson JS, Hara AK, et al. Volvulus of the gastrointestinal tract: appearances at multimodality imaging. Radiographics. 2009;29: 1281–93.

92. Pickhardt PJ, Bhalla S. Unusual nonneoplastic peritoneal and subperitoneal conditions: CT findings. Radiographics. 2005;25:719–30.

93. Pickhardt PJ, Bhalla S. Primary neoplasms of the peritoneal and subperitoneal origin: CT findings. Radiographics. 2005;25:983–95.

94. Pickhardt PJ, Levy AD, Rohrmann CA, et al. Primary neoplasms of the appendix: radiologic spectrum of disease with pathologic correlation. Radiographics. 2003;23:645–62.

95. Pickhardt PJ, Levy AD, Rohrmann Jr CA, Kende Maj AI. Primary neoplasms of the appendix as acute appendicitis: CT findings with pathologic comparison. Radiology. 2002;224:775–81.

96. Power N, Bent C, Chan O. Imaging of cystic liver lesions in the adult. Appl Radiol. 2007;36:24–32.

97. Prando A, Prando P, Prando D. Urothelial cancer of the renal pelvicaliceal system: unusual imaging manifestations. Radiographics. 2010;30:1553–66.

98. Prasad SR, Humphrey PA, Catena JR, et al. Common and uncommon histologic subtypes of renal cell carcinoma: imaging spectrum with pathologic correlation. Radiographics. 2006;26:1795–810.

99. Procacci C, Megibow SJ, Carbognin G, et al. Intraductal papillary mucinous tumor of the pancreas: a pictorial essay. Radiographics. 1999;19:1447–63.

100. Purysko AS, Remer EM, Coppa CP, et al. LI-RADS: a case-based review of the new categorization of liver findings in patients with end-stage liver disease. Radiographics. 2012;32:1977–95.

101. Rao PM, Wittenberg J, Lawrason JN. Primary epiploic appendagitis: evolutionary changes in CT appearance. Radiology. 1997;204:713–7.

102. Rha SE, Ha HK, Kim AY, et al. Peritoneal leiomyosarcomatosis originating from gastrointestinal leiomyosarcomas: CT features. Radiology. 2003;227:385–90.

103. Rha SE, Ha HK, Lee SH, et al. CT and MR imaging findings of bowel ischemia from various primary causes. Radiographics. 2000;20:29–42.

104. Roggeveen MJ, Tismenetsky M, Shapiro R. Ulcerative colitis. Radiographics. 2006;26:947–51.

105. Rozenblit A, Morehouse HT, Stephen Amis Jr E. Cystic adrenal lesions: CT features. Radiology. 1996;201: 541–8.

106. Rybicki FJ. The WES, sign. Radiology. 2000;214: 181–2.

107. Sahani DV, Kadavigere R, Saokar A, et al. Cystic pancreatic lesions: a simple imaging-based classification system for guiding management. Radiographics. 2005; 25:1470–84.

108. Scarsbrook AF, Thakker RV, Wass JAH, et al. Multiple endocrine neoplasia: spectrum of radiologic appearances and discussion of a multitechnique imaging approach. Radiographics. 2006;26:433–51.

109. Sebastia C, Quiroga S, Espin E, et al. Portomesenteric vein gas: pathologic mechanisms, CT findings, and prognosis. Radiographics. 2000;20:1213–24.

110. Seo BK, Ha HK, Kim AY, et al. Segmental misty mesentery: analysis of CT features and primary causes. Radiology. 2003;226:86–94.

111. Shanbhogue AKP, Fasih N, Surabhi VR, et al. A clinical and radiologic review of uncommon types and causes of pancreatitis. Radiographics. 2009;29: 1003–26.

112. Shanmuganathan K, Chen JD, Mirvis SE. Imaging blunt hepatic trauma. Appl Radiol. 2000;29:14–22.

113. Sheth S, Ali S, Fishman E. Imaging of renal lymphoma: patterns of disease with pathologic correlation. Radiographics. 2006;26:1151–68.

114. Sheth S, Horton KM, Garland MR, et al. Mesenteric neoplasms: CT appearances of primary and secondary tumors and differential diagnosis. Radiographics. 2003;23:457–73.

115. Silva AC, Beaty SD, Hara AK, et al. Spectrum of normal and abnormal CT appearances of the ileocecal valve and cecum with endoscopic and surgical correlation. Radiographics. 2007;27:1039–54.

116. Silverman SG, Mortele KJ, Tuncali K, et al. Hyperattenuating renal masses: etiologies, pathogenesis, and imaging evaluation. Radiographics. 2007;27:1131–43.

117. Singh AK, Gervais DA, Hahn PF, et al. Acute epiploic appendagitis and its mimics. Radiographics. 2005;25:1521–34.

118. Takahashi N, Brown JJ. MRI of the pancreas. Appl Radiol. 2002;31:17–25.

119. Takeyama N, Gokan T, Ohgiya Y, et al. CT of internal hernias. Radiographics. 2003;25:997–1015.

120. Tan L, Stoker J, Zwamborn AW, et al. Female pelvic floor: endovaginal MR imaging of normal anatomy. Radiology. 1998;206:777–83.

121. Theoni RF. The revised Atlanta classification of acute pancreatitis: its importance for the radiologist and its effect on treatment. Radiology. 2012;262(3):751–64.

122. Thoeni RF, Cello JP. CT imaging of colitis. Radiology. 2006;240:623–38.

123. Torrisi JM, Schwartz LH, Gollub MJ, et al. CT findings of chemotherapy-induced toxicity: what radiologist need to know about clinical and radiologic manifestations of chemotherapy toxicity. Radiology. 2011;258:41–6.

124. Turner MA, Fulcher AS. The cystic duct: normal anatomy and disease processes. Radiographics. 2001;21:3–22.

125. Urrutia M, Mergo PJ, Ros LH, et al. Cystic masses of the spleen: radiologic-pathologic correlation. Radiographics. 1996;16:107–29.

126. van Breda Vriesman AC. The hyperattenuating ring sign. Radiology. 2003;226:556–7.

127. Vikram R, Ng CS, Tamboli P, et al. Papillary renal cell carcinoma: radiologic-pathologic correlation and spectrum of disease. Radiographics. 2009;29:741–57.

128. Wagner BJ, Wong-You-Cheong JJ, Davis CJ. Adult renal hamartomas. Radiographics. 1997;17:155–69.

129. Warshauer DM, Lee JKT. Imaging manifestation of abdominal sarcoidosis. Am J Roentgenol. 2004;182:15–28.

130. Wiesner W, Khurana B, Ji H, et al. CT of acute bowel ischemia. Radiology. 2003;226:635–50.

131. Wittenberg J, Harisinghani MG, Jhaveri K, et al. Algorithmic approach to CT diagnosis of the abnormal bowel wall. Radiographics. 2002;22:1093–109.

132. Wong-You-Cheong JJ, Wagner BJ, Davis CJ. Transitional cell carcinoma of the urinary tract: radiologic- pathologic correlation. Radiographics. 1998;18:123–42.

133. Yamakado K, Tanaka N, Nakagawa T, et al. Renal angiomyolipoma: relationships between tumor size, aneurysm formation, and rupture. Radiology. 2002;225:78–82.

134. Yoo E, Kim JH, Kim MJ, et al. Greater and lesser omenta: normal anatomy and pathologic processes. Radiographics. 2007;27:707–20.

135. Yoon W, Jeong YY, Kim JK, et al. CT in blunt liver trauma. Radiographics. 2005;25:87–104.

136. Yu JS, Kim KW, Lee HJ, et al. Urachal remnant diseases: spectrum of CT and US findings. Radiographics. 2001;21:451–61.

Part IV

Reproductive System

Female

18

Contents

R. Agarwala, *Atlas of Emergency Radiology:*
Vascular System, Chest, Abdomen and Pelvis, and Reproductive System,
DOI 10.1007/978-3-319-13042-2_18, © Springer International Publishing Switzerland 2015

Infection

Diagnosis
Pelvic Inflammatory Disease (Infection of the Upper Female Genital Tract: Endometrium, Fallopian Tubes, and Ovaries)

Imaging Features
Salpingitis, pyosalpinx, tubo-ovarian abscess, and endometritis

Early:

1. Mild pelvic edema with haziness of the pelvic fat and thickening of the uterosacral ligaments.
2. Salpingitis—inflammatory thickening, enhancing fallopian tubes which are not dilated.
3. Oophoritis—enlarged ovaries with indistinct contours and periovarian fluid or polycystic appearance.

4. Endometritis—thick hypoechoic endometrium with increased vascularity by US. CT also shows thick endometrium with increased enhancement.

Advanced:

1. Pyosalpinx—distention of obstructed fallopian tubes with echogenic fluid by US and enhancing walls by CT.
2. Tubo-ovarian and pelvic abscess—thick-walled solid-cystic mass, septations, complex fluid, and rarely gas collection.
3. Reactive changes in the adjacent sigmoid colon and small bowel with wall thickening and ileus. The ureters may be obstructed.

Diagnosis
Early PID

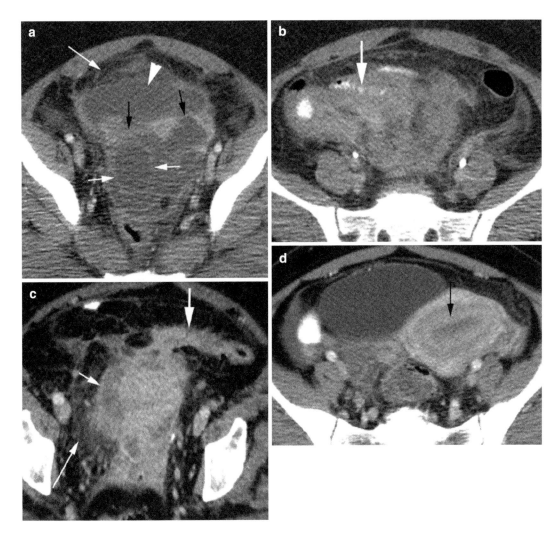

Fig. 18.1 Early pelvic inflammatory disease in different patients. Axial CT (**a**) shows thickening of the broad ligaments (*black arrows*), oophoritis of the right ovary (*short white arrows*) which is enlarged with indistinct borders, diffuse pelvic fluid collection (*arrowhead*), and diffuse haziness of pelvic fat (*long white arrow*). (**b**) Reactive wall thickening of the distal small bowel (*thick arrow*). (**c**) Reactive wall thickening of the sigmoid colon (*thick arrow*). Mild salpingitis as seen by dilated, thick-walled right fallopian tube (*short arrow*) and diffuse inflammatory changes with haziness of pelvic fat (*long arrow*). (**d**) Endometritis with thick enhancing endometrium (*arrow*) with simple endometrial fluid

Diagnosis

Hydrosalpinx and Pyosalpinx

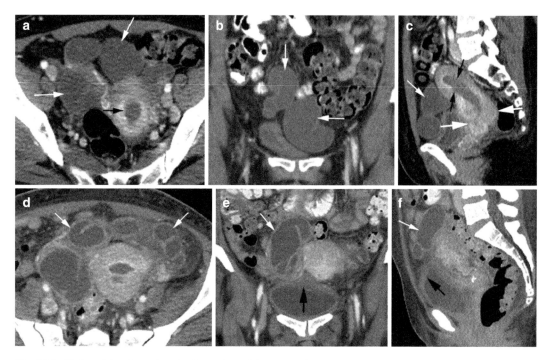

Fig. 18.2 Hydrosalpinx from chronic obstruction of the cervix by adenosquamous carcinoma. CECT (**a**) axial, (**b**) coronal, and (**c**) sagittal reformatted images show dilated bilateral fallopian tubes without wall thickening or enhancement (*white arrows*). Fluid distending the endometrial canal (*black arrows*) due to outlet obstruction. Soft tissue mass is identified constricting the cervical canal (*thick white arrows*). (**d–f**) Pyosalpinx with leuko-cytosis and clinical signs of infection following chemo- and radiation therapy of the same patient. CECT (**d**) axial, (**e**) coronal, and (**f**) sagittal reformatted images show PID with wall thickening of the previously seen hydrosalpinx (*white arrows*), diffuse increased density of pelvic adipose tissue between the fallopian tubes, and cystitis with thick-walled bladder (*thick arrow*)

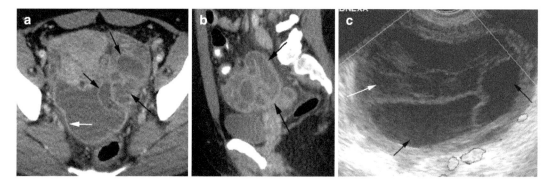

Fig. 18.3 Advanced PID with pyosalpinx and focal peritonitis. CT axial (**a**) and sagittal reformatted (**b**) images show conglomeration of the dilated left fallopian tube (*black arrows*) with enhancing thick wall and fluid in posterior cul-de-sac surrounded by enhancing peritoneum (*white arrow*). (**c**) Endovaginal ultrasound of the left adnexa shows dilated fallopian tube (*black arrows*) with adjacent echogenic fluid (*white arrow*) as seen in CT

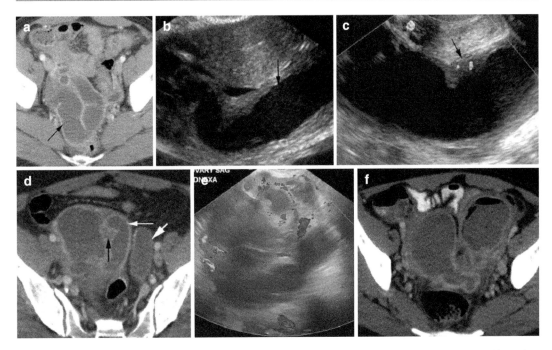

Fig. 18.4 Pyosalpinx in three patients. (**a–c**) First patient with gonorrhea: (**a**) Axial CT shows dilated right fallopian tube with thick enhancing wall (*arrow*). (**b**) Endovaginal grayscale US examination shows the right fallopian tube is distended with echogenic fluid (*arrow*). (**c**) Color Doppler study shows increase color flow within the thickened tubal wall. (**d–f**) Second patient with right lower quadrant pain: (**d**) Axial CT shows right-sided pyo-salpinx with dilated thick enhancing walls (*thin white arrow*) and increased fat stranding (*black arrow*). The left fallopian tube shows hydrosalpinx (*thick arrow*) with no wall enhancement. (**e**) Color Doppler US of the right adnexa shows dilated right fallopian tube with increased flow around it. Third patient: (**f**) Axial CT shows bilateral pyosalpinx with gas and fluid in the left fallopian tube post chromopertubation

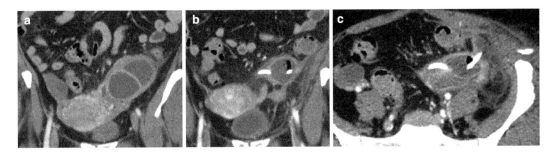

Fig. 18.5 Pyosalpinx with drain. (**a**) Coronal reformatted CT shows dilated thick-walled left fallopian tube. (**b, c**) Coronal reformatted and axial CT at a later date show insertion of drainage tube with gas within the fallopian tube

Diagnosis

TOA

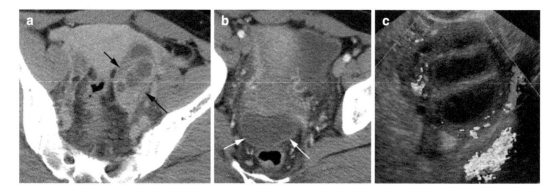

Fig. 18.6 Tubo-ovarian abscess from advanced PID. CT axial (**a**) shows multiple thick-walled fluid collections in the left adnexa (*arrows*). (**b**) shows posterior cul-de-sac fluid collection with enhancing peritoneum (*arrows*). (**c**) Endovaginal color Doppler US shows thick-walled cystic collection with thick septations in the left adnexa with increased vascularity

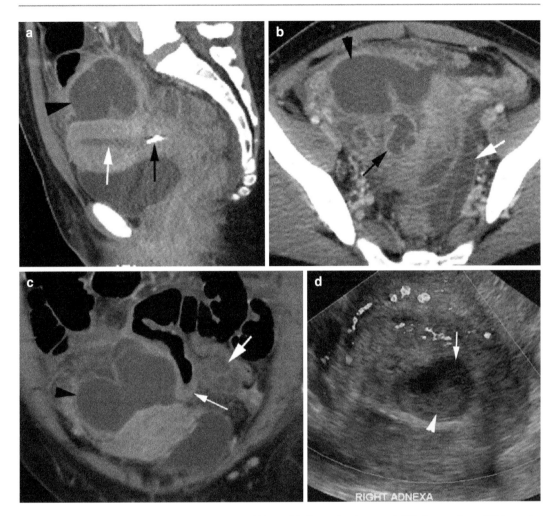

Fig. 18.7 Tubo-ovarian abscess (TOA) following IUD removal and retained fragment. (**a**) Sagittal reformatted CT shows a piece of retained IUD in the lower uterine segment (*thin black arrow*) with fluid (*thin white arrow*) in the endometrial cavity. (**b**) Axial CT shows large TOA with complex fluid collection in the right adnexa (*arrowhead*) surrounding the pyosalpinx (*black arrow*). Pyosalpinx on the left side (*white arrow*) is more dilated. (**c**) Coronal reformatted CT shows a large TOA on the right side (*arrowhead*) and a smaller one on the left (*thick white arrow*) with thick-walled small bowel (*thin white arrow*) in between. (**d**) Color Doppler ultrasound shows increased vascularity of the solid area in the right adnexa surrounding the abscess cavity (*thin arrow*) with echogenic debris (*arrowhead*)

Diagnosis
Endometritis

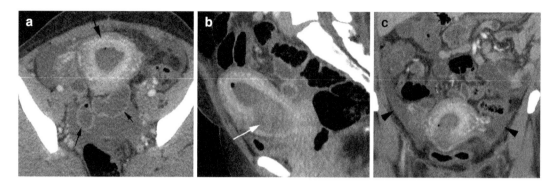

Fig. 18.8 Endometritis with septic shock post dilatation and curettage. CT axial (**a**), sagittal (**b**), and coronal (**c**) reformatted images show thickened avidly enhancing endometrium (*thick black arrow*). The endometrial cavity is distended with heterogeneous hemorrhagic fluid (*white arrow*) and small focus of gas. Surrounding small bowel loops show reactive ileus (*thin black arrows*). A small amount of ascites is seen in the lower abdomen and pelvis, but the peritoneum is not enhancing (*arrowhead*), indicating absence of peritonitis

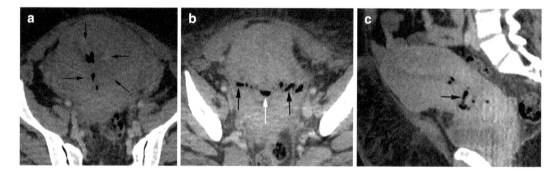

Fig. 18.9 Endometritis. Patient with chorioamnionitis had crash C-section with wound and endometrial infection following surgery. CT axial image (**a**) shows gas and irregular heterogeneous fluid collection in the endometrial cavity (*arrows*). (**b**) The gas linearly arranged in the surgical myometrial wound (*black arrows*) is continuous with endometrial gas (*white arrow*). Sagittal reformatted image (**c**) shows gas and fluid in the endometrial cavity extending to the anterior myometrium in the lower uterine segment (*arrow*)

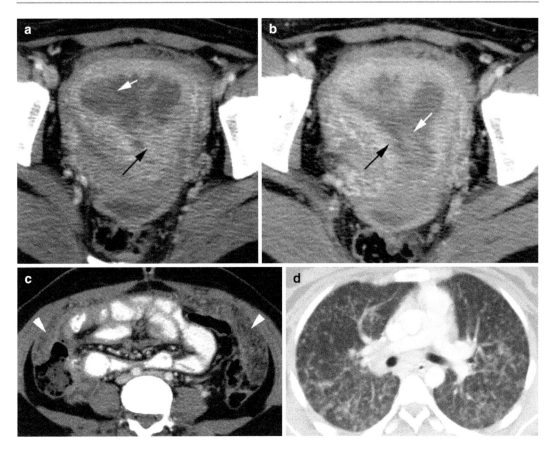

Fig. 18.10 Tuberculous endometritis: Axial CT (**a**, **b**) of uterus at different levels shows distended endometrial cavity with heterogeneous fluid (*white arrow*). The endometrium is thick and irregular (*black arrow*). (**c**) Axial CT in the mid-abdomen shows thick omentum with increased markings (*arrowheads*). (**d**) Lung bases show miliary TB in random distribution of nodules

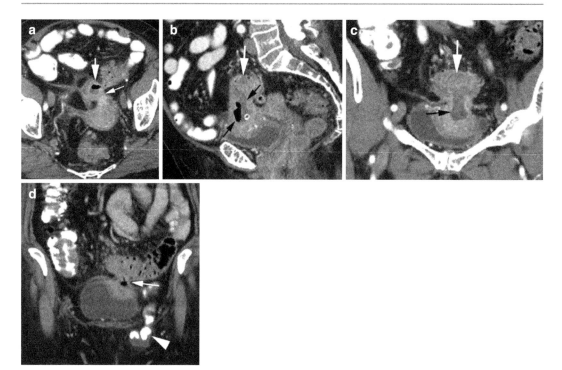

Fig. 18.11 Diverticulitis with fistula to uterus. CT axial (**a**), sagittal (**b**), and coronal (**c**, **d**) reformatted images show large fistula (*thin white arrow* in **a**, **d**) with fluid and gas (*black arrows*) extending from the sigmoid colon (*thick white arrows*) to the fundus of the uterus. Small bowel hernia is seen in the left inguinal canal (*arrowhead* in **d**)

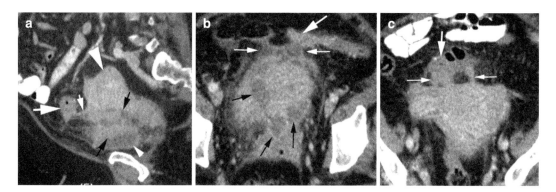

Fig. 18.12 Diverticulitis resembling PID in uterovesical pouch. Sagittal reformatted CT (**a**) shows a tract (*thin white arrow*) from the sigmoid colon (*thick white arrow*) into the anterior cul-de-sac, the space between the uterus (*thick arrowhead*) and bladder (*thin arrowhead*) which is filled with irregular soft tissue density and fluid (*thin black arrows*). (**b**, **c**) Axial CT shows the same heterogeneous multiloculated fluid collection (*black arrows*) in the anterior cul-de-sac. Linear tracts (*thin white arrows*) are again seen from the colon (*thick arrow*) extending inferiorly to the fundus of the uterus

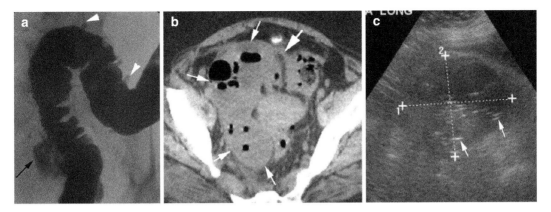

Fig. 18.13 Diverticulitis with fistulous communication with ovarian cyst. (**a**) Barium enema examination shows extravasation of contrast from the distal sigmoid colon (*black arrow*). Multiple diverticula are also present in the rest of the sigmoid colon (*arrowheads*). (**b**) Axial CT shows a large mass in the right adnexa with multiple air-fluid collections (*thin arrows*) with a connection to the colon (*thick arrow*). (**c**) Grayscale endovaginal US reveals a large heterogeneous mass in the right adnexa (*cursors*) with numerous echogenic foci of gas collection (*arrows*). At surgery, a 5 cm right adnexal inflammatory cystic mass replacing the ovary was seen with fistula with the sigmoid colon

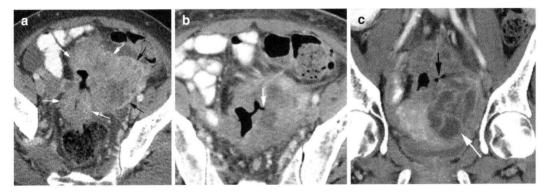

Fig. 18.14 Sigmoid cancer infiltrating to the left ovary with TOA. (**a**) Axial CT shows sigmoid colon cancer with wall thickening (*white arrows*). The sigmoid mass is extending to the left ovary (*black arrows*) with central necrosis and displaced follicles. (**b**) Axial CT shows fistulous tract to the left ovary (*arrow*) from the affected sigmoid colon. (**c**) Coronal reformatted image shows the fistula (*black arrow*) over the left TOA (*white arrow*)

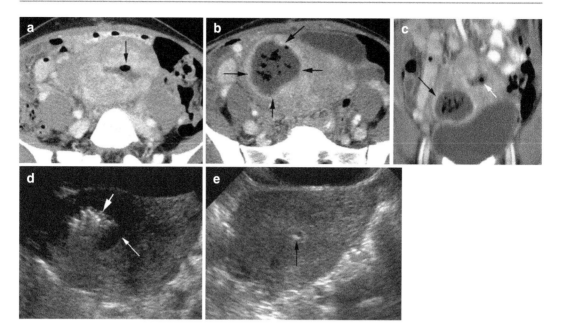

Fig. 18.15 Post-myomectomy infection and endometritis. CT (**a**) axial image shows fluid and gas collection in the endometrial cavity (*arrow*). (**b**) Axial image at a lower plane and (**c**) coronal reformatted image show a thick-walled intramural abscess with fluid and gas collection at the myomectomy site (*black arrows*) in the anterior body of the uterus separate from the endometrial fluid and gas (*white arrow* in **c**). Grayscale endovaginal US (**d**) shows intramural pocket of fluid (*thin arrow*) and high echogenic gas collection (*thick arrow*) within the uterus on the right. (**f**) Echogenic focus in the endometrial cavity (*arrow*) due to gas as seen in the CT study

Diagnosis
Hemorrhagic Ovarian Cyst

Imaging Features

US:

1. Can appear as solid nodule with concave outer margin and with no internal vascularity
2. Reticular pattern from fibrin strands
3. Can have a fluid level

CT:

1. High density within cyst, homogeneous or heterogeneous
2. Can have hematocrit level
3. Can rupture into the peritoneal cavity and cause hemoperitoneum

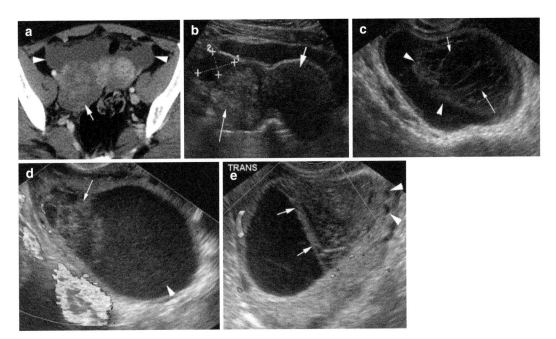

Fig. 18.16 Acute hemorrhage in the ovary in two patients with acute pelvic pain. Patient 1: (**a**) Axial CT shows heterogeneous density of the right ovary cyst (*arrow*) with small hemoperitoneum (*arrowheads*). (**b**) Transverse grayscale US is similar to the CT image. The right ovary is filled with echogenic clot (*thin arrow*) with small adjacent hemorrhagic fluid (*cursors*). The uterus (*thick arrow*) is less echogenic than the hemorrhage. Second patient with bilateral acute hemorrhage in ovary cysts: (**c**) Grayscale US shows retracted clot (*arrowhead*) with fibrin strands giving a lacy pattern (*arrow*) in the right ovary. (**d**) Color Doppler study shows no flow within the clot. The retracted portion has heterogeneous echogenicity (*arrow*) while the rest of the cyst has low echogenic hemorrhage (*arrowhead*). (**e**) The left ovary shows clot retraction with flat-free surface (*arrow*). The hemorrhagic cyst is displacing the follicles (*arrowheads*) of the rest of the ovary

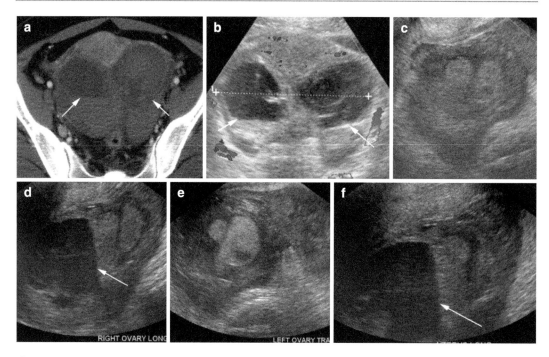

Fig. 18.17 Acute hemorrhagic ovarian cyst in a patient with systemic lupus erythematosus. (**a**) Axial CT image shows high-attenuating acute hemorrhagic fluid with hematocrit level in both ovaries (*arrows also in b*). (**b**) A transverse image from endovaginal sonogram shows simi-lar findings to the CT. (**c–f**) Transverse and longitudinal images of the right and left ovaries, respectively, show heteroechoic hemorrhage in both ovaries with hematocrit level (*arrows*)

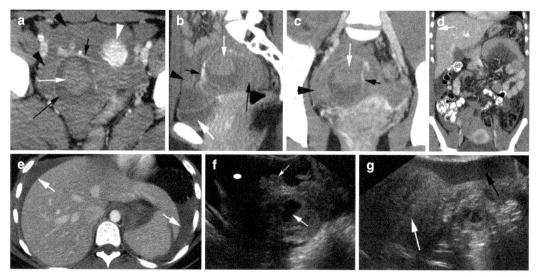

Fig. 18.18 Ruptured corpus luteum cyst in two patients. Patient 1: CT axial (**a**), sagittal (**b**), and coronal (**c**) refor-matted views show a large corpus luteum cyst with promi-nent vessels on the cyst wall (*short black arrow*) which are continuous with the uterine artery (*short black arrow* in **b**, **c**). Large thrombus is within the cyst (*thin white arrow*) and hemorrhagic fluid posterior to the thrombus (*long black arrow*). Sentinel clot (*black arrowheads*) is sur-rounding the uterus (*white arrowhead*) and corpus luteum cyst and is of higher density than urine in the bladder (*thick white arrow*). Coronal reformatted (**d**) and axial (**e**) CT show hemoperitoneum in both paracolic gutters (*arrows*) extending to the subphrenic spaces. Patient 2: Endovaginal US (**f**) shows the corpus luteum cyst (*thick white arrow*) surrounded by echogenic thrombus (*thin arrow*) with peripheral sonolucent fluid (*ellipse*). (**g**) Sentinel echogenic clot (*white arrow*) is surrounded by low-level echogenic hemoperitoneum (*black arrow*)

Diagnosis
Endometrioma

Imaging Features

1. Complex cyst with diffuse low- to medium-level internal echoes with ground-glass appearance
2. Can have fluid/fluid or fluid-debris levels
3. Unilocular or multilocular with thin or thick septations
4. Can have mural irregularity and echogenic foci in the walls, rarely with internal vascularity from endometrial tissue
5. Rarely can be anechoic, heterogeneous echogenicity or calcification

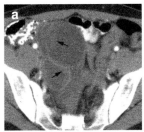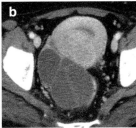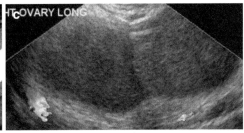

Fig. 18.19 Endometriomas in three different patients. Axial CT (**a**, **b**) shows multilocular cyst in the right adnexa with mural irregularity from adherent thrombus or fibrin in the walls (*arrows* in **a**). (**c**) Endovaginal US shows multilocular cyst with uniform low-level echoes

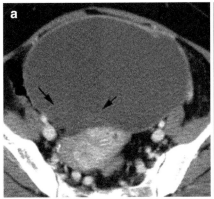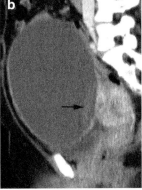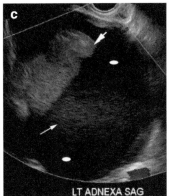

Fig. 18.20 Endometrioma with heterogenicity. CT (**a**) axial and (**b**) sagittal reformatted images show a large low-density cyst with focal-dependent higher-density (*arrows*) debris. (**c**) Endovaginal US shows complex cyst in the left adnexa with nonvascular solid area (*thick arrow*) like dermoid, low-level echoes (*thin arrow*) and anechoic regions (*ellipse*)

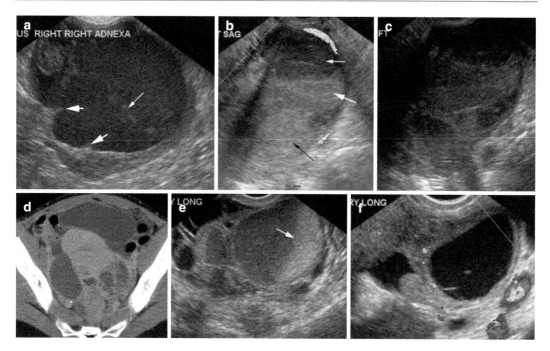

Fig. 18.21 Endometriomas. Case 1: (**a**) endovaginal US shows a large complex cyst with septation (*thin arrow*) and wall nodularity (*thick arrow*). Case 2: US (**b–d**) axial CT show multilocular left adnexal endometrioma with varying degrees of echogenicity (*arrows*). Case 3: endovaginal US (**e, f**) images show an echogenic endometrioma with fluid/fluid level in the right adnexa (*arrow*) and anechoic endometrioma in the left adnexa

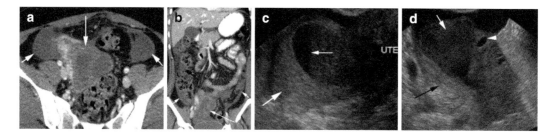

Fig. 18.22 Ruptured endometrioma. (**a, b**) Axial and coronal reformatted CT show multiloculated cyst of the right adnexa (*long arrow*) with hemoperitoneum in bilateral paracolic gutters (*short arrows*). Endovaginal US (**c**) shows fluid/fluid level in the endometrioma (*thin arrow*) with surrounding echogenic hemorrhage (*thick arrow*). (**d**) Low-level internal echoes in the endometrioma (*white arrow*) displacing follicles in the ovary to the left (*arrowhead*) and echogenic hemorrhage posterior to it (*black arrow*)

Diagnosis

Mature Teratoma or Dermoid

Imaging Features

1. Can be purely cystic, mixed mass with components of all three germ layers, noncystic mass mainly with fatty tissue
2. US:
   (a) Cystic mass with densely echogenic mural nodule (dermoid plug) which may produce distal shadowing
   (b) Diffusely or partially echogenic mass may cause air-fluid level
   (c) Curvilinear interface resulting in "tip-of-the-iceberg" sign
   (d) Hyperechoic dots and lines causing dermoid mesh
3. CT—fat attenuation with or without calcification
4. Avascular mass

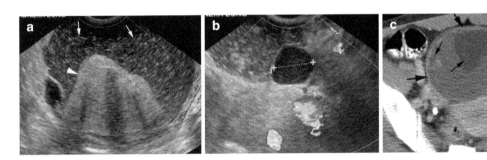

Fig. 18.23 Mature cystic teratoma. Endovaginal color Doppler US (**a**) shows a large cystic mass. Focal increased echogenic area within the posterior aspect is the floating hair ball giving the "tip-of-the-iceberg" sign (*arrowhead*). Diffuse echogenic dots or "dermoid mesh" (*arrows*) are seen scattered throughout the cyst. (**b**) Focal hypoechoic region (*calipers*) with low-level echoes is the loculated sebum. (**c**) Axial CT shows dermoid (*thick arrows*) containing the loculated areas of the sebum with fat attenuation (*thin arrows*)

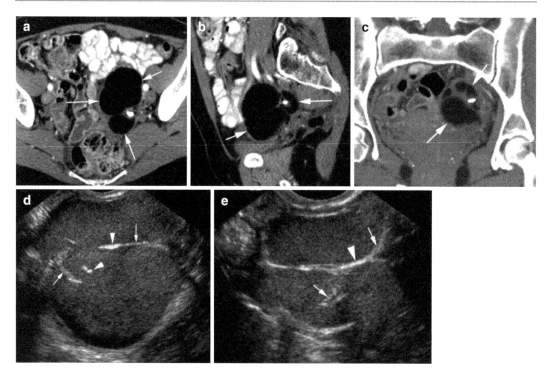

Fig. 18.24 Dermoid. CT axial (**a**), sagittal (**b**), and (**c**) coronal reformatted images show a well-capsulated fatty mass with coarse calcification and septations (*arrows*). US (**d**, **e**) shows the large mass with diffuse low-level echogenicity and thick septations (*arrows*) containing focal areas of calcification with higher echogenicity (*arrowheads*)

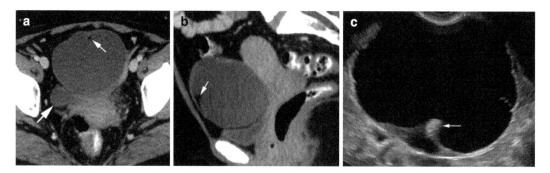

Fig. 18.25 Cystic dermoid. CT axial (**a**) and sagittal reformatted (**b**) images show a large cyst with small focal fatty tissue (*arrow*) arising from the left adnexa. The separate right ovary is seen (*thick arrow*). (**c**) Grayscale US shows a large cyst. Focal echogenicity (*arrow*) corresponds to the focal fatty tissue in the CT study

Complications of Dermoid
1. Malignant transformation
2. Rupture
3. Torsion
4. Infection

Diagnosis
Squamous Cell Carcinoma in Mature Teratoma

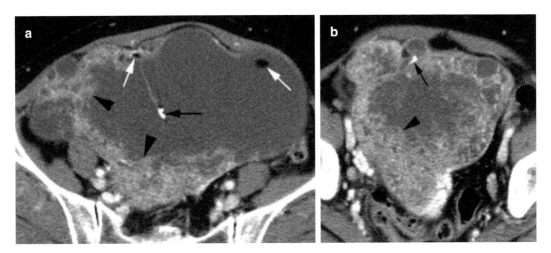

Fig. 18.26 Squamous cell carcinoma in mature cystic teratoma of the ovary. Axial CT at the upper (**a**) and lower (**b**) pelvis shows a large cystic teratoma with focal calcification (*thin black arrows*) and fat globules (*white arrows*).

Diffuse enhancing soft tissues are seen at the periphery (*arrowhead*) more in the lower portion due to malignant transformation

Diagnosis
High-Grade Immature Teratoma

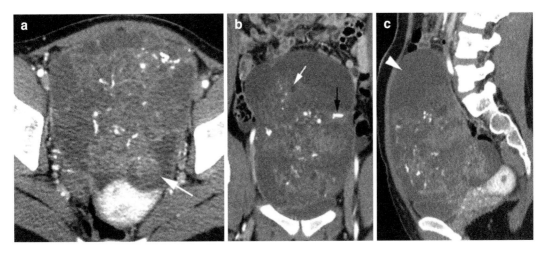

Fig. 18.27 High-grade immature teratoma. CT axial (**a**), coronal (**b**), and sagittal (**c**) reformatted images show a large complex mass arising from the left ovary (*thick arrow*) with cystic spaces (*arrowhead*), scattered calcification (*black arrow*), fatty tissue (*white arrow*), and lobular enhancing soft tissue

Diagnosis
Intraperitoneal Rupture of the Dermoid

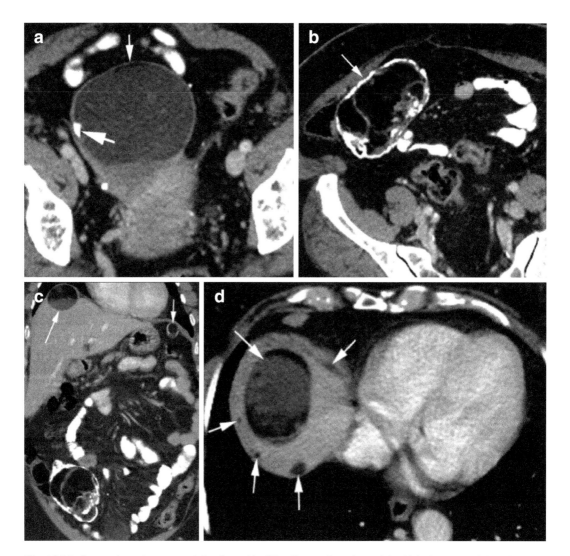

Fig. 18.28 Intraperitoneal rupture of the dermoid. CT axial (**a**) shows a cystic teratoma in the right adnexa with focal calcification (*thick arrow*) and small rim of fat under the capsule (*thin arrow*). (**b**) shows dermoid in the ileocecal region with thick-rimmed calcification and more fatty tissue (*arrow*). (**c**) Coronal reformatted and (**d**) axial CT show multiple dermoids under both hemidiaphragms more on the right side (*arrows*)

Diagnosis
Infected Dermoid

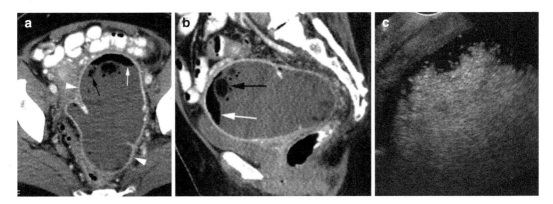

Fig. 18.29 Infected dermoid surgically proven. History of pelvic pain. (**a**) AxialCT and (**b**) sagittal reformatted images show a large dermoid in the left adnexa with thick enhancing capsule (*arrowhead*), layered and speckled gas (*long white arrow*), and also small pockets of fat within this mass (*black arrow*). (**c**) US shows the dermoid as a large cystic mass with echogenic "tip-of-the-iceberg" sign

Paraovarian Cyst

Imaging Features
1. Simple cysts within the broad ligament
2. Separate from the ovary

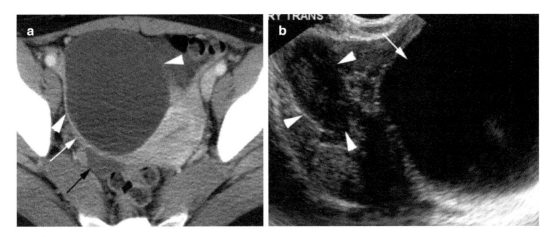

Fig. 18.30 Paraovarian cyst. (**a**) Axial CT shows a large simple cyst (*arrowheads*) in the right side of the pelvis separate from the ovary (*black arrow*) by the round ligament (*white arrow*). (**b**) Ultrasound of the pelvis shows the ovary (*arrowheads*) separate from the anechoic simple cyst (*arrow*). Findings were confirmed at surgery

Ovarian Torsion

Imaging Features

US:

1. Enlarged heterogeneous ovary
2. Displaced follicles to the periphery
3. Little or no arterial flow in the ovary, absent or reversed diastolic flow, normal flow if dual blood supply, and absent central venous flow in nonviable ovary
4. May have underlying ovarian lesion

CT:

1. Fallopian tube thickening or twisted vascular pedicle
2. Wall thickening of torsed cystic ovarian mass which can also have hemorrhage or gas
3. Ipsilateral deviated uterus, ascites

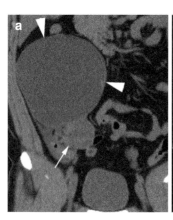 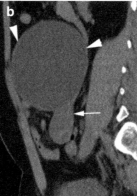 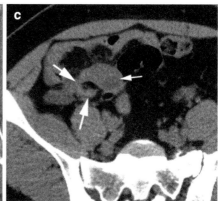

Fig. 18.31 Ovarian torsion. CT (**a**) coronal and (**b**) sagittal reformatted images show a large exophytic cyst (*arrowheads*) from the right ovary (*arrow*). (**c**) Axial CT shows the thick fallopian tube (*thick arrows*) attached to the right side of the ovary (*thin arrow*) with a C-shaped twist. At surgery, the ovary with the fallopian tube had twisted three times and was thrombosed. The cyst was black and hemorrhagic

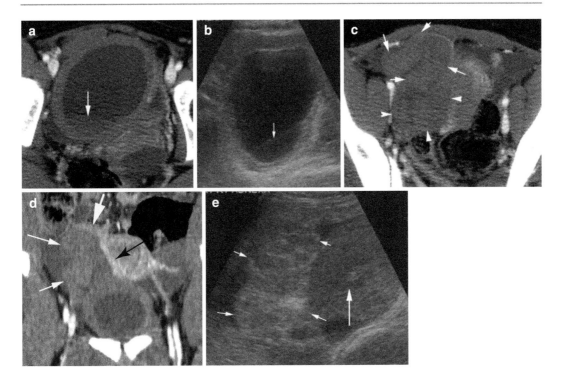

Fig. 18.32 Ovarian torsion. The right ovary was seen at surgery to be posterior to the uterus with unusually long infundibulopelvic ligament which was thick and thrombosed and twisted twice. The ovary and fallopian tube were black. CT axial (**a**) and grayscale US (**b**) show a thick-walled cyst with fluid-debris level (*arrow*). Axial CT (**c**) shows a thick tubular structure with heterogeneous density on the right side of the pelvis (*white arrows*) continuous with the oval area of similar density (*arrowheads*) caused by infarcted fallopian tube and ovary. Coronal reformatted image (**d**) shows infarcted fallopian tube and ovary (*thin white arrows*) with a cyst distally causing extrinsic pressure on the round ligament (*thick white arrow*) and uterus. (**e**) Ultrasound shows the thick echogenic area (*short arrows*) adjacent to the right side of the ovary (*long arrow*) as the conglomeration of the infarcted fallopian tube and ovary (*arrow*)

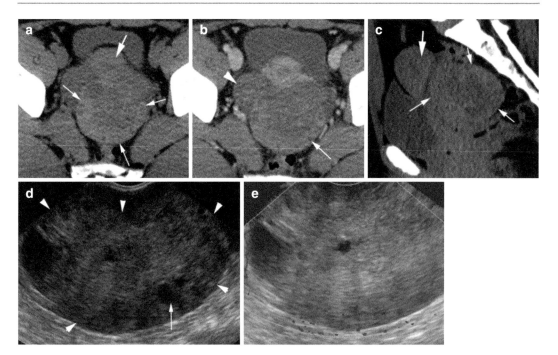

Fig. 18.33 Torsion of the ovary. A patient with left lower pelvic pain. Axial CT (**a**) unenhanced and (**b**) postcontrast study shows a large left ovary (*thin arrows*) with no enhancement and peripherally displaced follicles and central low density posterior to the uterus (*thick arrow*). The ovary has higher attenuation appreciated in the noncontrast study from acute hemorrhage (*arrow head right ovary*). (**c**) Sagittal reformatted image shows large left ovary (*thin arrows*) posterior to the uterus (*thick arrow*). US (**d**) done after the CT shows a large ovary with inhomogeneous echogenicity (*arrowheads*) and displaced follicle (*arrow*). (**e**) Color Doppler study and spectral study (not shown) showed no internal flow. At surgery, the left fallopian tube had twisted twice and the ovary was 10 cm in size and black in color

Ovarian Hyperstimulation Syndrome

Imaging Features
1. Bilaterally enlarged ovaries with multiple cysts of varying size
2. Can have ascites and pleural effusion
3. Can have thromboembolism

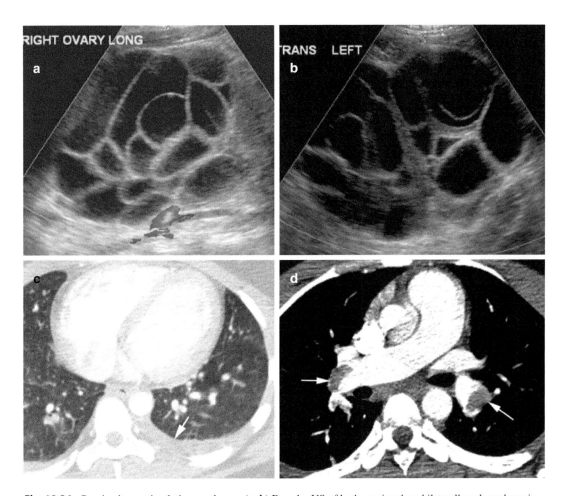

Fig. 18.34 Ovarian hyperstimulation syndrome. (**a, b**) Doppler US of both ovaries show bilaterally enlarged ovaries with multiple cysts and no vascularity of the cyst walls. Axial CT (**c**) shows a small left pleural effusion (*arrow*). (**d**) Axial CT angiogram shows bilateral pulmonary emboli (*arrows*)

Abnormal First Trimester Gestation

Ectopic Pregnancy

Location in decreasing order of frequency—
ampullary, isthmic, fimbrial, interstitial (cornual),
and ovarian sites. Also abdominal, cervical, and
scar pregnancies

Diagnosis
Tubal Pregnancy

Imaging Features
1. Extraovarian adnexal mass
2. Tubal ring with yolk sac and embryo, tubal
   ring with yolk sac, only tubal ring, and
   complex adnexal mass separate from the
   ovary

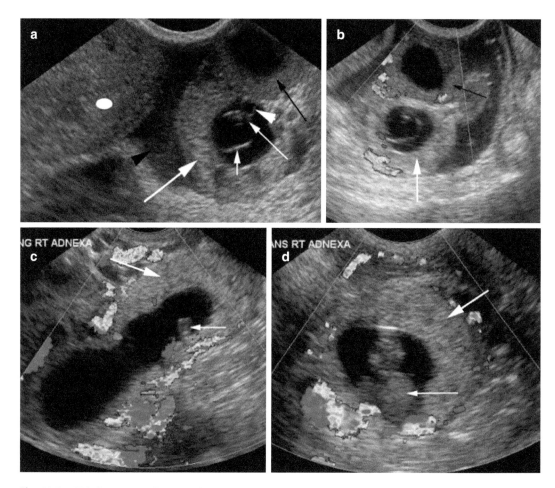

Fig. 18.35 Tubal pregnancy in two patients. Patient 1:
Endovaginal US (**a**, **b**) shows a thick-walled tubal ring
(*thick white arrow*) containing gestational sac with fetal
pole (*thin white arrow*), amnion (*short arrow*), and yolk
sac (*white arrowhead*) separate from the uterus (*ellipse*)
and ovary with corpus luteum cyst (*black arrow*). A small
hemorrhagic fluid with low-level echoes is seen between
the tubal ring and uterus (*black arrowhead*). The corpus

luteum cyst is less echogenic than the tubal ring but more
vascular. At surgery, the tubal pregnancy was partially
ruptured. Patient 2: (**c**, **d**) Color Doppler study shows
dilated thick-walled fallopian tube (*thick arrow*) with
increased vascularity around the fallopian tube. The gestational sac with fetal pole (*thin arrow*) is at the tip of the
tube

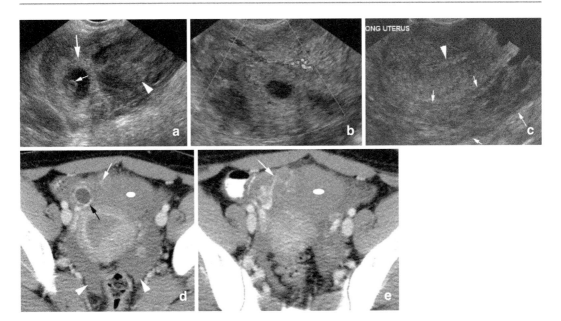

Fig. 18.36 Ruptured tubal ectopic pregnancy. US (**a**) shows the adnexal tubal ring (*thick arrow*) with yolk sac (*thin arrow*) and surrounding echogenic hemorrhage (*arrowhead*). (**b**) Doppler study shows increase vascularity in and around the tubal ring. (**c**) shows hemorrhagic fluid in the posterior cul-de-sac (between *arrows*) with empty endometrium (*arrowhead*). Axial CT shows (**d**, **e**) wall enhancement of the gestational sac (*black arrow*), active extravasation of contrast into the peritoneum (*white arrow*), hemorrhagic fluid in pelvis (*arrowhead*), and high-density sentinel clot around the gestation (*ellipse*)

Diagnosis
Interstitial Pregnancy

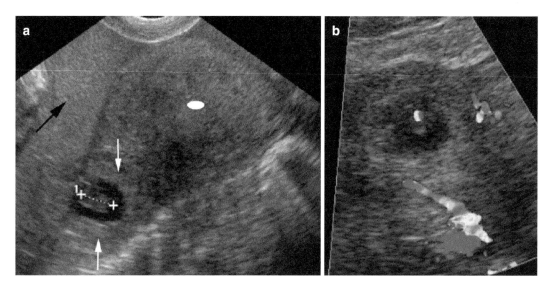

Fig. 18.37 Interstitial pregnancy with rupture. (**a**) Endovaginal US shows an eccentrically located thick-walled gestational sac with fetal pole (*calipers*) surrounded by a thin mantle of myometrium (*arrows*) at the fundus of the uterus (*ellipse*). The hemorrhagic fluid (*black arrow*) surrounds the empty uterus (*ellipse*). (**b**) Doppler study shows flow within the fetal pole

Diagnosis
Cervical Ectopic

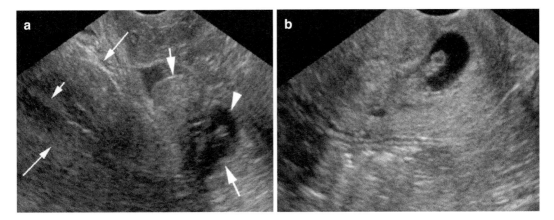

Fig. 18.38 Cervical ectopic gestation. US (**a**) shows hourglass-shaped uterus (*long thin arrows*) with normal endometrial stripe (*short arrow*) and expansion of the cervix (*thick arrows*) with gestational sac (*arrowhead*). (**b**) shows a gestational sac with fetal pole and yolk sac in the cervix

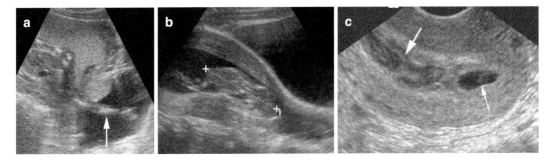

Fig. 18.39 Inevitable abortion in three patients. (**a**) Patient 1: longitudinal US of the uterus shows a 16-week gestation with lower extremity protruding into the vagina (*arrow*) and with little amniotic fluid. (**b**) Patient 2: longitudinal US shows a 13-week fetus (*calipers*) in the cervical canal. (**c**) Patient 3: longitudinal US shows the gestational sac (*thin arrow*) in the cervical canal and the endometrial canal proximal to it distended with hemorrhagic echogenic fluid (*thick arrow*)

Diagnosis
Scar Ectopic

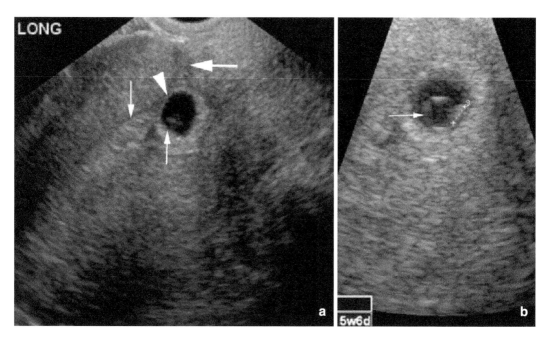

Fig. 18.40 Scar ectopic. Longitudinal ultrasound of the lower uterine segment shows a linear scar tissue (*thick arrow*) anterior to the gestational sac (*arrowhead*). The sac is extrinsic to the endometrium (*thin arrows*) at this site. (**b**) Gestational sac showing yolk sac (*arrow*) and fetal pole (*calipers*)

Diagnosis
Ovarian Ectopic

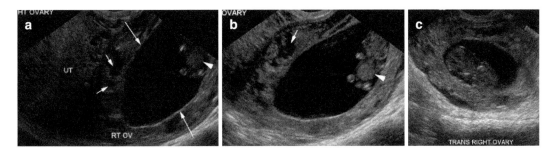

Fig. 18.41 Ovarian ectopic gestation. US (**a**, **b**) shows large gestational sac (*long arrows*) with embryo (*arrowhead*) separate from the uterus. The sac is surrounded by follicles (*short arrows*). (**c**) Gestational sac with embryo in the ovary

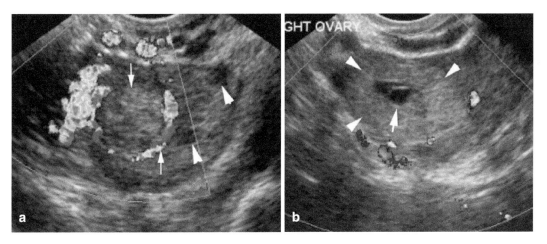

Fig. 18.42 Ovarian ectopic pregnancy: (**a**) Longitudinal US shows a focal echogenic area with surrounding "ring of fire" (*arrows*) within the less echogenic ovary with follicles (*arrowheads*). (**b**) Transverse view shows thick echogenic wall (*arrowheads*) of the gestational sac containing yolk sac (*white arrow*)

Diagnosis
Heterotrophic Gestation

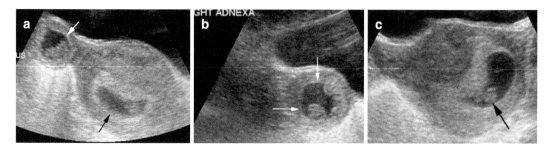

Fig. 18.43 Heterotrophic pregnancy. Transverse US (**a**) shows an intrauterine gestational sac (*black arrow*) and gestational sac in the right adnexa (*white arrow*). (**b**) US of the right adnexa shows ectopic gestation with tubal ring sign (*white arrows*). (**c**) Intrauterine pregnancy with fetal pole (*black arrow*)

Molar Gestation

Diagnosis
Complete Molar Gestation

Imaging Features
1. Central fluid collection in the uterus mimicking anembryonic gestation and missed or incomplete abortion.
2. Complex intrauterine echogenic mass with numerous cystic spaces.
3. Echogenic mass filling the uterine cavity without vesicular appearance.
4. Increased vascularity with venous and low resistance arterial flow.
5. Coexistence of the fetus (dizygotic twin) is rare.
6. In partial mole, the placenta is enlarged with diffuse anechoic lesions; the fetus is usually nonviable or abnormal.
7. Ovarian enlargement with bilateral theca lutein cysts.

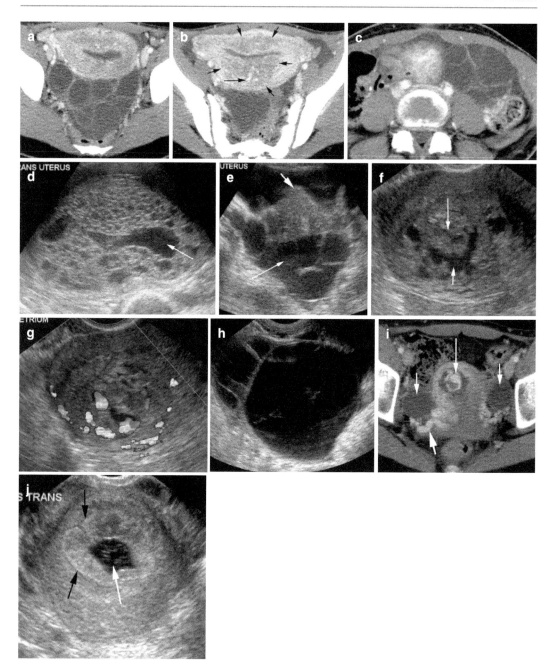

Fig. 18.44 Complete molar gestation and theca lutein cysts (hyperreactio luteinalis) in different patients. Patient 1: Axial CT (**a–c**) shows multiple large cysts in both ovaries. The thick endometrium has low density (*short arrows*) and increased vascularity (*long arrow*). (**d, e**) Endovaginal US of the same patient: (**d**) shows the thickened endometrium filled with multiple anechoic cysts. The endometrial canal contains low echogenic fluid (*arrow*). (**e**) Enlarged right ovary with multiple cysts (*thin arrow*) behind the cervix (*thick arrow*). Patient 2: Endovaginal US (**f**) shows thickened heteroechoic endometrium (*long arrow*) with anechoic fluid in the canal (*short arrow*). (**g**) Color Doppler US shows dilated vessels in the endometrium. (**h**) Multiple large cysts of varying sizes in enlarged left ovary. (**i**) Axial CT shows distended endometrial cavity with dilated vessel (*long arrow*), large right uterine vessels (*thick arrow*), and large cysts in bilateral ovaries (*short arrow*). Patient 3: (**j**) Endovaginal ultrasound shows thick heterogeneous endometrium (*black arrows*). Intermediate echoes in the endometrial fluid (*white arrow*)

Diagnosis
Partial Molar Gestation

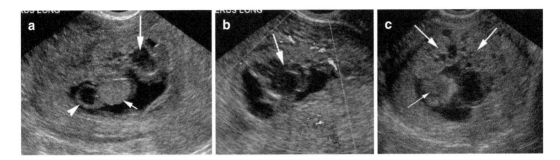

Fig. 18.45 Partial molar gestation. Endovaginal US (**a**, **b**) shows deformed echogenic embryo (*short arrow*) with a thick-walled yolk sac (*arrowhead*). The placenta is heterogeneous with cystic spaces (*long arrow*). The endometrium shows increased vascularity. (**c**) Follow-up US shows increased deformity of the embryo (*thin arrow*) and increased size of placenta with cystic spaces (*thick arrows*)

Anembryonic Gestation

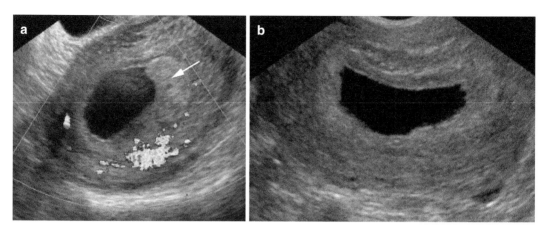

Fig. 18.46 Anembryonic gestation: Endovaginal US in two patients. (**a**) shows normal placenta (*arrow*) with no embryo. (**b**) US on a different patient shows a large gesta-tional sac more than 7 weeks of gestation with empty sac and diffusely thickened endometrium. Beta-hCG levels were not increased

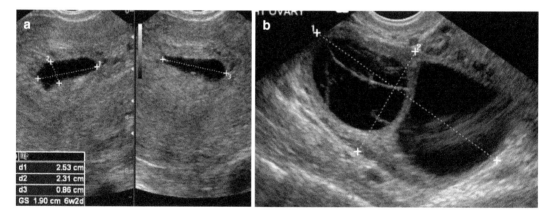

Fig. 18.47 Empty sac with theca lutein cyst of the right ovary and normal beta-hCG levels. Patient was bleeding heavily and passing tissue. Subsequent US showed complete abortion. Endovaginal US (**a**) shows a single gesta-tional sac (*calipers*) more than 6 weeks with no fetal pole and thick endometrium. (**b**) US of the right ovary shows large cysts in the right ovary (*calipers*)

Retained Products of Conception (RPOC)

Imaging Features
1. Thickened endometrial echo complex (EEC) more than 10 mm

2. Higher likelihood of RPOC with endometrial or intrauterine mass
3. Vascularity in EEC or endometrial mass

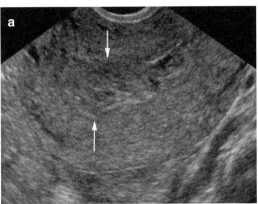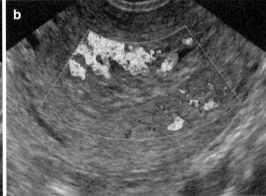

Fig. 18.48 Retained products of conception. A patient with history of recent abortion. (**a**) Endovaginal US shows thick endometrial echo complex (*arrows*). (**b**) Color Doppler image shows increased vascular flow into the EEC

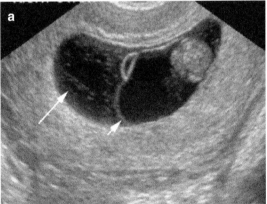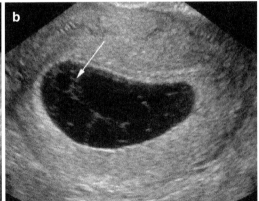

Fig. 18.49 Hemorrhage in the gestational sac. History of painful uterine contractions and vaginal bleeding. (**a**) Longitudinal and (**b**) transverse grayscale US show scattered low-level echoes (*long arrow*) in the gestational sac outside the amnion (*short arrow*) from hemorrhage. The gestation did abort a few hours later. Sac size is 8 weeks 6 days

Traumatic Rupture of Gravid Uterus

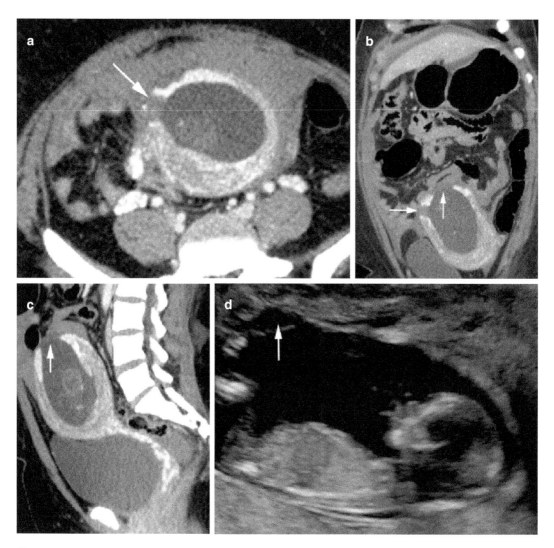

Fig. 18.50 Traumatic rupture of a gravid uterus. CT (**a**) axial, (**b**) coronal, and (**c**) sagittal reformatted images show rupture of the fundus of the uterus at two sites (*arrows*). Small amount of fluid is seen in the subphrenic spaces and right paracolic gutter. (**d**) Longitudinal US shows outward bulging of the anterior wall of the gestational sac (*arrow*)

IUP with IUD

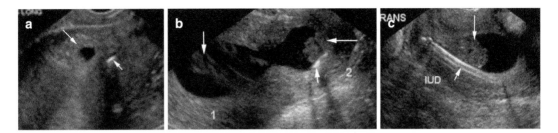

Fig. 18.51 Intrauterine contraceptive device with intrauterine pregnancy in two patients. Patient 1: (**a**) US shows a single gestational sac (*long arrow*) and echogenic IUD inferior to the sac (*short arrow*). Patient 2: (**b, c**) monoamniotic monochorionic twin gestation (*long arrows*) with linear echogenic IUD (*short arrow*) posterior to the sac

Benign Lesions of the Uterus

Diagnosis

Aborting Leiomyoma

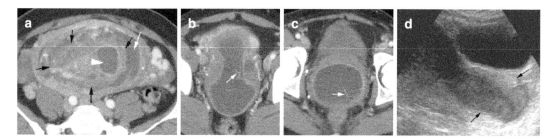

Fig. 18.52 Aborting leiomyoma. Axial CT (**a**) at the upper pelvis shows a large fibroid at the fundus of the uterus with dilated vessels (*black arrows*) and focal circumscribed necrosis (*arrowhead*). Small fluid is seen in the endometrial cavity (*white arrow*). (**b**) At the level of the cervix, the necrotic fibroid with peripheral vessel (*arrow*) distends the cervical canal and protrudes into the vagina. (**c**) At a lower level, the vagina is distended by the necrotic fibroid with a peripheral vessel (*arrow*). (**d**) Longitudinal US shows the cervix to be distended (*arrows*) with heteroechoic degenerating fibroid. At surgery, the aborting fibroid was found

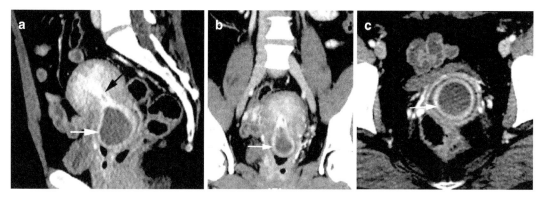

Fig. 18.53 Fibroid prolapse. CT sagittal (**a**), coronal (**b**) reformatted, and axial (**c**) images show a degenerating fibroid with rim enhancement and central necrosis in the vagina (*white arrow*). An enhancing stalk (*black arrow*) is extending from the fibroid to the fundus of the uterus

Diagnosis
Hematocolpos

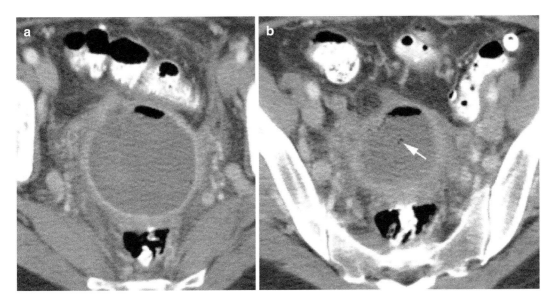

Fig. 18.54 Hematocolpos. Patient had a recent total abdominal hysterectomy with vaginal bleeding and foul-smelling solid material discharge. Axial CT (**a**) and (**b**) at a higher level shows high-density fluid distending the vaginal cuff with air-fluid levels and small gas specks (*arrow*) in the hematoma

Diagnosis
Hematometra

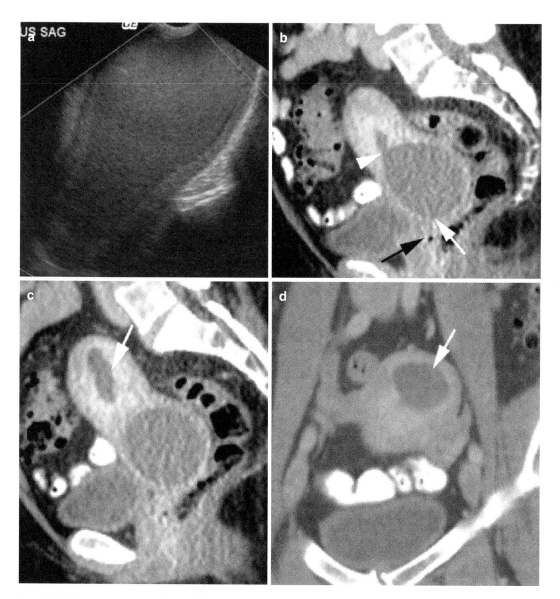

Fig. 18.55 Hematometra. (**a**) Sagittal US views of the uterus show diffuse low-level echoes distending the endometrial cavity. Patient had cervical stenosis from previous biopsy. (**b–d**) CT on a different patient with history of vaginal bleeding. (**b**) Sagittal reformatted CT shows dilated cervical canal above the vagina (*black arrow*) with stenosis at external os (*white arrow*) and internal os (*arrowhead*). (**c, d**) Sagittal and coronal reformatted views show dilated endometrial cavity (*arrow*) above the narrowed internal os. Patient had squamous cell carcinoma in situ at the cervix

Malignant Lesions of the Uterus

Endometrial Malignancy

Diagnosis
Prolapsing Endometrial Stromal Sarcoma

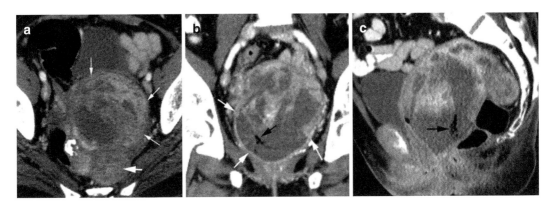

Fig. 18.56 Prolapsing endometrial stromal sarcoma. CT axial (**a**), coronal (**b**), and sagittal (**c**) reformatted images show large necrotic mass (*thin arrows*) in the endometrial cavity protruding into the vagina (*thick arrow*). Gas collections within the mass (*black arrow*) are from recent biopsy

Diagnosis
Endometrial Carcinoma with Bilateral Salpingitis

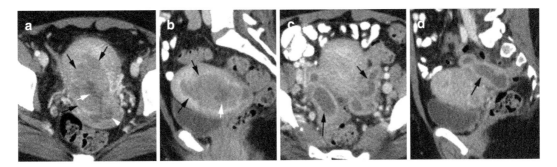

Fig. 18.57 Endometrial carcinoma with bilateral salpingitis. CT axial (**a**) and sagittal reformatted images (**b**) show a low-attenuated soft tissue mass thickening the endometrium (*black arrows*) causing irregularity of the fluid-filled endometrial canal (*white arrow*). Endometrial fluid is flowing into the vagina (*arrowhead*). (**c**) Axial and (**d**) sagittal images at different levels show salpingitis with dilated fallopian tubes showing enhancement of the thick walls (*arrows*)

Diagnosis
Endometrial Carcinoma with Infection

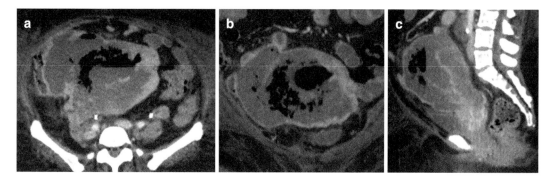

Fig. 18.58 Endometrial carcinoma with *E.coli* infection. CT axial (**a**), coronal (**b**), and sagittal (**c**) reformatted images show enlarged irregular uterus filled with necrotic and heterogeneously enhancing mass with gas collection

Diagnosis
Endometrial Carcinoma with Peritoneal Metastasis

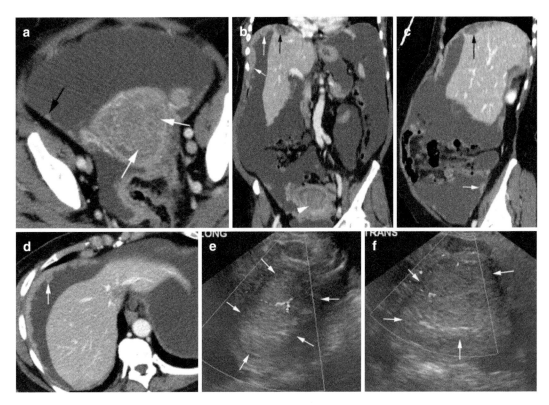

Fig. 18.59 Endometrial cancer with peritoneal metastasis. CT (**a**) axial image shows a mass with increased vascularity thickening the endometrium (*white arrows, arrowhead in b*). Large ascites is seen with small nodular peritoneal metastasis (*black arrow*). (**b**) Coronal, (**c**) sagittal reformatted, and (**d**) axial images show peritoneal nodules at the lower abdominal and pelvic peritoneum (*white arrows*), nodular thickening of the undersurface of the right hemidiaphragm (*white arrows*), and subcapsular nodules of the adjacent liver (*black arrow*). (**e**, **f**) Longitudinal and transverse US views of the uterus show very thick echogenic endometrium with increased vascular flow (*arrows*)

Cervical Carcinoma

Diagnosis
Squamous Cell Cervical Cancer with Outlet
Obstruction

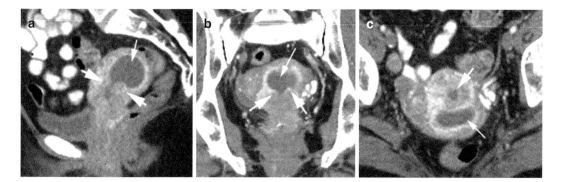

Fig. 18.60 Outlet obstruction of the uterus by squamous cell carcinoma of the cervix. CT sagittal (**a**), coronal (**b**) reformatted, and axial (**c**) images show fluid distending the endometrial cavity (*thin arrow*) of the retroverted uterus due to circumferential constriction of the cervical canal by enhancing mass (*thick arrow*) causing uterine outlet obstruction

Diagnosis
Cervical Cancer with Bladder Invasion

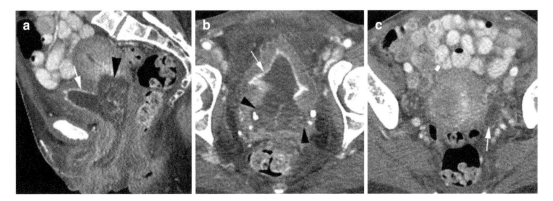

Fig. 18.61 Carcinoma of the cervix with extension to the bladder and left ureteral obstruction. CT (**a**) sagittal reformatted image shows a large necrotic mass in the cervix (*arrowhead also in b*) with extension into the collapsed bladder (*thin arrow*). (**b**) Axial image shows the necrotic mass at the cervix showing rim enhancement (*arrow*) in the bladder extension. (**c**) Axial CT at a higher level shows dilated obstructed ureter (*arrow*)

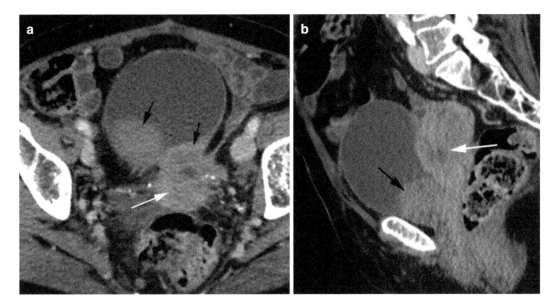

Fig. 18.62 Carcinoma of the cervix invading the urinary bladder. CT (**a**) axial and (**b**) sagittal reformatted images show mass in the cervix (*white arrow*) which is invading into the adjacent bladder (*black arrows*). The bladder is distended with lobulated soft tissue mass at the base (*black arrows*)

Diagnosis

Squamous Cell Cervical Carcinoma with Small
Bowel and Ureteral Fistula

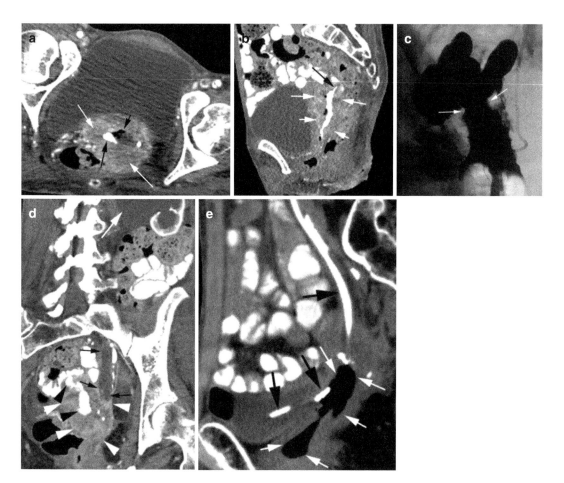

Fig. 18.63 Squamous cell carcinoma of the cervix with small bowel and ureteral fistula. Patient complained of leakage of urine from the vagina. CT (**a**) axial shows a large cervical mass (*long white arrows*). Gas (*short black arrow*) and enteric contrast (*long black arrow*) within the mass are from the enteric fistula. (**b**) Sagittal reformatted image shows enteric contrast leaking from a small bowel loop (*black arrow*) into the necrotic cervical mass (*white arrows*). (**c**) Fistulogram done through rectal tube in the vagina shows a wide neck fistula (*arrows*) between the vagina and small bowel. (**d**) Coronal reformatted image shows the dilated left ureter (*black arrows*) up to the cervical mass (*white arrowheads*) with hydronephrosis (*white arrow*) and the enteric fistula (*black arrowheads*). (**e**) Sagittal reformatted image at later date shows the stent in the ureter (*black arrows*) traversing the gas-filled fistulous space which is continuous with the vagina (*white arrows*)

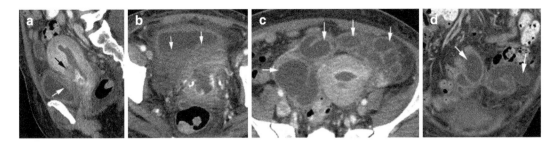

Fig. 18.64 Adenosquamous carcinoma of the cervix with bladder invasion and salpingitis. CT sagittal reformatted (**a**) and axial (**b**) image shows low-density soft tissue mass extending from the lower part of the uterus (*black arrow*) invading the urinary bladder resulting in thickening of the affected bladder wall (*white arrow*). (**c**) Axial and coronal reformatted images (**d**) show bilateral salpingitis with dilated thick-walled fallopian tubes (*arrows*) and haziness of the surrounding fat

Adnexal Lesions

Endometrioid Endometrial Cancer

Diagnosis
Endometrioid   Endometrial   Cancer   of   the
Fallopian Tube

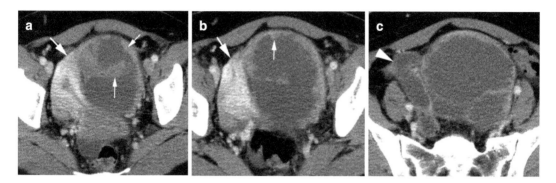

Fig. 18.65 Endometrioid adenocarcinoma of the fallopian tube. History of left lower abdominal pain and dys-
uria. (**a–c**) CT axial images at different levels show the
distal left fallopian tube to be dilated with irregular mural
nodules (*thin arrows*). The proximal part of the tube is
dilated with no nodules (*arrowhead*). The uterus is pushed
to the right (*thick arrow*)

Diagnosis
Endometrioid Endometrial Cancer of the Uterus

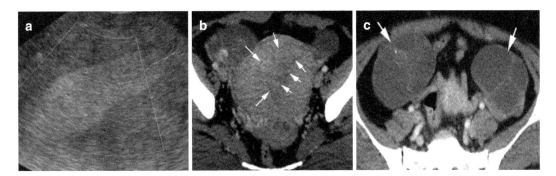

Fig. 18.66 Endometrioid endometrial carcinoma stage IA with concomitant bilateral ovarian benign mucinous cystadenoma, pathology proven. History of lower abdominal pain and weight loss. (**a**) Longitudinal Doppler US of the uterus shows a marked thickening of the endometrium with no vascular flow. (**b**) Axial CT shows a thick endometrium (*short arrows*) with a thin linear lucent line separating the myometrium (*long arrows*). (**c**) Axial CT at a higher level shows complex cysts in both ovaries with thick septations and a punctate calcification in the right ovary (*arrow*)

Ovarian Tumor

Diagnosis
Brenner Tumor of the Ovary

Imaging Features
1. Hypoechoic solid mass of the ovary with high incidence of calcification.
2. Solid component may show mild enhancement.

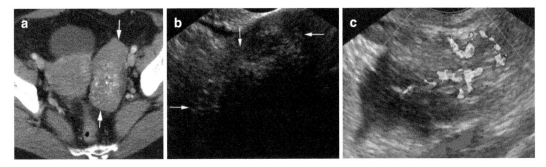

Fig. 18.67 Brenner tumor, benign. (**a**) Axial CT image shows a large solid mass in the left ovary with multiple calcifications (*arrows*). (**b**) Ultrasound shows echogenic punctate calcification in the left ovary (*arrows*) with posterior echo shadowing. (**c**) Doppler study shows increased vascularity of the mass

Cystic Ovarian Malignancy

Imaging Features
1. Cysts with thick septations (>3 mm)
2. Vascularized areas of focal wall thickening of the cyst
3. Irregular solid mass with centrally located flow
4. Ascites, peritoneal, omental, and other organ metastasis

Diagnosis
Collision Tumor

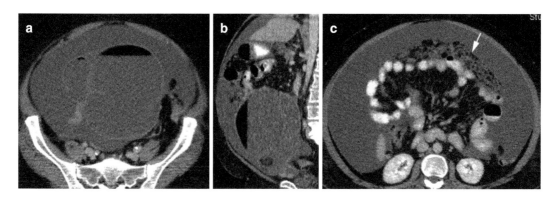

Fig. 18.68 Collision tumor of mature teratoma and serous adenocarcinoma of the ovary. (**a, b**) CT axial and sagittal reformatted images show a large cystic mass with fat-fluid levels and multiple septations. (**c**) Axial CT shows omental metastasis (*arrow*) with reticular pattern. Large ascites is seen in all images

Diagnosis
Adenocarcinoma of the Ovary with Psammoma Bodies

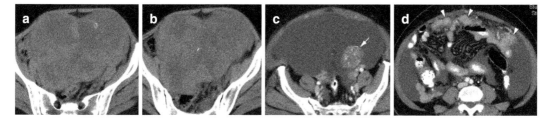

Fig. 18.69 Adenocarcinoma of the ovary with psammoma bodies in two patients. Axial CT in patient 1: (**a, b**) large heterogeneous mass in the pelvis with necrotic low-density areas and a few scattered calcifications. Axial CT in patient 2: (**c, d**) small mass on the left ovary with diffuse calcification, large ascites, and nodular omental metastasis (*arrowheads*)

Diagnosis
Serous Cystadenoma

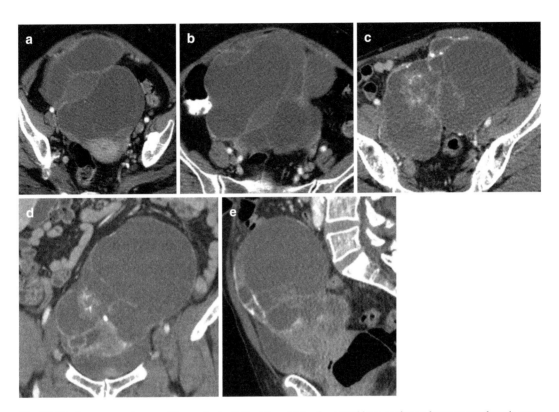

Fig. 18.70 Serous cystadenoma. Two patients. Patient 1: (**a**, **b**) Axial CT at different levels shows a large septated cystic ovarian mass had low malignant potential by pathology. Patient 2: CT (**c**) axial, (**d**) coronal, and (**e**) sagittal reformatted images show a large septated cystic mass with a misty soft tissue around some of the septations and calcification in some septations. This was borderline tumor by pathology

Diagnosis

Serous Mucinous Borderline Tumor

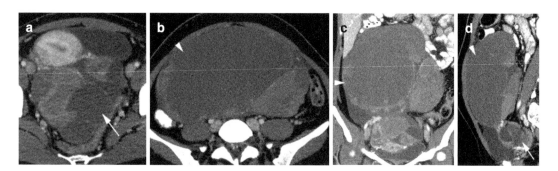

Fig. 18.71 Serous mucinous borderline tumor. CT (**a**, **b**) axial, (**c**) coronal, and (**d**) sagittal reformatted images show complex cystic masses in the right (*arrowhead*) and left ovary (*arrow*) with septations and prominent enhancing solid component

Diagnosis
High-Grade Papillary Serous Carcinoma

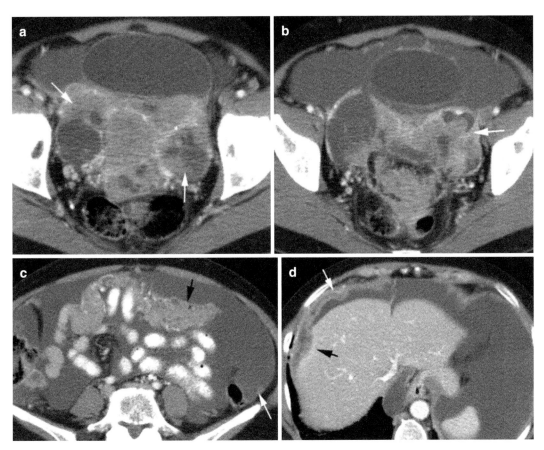

Fig. 18.72 High-grade papillary serous carcinoma. Axial CT of pelvis (**a**) and (**b**) at higher level shows bilateral complex ovarian cystic masses with solid nodules (*arrows*) and large ascites. (**c**) Axial CT at mid-abdomen shows diffusely thickened omentum from metastasis (*black arrow*) and small peritoneal implant (*white arrow*). (**d**) Axial CT at the level of the diaphragm shows peritoneal metastasis to the parietal peritoneum under the diaphragm (*white arrow*) and also the visceral peritoneum over the liver and with subcapsular involvement of the liver (*black arrow*) causing liver parenchymal indentation

Diagnosis
Papillary Serous Ovarian Carcinoma

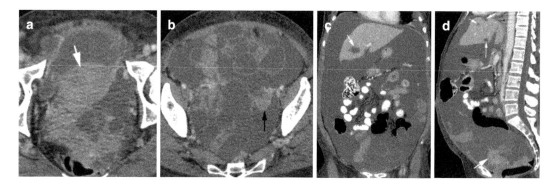

Fig. 18.73 Papillary serous ovarian carcinoma, stage IV. CT axial (**a**, **b**) at a higher level shows large multiloculated cystic mass with irregular enhancing solid component adherent to the septa (*black arrow*). It extends from the posterior cul-de-sac to the level of the umbilicus on the right side of the uterus (*white arrow*). (**c**) Coronal and (**d**) sagittal reformatted images show large ascites, ovarian mass in the lower abdomen, and liver metastasis (*thin arrow*)

Diagnosis
Granulosa Cell Tumor

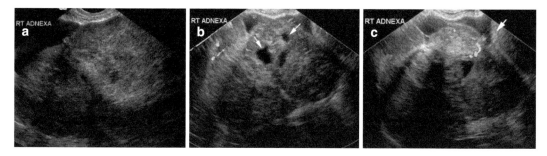

Fig. 18.74 Granulosa cell tumor. US (**a**) shows a large heterogeneous mass in the right adnexa. (**b**, **c**) Color Doppler US shows some cystic spaces (*arrows*) within the solid tissue and a focal area of increased vascularity in the solid area. The uterus is displaced to the left (*arrow* in **c**)

Diagnosis
Mixed Germ Cell Tumor

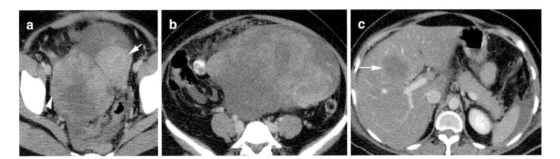

Fig. 18.75 Mixed germ cell tumor. Contrast-enhanced axial CT (**a**, **b**) shows a large heterogeneous ovarian mass (*arrowhead*) displacing the uterus to the left (*arrow*), (**c**) a low-density liver metastasis (*arrow*), and small ascites

Diagnosis
Krukenberg Tumor

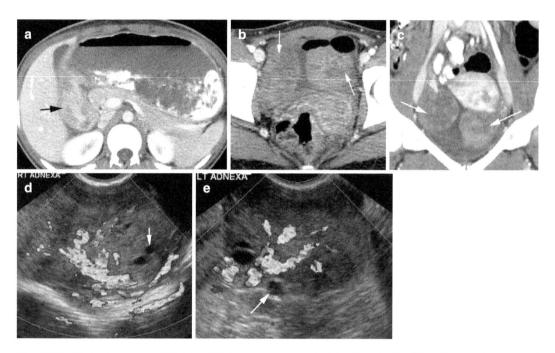

Fig. 18.76 Krukenberg tumor. CT (**a**) axial shows an enhancing mass (*arrow*) at the antrum of the stomach with gastric outlet obstruction. (**b**) Axial and (**c**) coronal reformatted CT of the pelvis show enlarged ovaries bilaterally (*arrow*). Color Doppler US (**d**, **e**) shows enlargement of both ovaries with echogenic solid vascular tissue displacing the follicles (*arrow*) to the periphery

Male

19

Contents

R. Agarwala, *Atlas of Emergency Radiology:*
Vascular System, Chest, Abdomen and Pelvis, and Reproductive System,
DOI 10.1007/978-3-319-13042-2_19, © Springer International Publishing Switzerland 2015

Trauma

Diagnosis
Testicular Rupture

Imaging Features
1. Discontinuity of the tunica albuginea
2. Poorly defined testicular margins
3. Hypoechoic or hyperechoic areas in the testicular parenchyma from hematoma or infarction
4. Decreased or no flow in affected areas
5. Hematocele

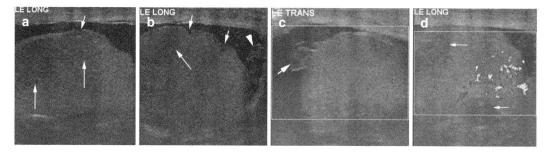

Fig. 19.1 Testicular rupture from gunshot injury. US of the right testis (**a**, **b**) shows discontinuity of the tunica albuginea (*short thin arrows*), hypoechoic regions of hematoma, and edema within the testes (*long thin arrows*) and surrounding hematocele (*arrowhead*). (**c**) The appendix of the testes also has areas of hematoma with decreased echogenicity (*arrow*). (**d**) Color Doppler US shows flow in the normal testicular parenchyma and no flow in the areas of hematoma (*arrows*)

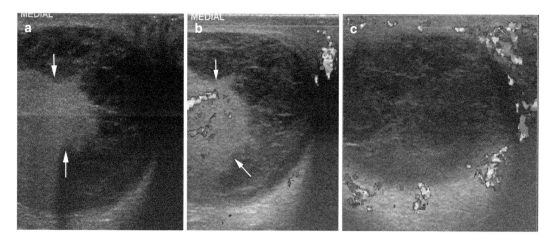

Fig. 19.2 Testicular rupture with hematocele. History of blunt trauma 10 days prior. Grayscale and color Doppler US of the right testis (**a**, **b**) show extrusion of the testicular parenchyma outside the tunica albuginea (between *arrows*) with intact vasculature. Heteroechoic hemorrhagic fluid is seen in the tunica vaginalis space surrounding the protruding testicular contents. (**c**) Scrotal wall shows increased vascularity due to reactive changes from trauma

Diagnosis
Hematocele

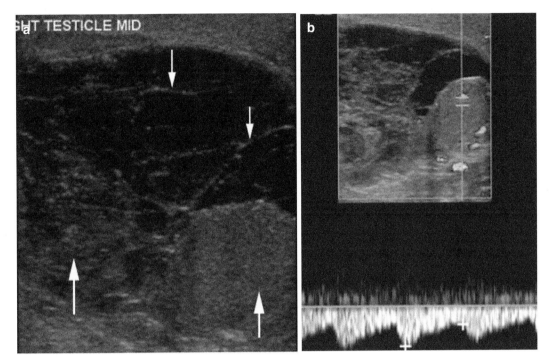

Fig. 19.3 Hematocele. History of gunshot injury of the upper thigh and perineum 2 weeks prior. Sonogram of the right scrotum (**a**, **b**) shows hematocele with solid hematomas (*thick arrows*) and areas of fibrin strands (*thin arrow*).

(**b**) Doppler study shows minimal increase in diastolic flow in the testes from reactive changes with no clinical signs of infection

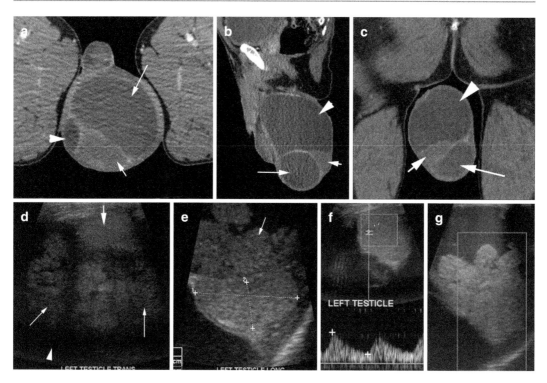

Fig. 19.4 Hydrocele with focal hematoma. History of the enlarging left scrotum with no known trauma. (**a**) Axial and (**b**) sagittal and (**c**) coronal reformatted CT images show high-density hemorrhagic fluid (*long arrow*) and hydrocele (*arrowhead*) surrounding the testes (*short arrow*). Sonogram (**d**, **e**) shows the left testis (*thick arrow* and *caliper*) surrounded by echogenic lobulated thrombus (*thin arrows*) with large hydrocele (*arrowhead*). (**f**) Spectral study (**g**) Color Doppler shows normal flow to the testes and no flow in the hematoma. Pathology showed no evidence of infection or tumor

Diagnosis

Testicular Fracture with Intratesticular Hematoma

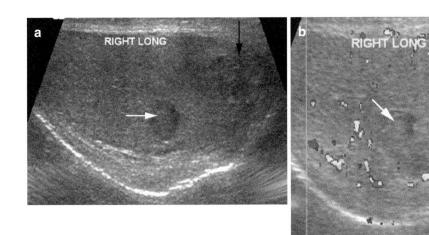

Fig. 19.5 Testicular fracture with intratesticular hematoma from gunshot injury to the penis. Grayscale US (**a**) shows two hematomas, one with increased echogenicity and is well marginated (*white arrow*) and the larger is ill-marginated with irregular low echogenicity (*black arrow*). Tunica albuginea is intact. (**b**) Color Doppler study shows flow around the hematomas (*white and black arrows*) and in the rest of the testicular parenchyma

Diagnosis

Post-trauma Intratesticular Gas

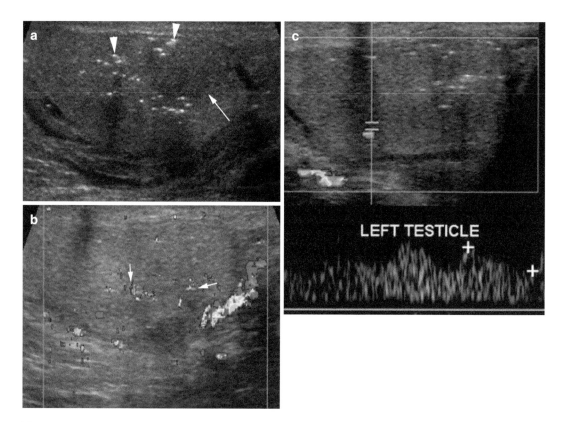

Fig. 19.6 Intratesticular gas post gunshot injury. Grayscale US (**a**) shows scattered punctate, increased echogenicity with faint posterior dirty shadowing from gas (*arrowhead*) in the testicular parenchyma mostly adjacent to the hematoma seen as area of decreased echogenicity (*arrow*). (**b**) Color Doppler US shows twinkling artifacts from the gas (*arrows*). (**c**) Spectral waves are seen to be preserved in the normal parenchyma

Diagnosis
Hematoma Epididymis

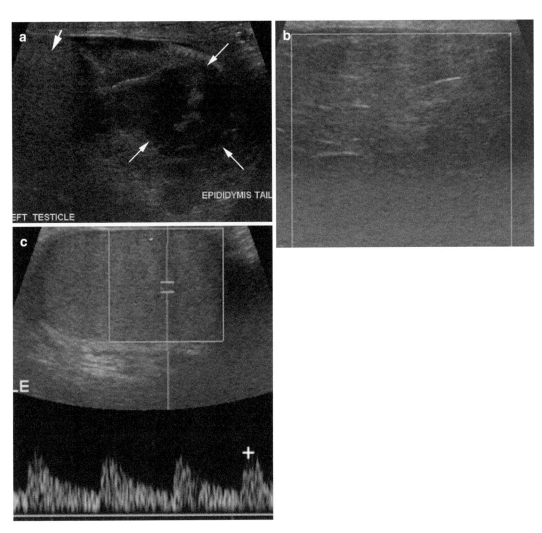

Fig. 19.7 Hematoma tail epididymis. History of blunt trauma. (**a**) Grayscale ultrasound shows a large tail of epididymis with heterogeneous density (*arrows*) with normal uniform echogenicity of the testes (*short arrow*). Color Doppler study (**b**) shows no flow in the epididymis with (**c**) normal spectral flow in the testes

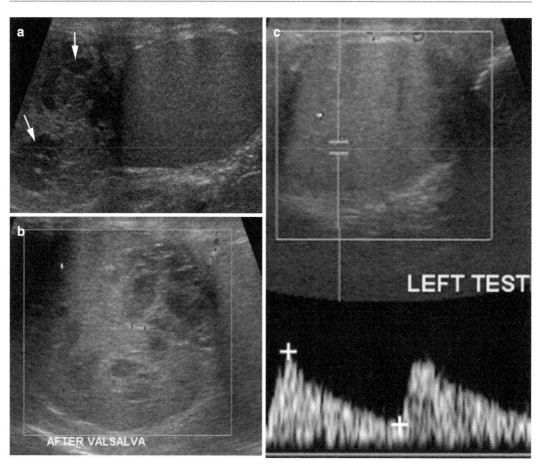

Fig. 19.8 Hematoma of the head of epididymis post-trauma. Sonogram of the left testis. (**a**) Grayscale study shows enlarged head of the left epididymis with multiple well-defined hematomas with low-level echoes (*arrows*). (**b**) Color Doppler shows very little flow is seen in the epididymis. (**c**) The testes shows normal echogenicity and normal spectral waves

Diagnosis

Post-trauma Gas Perineum

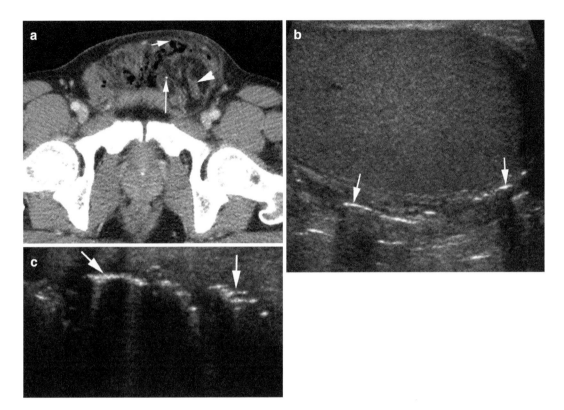

Fig. 19.9 Gas in soft tissue of the perineum from gunshot injury. (**a**) Axial CT shows gas (*short thin arrow*) in the perineum anteriorly. Herniation of the omentum and small bowel is seen in the left inguinal canal (*arrowhead*) and a small metallic fragment (*long arrow*). (**b**, **c**) Grayscale US shows multiple linear focal gas showing increased echogenicity with posterior dirty shadowing in the soft tissues outside the testes (*arrows*)

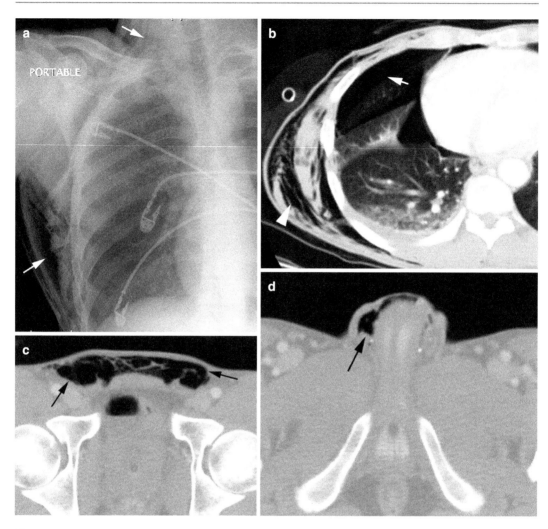

Fig. 19.10 Trauma of the right thorax with pneumothorax and thoracic wall emphysema tracking up to the scrotum. (**a**) Chest radiograph shows air in soft tissues of the thoracic wall (*arrows*). (**b**) CT of the chest shows pneumothorax (*arrow*) and air in the thoracic wall soft tissues (*arrowhead*). (**c**, **d**) Axial CT of the pelvis shows air dissecting down the subcutaneous tissue plane of the anterior abdominal wall (*arrows*) up to the scrotum, more on the right side (*arrow*)

Fig. 19.11 Fournier gangrene in three patients. Patient 1: (**a**) Longitudinal and (**b**) transverse grayscale US views of the scrotum show diffuse scrotal wall thickening with onion skin appearance due to layered edema (*long arrow*) in the fascial planes. Gas in the wall is seen as hyperechoic foci with dirty shadowing (*short arrow* also in **d**). Small hydrocele with strands (*thick arrow*) is also seen. (**c**, **d**) Color Doppler study shows increase flow to the scrotal wall due to cellulitis and to the testis bilaterally from epididymo-orchitis. Patient 2: (**e**) Radiograph of the pelvis shows streaky gas overlying the right scrotum (*arrow*). Patient 3: (**f**, **g**) Coronal and sagittal reformatted CT images show diffuse bilateral scrotal wall swelling with gas streaks (*white arrow*) and contrast-filled herniated small bowel (*arrowhead*)

Infection

Diagnosis
Fournier Gangrene

Imaging Features
1. CT—soft tissue inflammation, fluid and/or abscess, and gas collection
2. US:
   - Thickened and edematous scrotal wall with hyperemia

- Hyperechoic foci with dirty shadowing from gas collections
- May have reactive unilateral or bilateral hydrocele
- Testes and epididymis are often normal

3. Radiography—soft tissue air involving the scrotum or perineum, inguinal region, and anterior abdominal wall

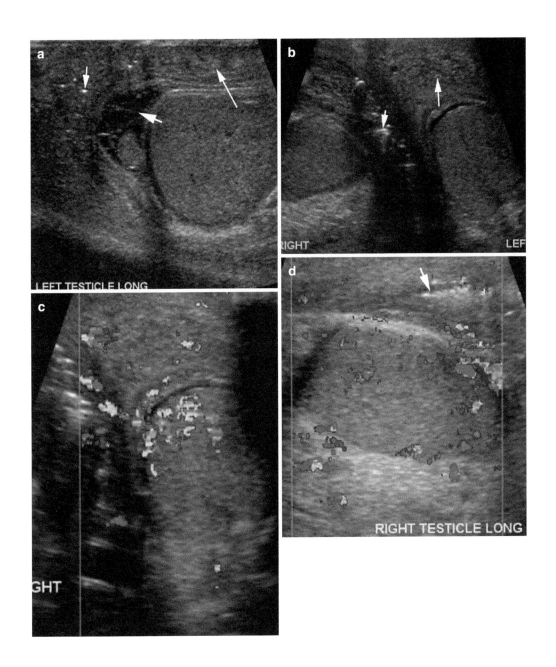

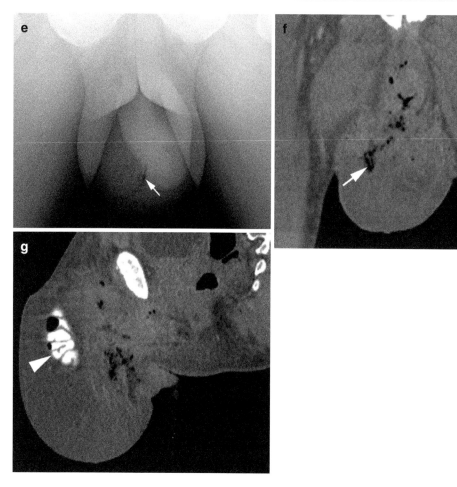

Fig. 19.11 (continued)

Diagnosis
Abscess Scrotal Wall

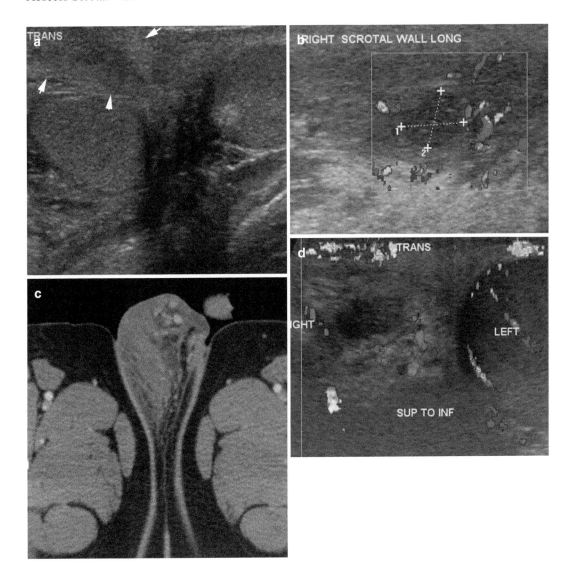

Fig. 19.12 Abscess scrotal wall in three patients. Patient 1: (**a**) Grayscale US shows diffuse wall thickening over the right testis (*arrows*). (**b**) Color Doppler shows increased flow around an avascular abscess (*calipers*) on the same area. (**c**) Axial CT shows increased edema and soft tissue thickening on the right side of the perineum and scrotal wall. Patient 2: (**d, e**) Color Doppler US in transverse and longitudinal views shows large low echogenic abscess (*arrow*) in the median raphe with increased flow around it. Patient 3: (**f**) Color Doppler US shows cellulitis of the left scrotal wall with hyperemia and focal heterogeneous low echogenic abscess with no vascular flow

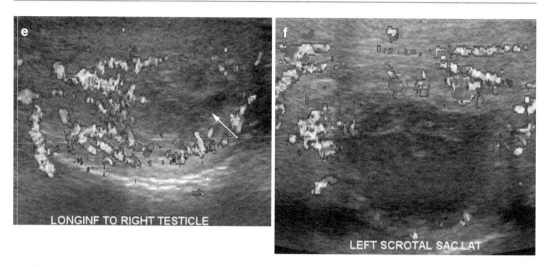

Fig. 19.12 (continued)

Epididymitis, Orchitis, Abscess, and Pyocele

Imaging Features
1. Epididymitis—enlarged epididymis, hypoechoic or hyperechoic, and hyperemia with high-flow, low resistance pattern
2. Orchitis—enlarged testes with heterogeneous echogenicity, hyperemia, and high-flow, low resistance pattern arterial flow and increased venous flow

3. Pyocele—septated or complex heterogeneous hydrocele
4. Abscess—complex heterogeneous fluid collection with surrounding hyperemia

Diagnosis
Intratesticular Abscess

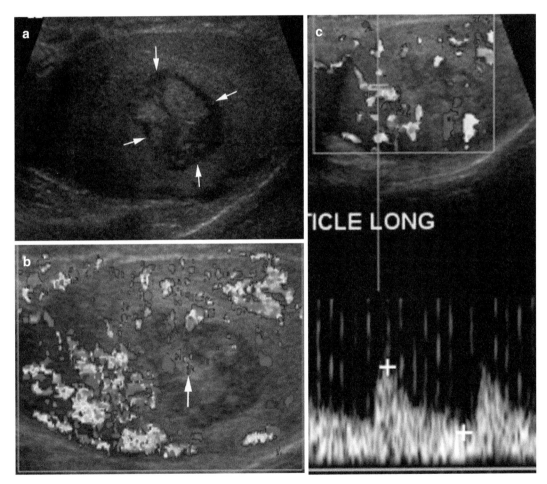

Fig. 19.13 Intratesticular abscess. History of gonorrhea and HIV infection. Grayscale US (**a**) shows a well-marginated intratesticular abscess with internal irregular echogenicity (*arrows*). (**b**) Color Doppler study shows increased vascularity of the testes from orchitis. The solid portion within the abscess is a granulation tissue showing vascularity (*arrow*). (**c**) Spectral study shows increased flow in the testes

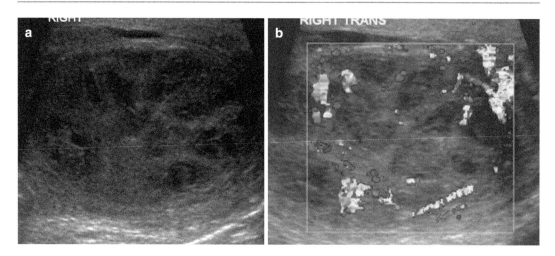

Fig. 19.14 Multiple intratesticular abscesses. A patient with intellectual disability and urethral stenosis. Grayscale (**a**) and color Doppler sonogram (**b**) of the right testis show multiple abscesses as focal fairly well-defined areas of heteroechoic decreased echogenicity having increased flow to the intervening testicular parenchyma

Diagnosis
TB Orchitis

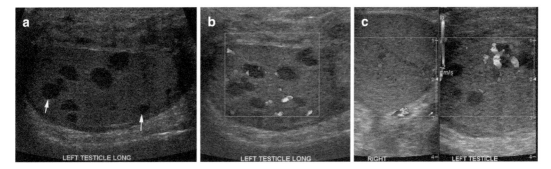

Fig. 19.15 Tuberculous orchitis, biopsy proven. History of scrotal pain and swelling not responding to antibiotic therapy. Grayscale and color Doppler sonogram (**a**, **b**) show diffuse discrete hypoechoic nodules (*arrows*) in the left testis rimmed by thin mildly echogenic wall. Increased vascularity is seen around the nodules. The scrotal wall is also thick on the left side. (**c**) The right testis shows normal echogenicity and vascularity

Diagnosis
TB Epididymitis

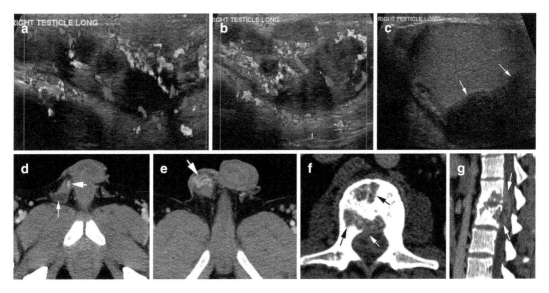

Fig. 19.16 Tuberculous epididymitis and spondylitis. (**a**, **b**) Color Doppler sonogram shows enlargement and hyperemia of the tail and body of the epididymis with multiple hypoechoic nodules. The head (not shown) was normal in size. (**c**) Grayscale US shows nodules at the tail causing extrinsic pressure on the testes (*arrows*). (**d**, **e**) Axial CT shows a low-density nodule (*thin arrow*) and dilated vessels in the thick right spermatic cord up to the tail of the epididymis (*thick arrow*). (**f**, **g**) Axial and sagittal reformatted CT show destructive changes in L1–L2 vertebral bodies (*black arrows*) and decrease in disk space, and epidural extension (*white arrows*) was proven to be TB spondylitis with epidural abscess

Diagnosis

Epididymo-orchitis with Epididymal Abscess

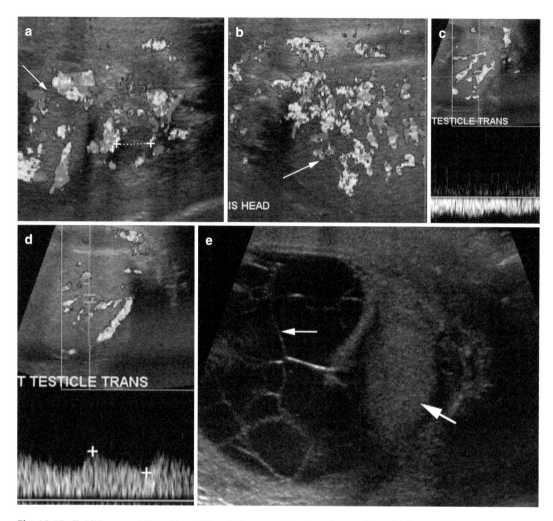

Fig. 19.17 Epididymo-orchitis with epididymal abscess and pyocele. (**a, b**) Color Doppler US shows enlarged epididymis with abscess at the tail (*caliper* in **a**) and increased vascularity of the testes (*arrow*) and epididymis. Spectral Doppler of testes shows (**c**) increased venous flow and (**d**) low-resistance arterial flow. (**e**) Grayscale US shows a pyocele with septations (*thin arrow*) compressing the left testis (*thick arrow*)

Diagnosis

Pyocele

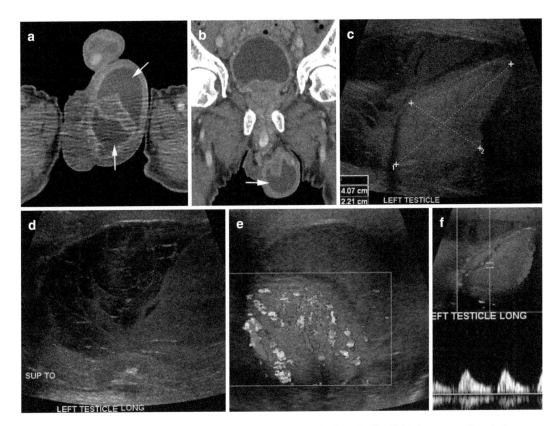

Fig. 19.18 Pyocele. A diabetic patient with scrotal swelling. (**a**, **b**) Axial and coronal reformatted CT images show infected hydrocele with large fluid collection in the left scrotum with enhancing rim (*arrows*). (**c**) Grayscale US shows tunica vaginalis space distended with low echoic heterogeneous fluid compressing the testes (*calipers*). The fluid shows septations in its upper part (**d**). (**e**) Color Doppler shows increased vascularity of the testes from orchitis. (**f**) Spectral study shows good systolic flow from the orchitis but absence of diastolic flow from venous compression by the large pyocele

Diagnosis
Seminal Vesicle Abscess

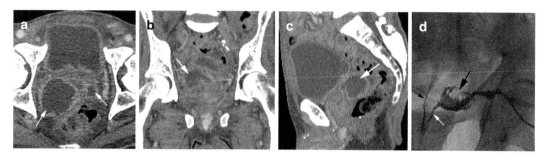

Fig. 19.19 Seminal vesicle abscess. Ten cc of pus was removed. Axial (**a**), coronal (**b**), and sagittal (**c**) reformatted CT images show seminal vesicle abscesses bilaterally, larger on the right side with rim enhancing fluid collections (*arrow*). (**d**) Abscessogram shows contrast in the seminal vesicle abscess (*thick black arrow*) draining into the prostatic urethra through the ejaculatory duct (*white arrow*) and contrast refluxing into the bladder (*thin black arrow*)

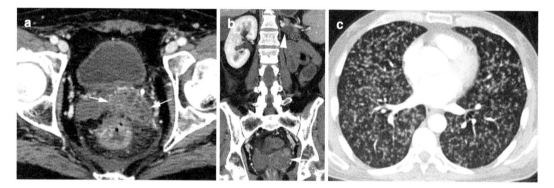

Fig. 19.20 Seminal vesicle metastasis from clear cell renal cell carcinoma. History of past left nephrectomy for RCC now with diffuse metastasis. (**a**) Axial CT shows enhancing mass in the left seminal vesicle with small cystic lesions (*arrows*). (**b**) Coronal reformatted image shows complex mass in the left seminal vesicle (*arrow*), cystic metastasis in the left adrenal gland (*arrowhead*), and absent left kidney. (**c**) Axial image of the chest shows diffuse miliary metastasis

Testicular Ischemia

Imaging Features

1. The spectral waveform varies depending on severity and duration of ischemia. It can be:
   (a) Monophasic wave with absence of dicrotic notch
   (b) Increased arterial flow resistance with decreased diastolic flow or reversal of diastolic flow
   (c) Absent arterial flow

2. Increase in size of both testis and epididymis
3. Homogeneous echotexture in mild ischemia, heterogeneous or hypoechic in complete necrosis, and hyperechogenic areas in hemorrhage
4. Torsion knot sign of twisted spermatic cord

Diagnosis

Chemical Orchitis with Ischemia

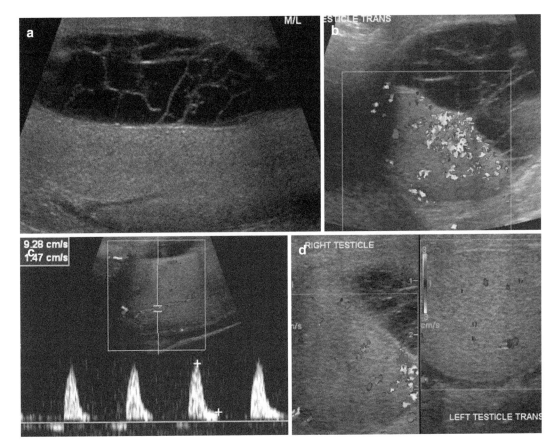

Fig. 19.21 Chemical orchitis with ischemia. History of chronic myelogenous leukemia, normal WBC count, negative urine analysis, and pain and swelling of the right testis. (**a**) Grayscale and (**b**) color Doppler US show the right testis to be compressed by a complex hydrocele with septations. Increased vascularity of the testes from orchitis. (**c**) Spectral study shows ischemia with risk of infarction with reversal of diastolic flow cause by compression by complex hydrocele. (**d**) Both testis have symmetrical uniform echogenicity

Diagnosis

Epididymitis with Testicular Infarction

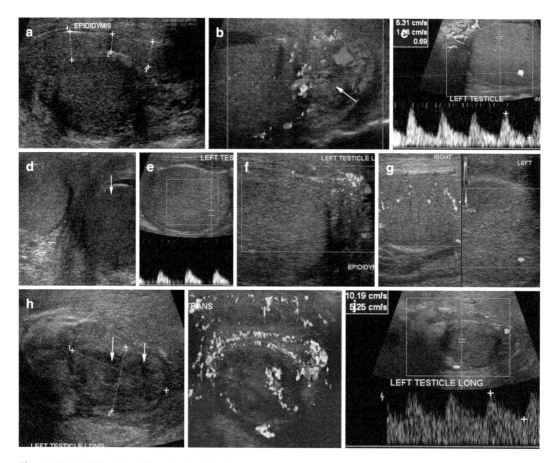

Fig. 19.22 Epididymitis with testicular infarction. (**a**, **b**) Grayscale and Color Doppler US show left epididymitis. The epididymis is diffusely enlarged (*calipers*) with increased vascularity (*arrow*). (**c**) Spectral flow in the testes shows monophasic flow with absence of dicrotic notch and with increased resistive index and normal echogenicity of the testes. (**d**–**g**) Follow-up study: (**d**, **e**) show severe ischemia with diffuse decreased echogenicity of the left testis and absent diastolic flow. (**f**, **g**) Color Doppler study at the same time shows unchanged increased vascularity of the epididymis but poor flow to the left testis and normal flow to the right side. (**h**–**j**) Subsequent sonogram (**h**) shows markedly shrunken left testis (*calipers*) with linear low echogenic segmental infarction (*arrows*). (**i**, **j**) Color Doppler and spectral study show increase diastolic flow within the intervening parenchyma due to new orchitis. The epididymis is still enlarged with engorged vessels. The wall of the left scrotum shows cellulitis with thickening and increased vessels

Diagnosis
Acute Hydrocele with Testicular Ischemia

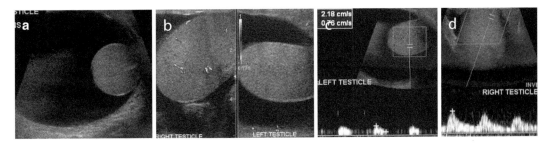

Fig. 19.23 Acute hydrocele with testicular ischemia. History of left scrotal swelling and pain. (**a**) Grayscale US shows large simple left scrotal hydrocele displacing the testes against the scrotal wall. (**b**) Color Doppler study shows decreased vascularity of the left testis and smaller hydrocele on the right side. (**c**) Spectral study shows high-resistance arterial waveform and absent diastolic flow from ischemia by the large hydrocele. (**d**) Normal flow to the right

Diagnosis
Testicular Torsion with Infarction

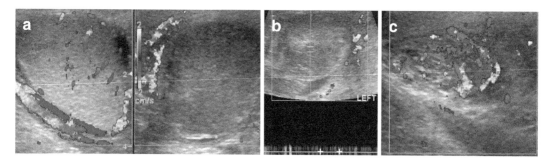

Fig. 19.24 Testicular torsion with infarction. (**a**) Color Doppler US shows no color flow to the left testis. Good flow is seen in the right testis. (**b**) Spectral study shows heterogeneous left testis with patchy areas of decreased echogenicity and with no spectral waves. (**c**) Color Doppler of the left inguinal region shows the knot of twisted spermatic cord with swirling of vessels

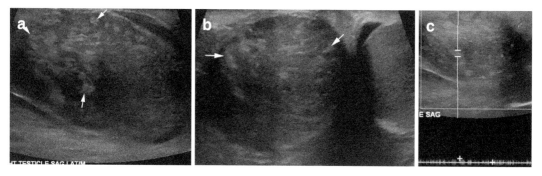

Fig. 19.25 Hemorrhagic infarction of the testes with 360° torsion. (**a**, **b**) Sonogram of the right testis shows heterogeneous density with multiple high echogenic foci (*arrows*) from hemorrhage and decreased echogenicity of the rest of the testicular parenchyma from necrosis. (**c**) Spectral study shows absence of flow

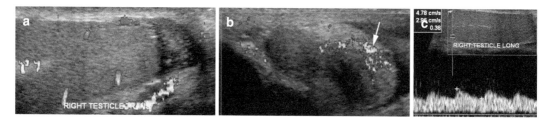

Fig. 19.26 Detorsion. Clinically a knot was felt which was untwisted. The patient had no pain during the sonogram examination. Color Doppler study of (**a**) the right testis shows normal vascularity. (**b**) Epididymis is thickened and shows increased vessels (*arrow*). Spectral study (**c**) shows high flow with low arterial resistance in the right testis due to vasodilatation from detorsion

Diagnosis

Torsion of the Appendix of the Testis

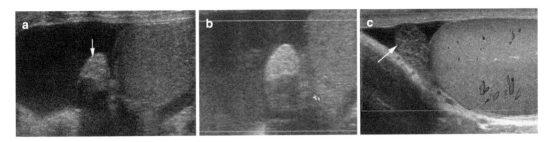

Fig. 19.27 Torsion of the appendix of the testes. (**a, b**) Patient 1 with situs ambiguous complained of diffuse abdominal and right testicular pain: (**a**) Grayscale and (**b**) Color Doppler US of the right testis show increased size and echogenicity of the appendix of the testes (*arrow*) with lack of vascularity. Large hydrocele is present. (**c**) Patient 2 with testicular pain: Color Doppler shows enlarged edematous appendix of the testis with no flow (*arrow*) and small hydrocele

Benign Lesions

Diagnosis
Giant Multilocular Spermatocele

Imaging Features
1. Most spermatoceles are unilocular cystic lesions in the region of the head of the epididymis with no symptoms.
2. Giant multilocular spermatocele can be very large in size with septations.

3. US shows multiple conglomerated cystic spaces near the head of the epididymis with no evidence of infection in the testis or rest of epididymis.
4. Intratesticular spermatocele communicates with seminiferous tubules.

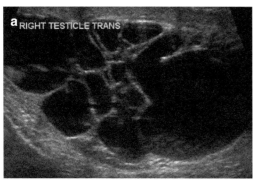 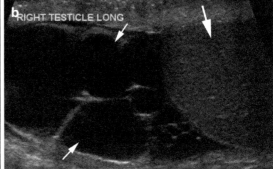

Fig. 19.28 Multilocular spermatocele. History of palpable mass. (**a, b**) Transverse and longitudinal sonogram of the right testis show a large multilocular cystic lesion at the head of the epididymis (*thin arrows*). The rest of the epididymis and the testes (*thick arrow*) had normal findings

Diagnosis
Spermatocele, Intratesticular, and Epididymal

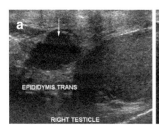 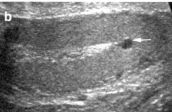 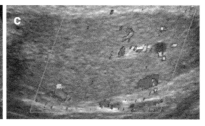

Fig. 19.29 Spermatocele, intratesticular, and epididymal. (**a**) Transverse grayscale US view of the testes shows a large spermatocele at the head of the epididymis with low-level internal echoes (*arrow*). (**b, c**) Grayscale and color Doppler US show intratesticular spermatocele in the mediastinum testes (*arrow*) as cystic lesion with no vascularity

Diagnosis
Tunica Albuginea Cyst

Imaging Features
1. Common extratesticular cyst
2. Usually small, unilocular, or multilocular with through transmission
3. Located usually in the upper anterior or lateral aspect of the testis
4. If large can compress testicular parenchyma and then difficult to differentiate from intra-testicular cyst
5. Can have low-level echoes or calcification

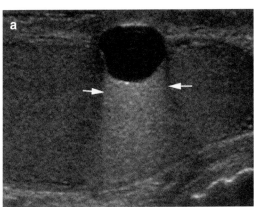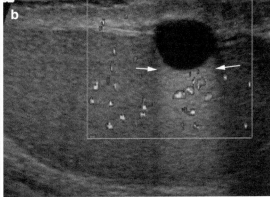

Fig. 19.30 Cyst of tunica albuginea. History of palpable mass. Grayscale US (**a**) shows a simple unilocular cyst in the upper anterior part of the testes with an increase through transmission (*arrows* in **a** and **b**). (**b**) Color Doppler US shows normal underlying testicular vascularity

Diagnosis
Testicular Adrenal Rest

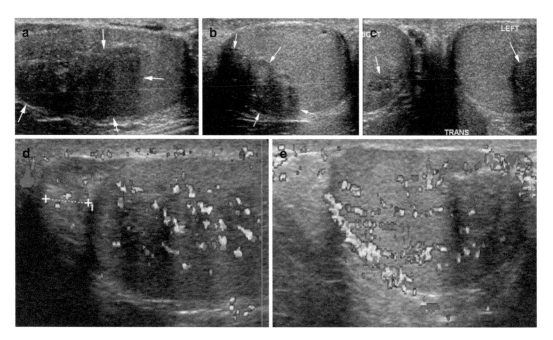

Fig. 19.31 Testicular adrenal rest. Patient with congenital adrenal hyperplasia and hypogonadism. Sonogram of both testes (**a–c**) shows lobulated area of decreased echogenicity (*arrows*) in the mediastinum bilaterally with no destructive change in the testicular parenchyma which shows normal echogenicity. (**d, e**) Color Doppler shows no discrete altered vascularity between the testes, the adrenal rests and head of epididymis (*calipers*)

Diagnosis
Epidermoid Cyst

Imaging Features
Varies with maturation and compactness and quantity of keratin in the cyst

1. Target appearance—halo with central echogenicity
2. Mass with rim calcification or focal mass with echogenic rim
3. Onion-ring appearance is the classic appearance
4. No blood flow by Doppler study

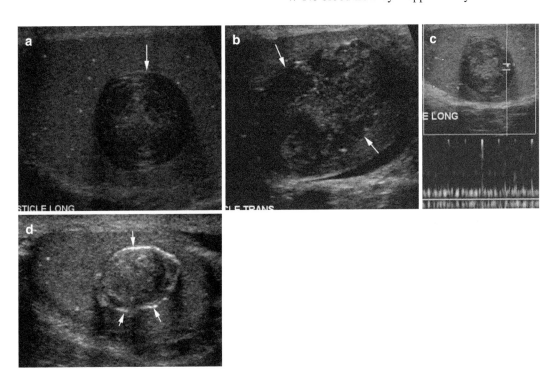

Fig. 19.32 Epidermoid cyst. Grayscale US shows (**a**) an onion-ring pattern in longitudinal view and (**b**) heterogeneous pattern in transverse view (*arrows* in **a**, **b**, **d**). Color Doppler (**c**) shows no internal vascularity. (**d**) Different patients show more solid mass with echogenic rim

Diagnosis
Lipoma of the Spermatic Cord

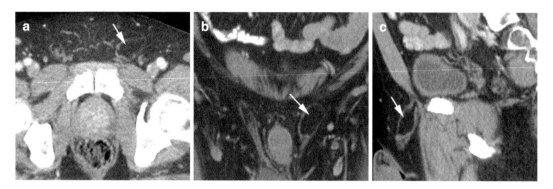

Fig. 19.33 Lipoma of the spermatic cord confirmed by surgery. (**a**) Axial, (**b**) coronal, and (**c**) sagittal CT images show small loculated lipoma with fat attenuation (*arrow*) in the left inguinal canal

Tumors of the Epididymis

Diagnosis
Leiomyosarcoma of the Epididymis

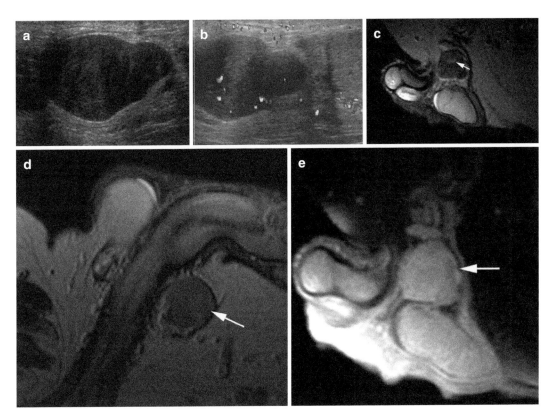

Fig. 19.34 Leiomyosarcoma of the epididymis. History of treated prostate cancer, now with mass on the left scrotum. (**a, b**) Sonogram of the left testis shows a well-defined mass with low echogenicity but with vascularity similar to the testis which is adherent to the epididymis. MRI of the mass superior to the left testis (**c**) T2-weighted fat-saturated sagittal image shows intermediate signal with central high signal (*thin arrow*). (**d**) Axial T1-weighted fat-saturated study shows low signal (*arrow*). (**e**) Postcontrast T1-weighted fat-saturated study shows enhancement (*arrow*). Pathology showed mass involving the epididymis

Diagnosis
Myofibroblastic Tumor of the Epididymis

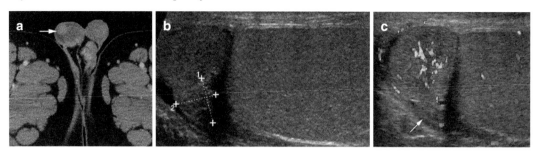

Fig. 19.35 Myofibroblastic tumor of the epididymis. History of palpable lump. (**a**) Axial CT shows a nodule in the region of the right epididymis (*arrow*). (**b**) Grayscale US shows an exophytic echogenic mass anterior to the head of the epididymis (*calipers*). (**c**) Color Doppler US shows poor vascularity of the mass (*arrow*). Pathology found the mass to be adherent to the epididymis with no invasion

Diagnosis
Adenomatoid Tumor of the Tail of the Epididymis

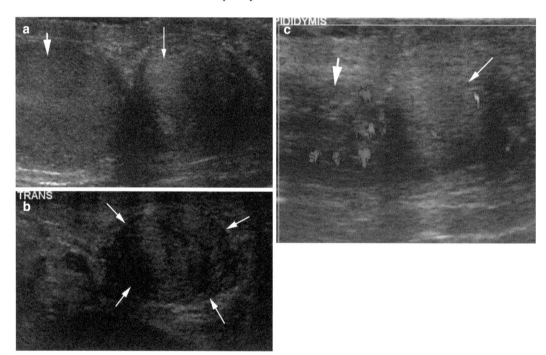

Fig. 19.36 Adenomatoid tumor of the tail of the epididymis. (**a**, **b**) Grayscale US shows a large solid well-marginated mass (*thin arrows*) at the tail of the epididymis, posterior to the testes (*thick short arrow*). (**c**) Color Doppler US shows a few prominent vessels in the mass (*thin arrow*) and is less vascular than the adjacent epididymis (*thick short arrow*)

Fig. 19.37 Inguinal herniation of the omentum. (**a**) Grayscale and (**b**) color Doppler US of the right inguinal region show a mass (*arrows*) of same echogenicity as the subcutaneous fat (*ellipse*) and with dilated vessels. (**c**, **d**) Different patient grayscale and color Doppler US show an herniated omentum (*arrows* in **c**) with dilated vessels up to the scrotum which shows pyocele (septations in the hydrocele) (*arrowhead*). (**e**) Color Doppler at different level shows pyocele and orchitis with increased vascularity of the testes (*arrow*), and the omentum lies posteriorly (*arrowhead*). (**f**, **g**) Axial and coronal CT show herniation of the omentum (*arrow*) medial to the spermatic cord (*arrowhead*). (**h**) Different patients show the omentum (*arrows*) floating in the simple hydrocele

Inguinoscrotal Hernia

Diagnosis
Omental Hernia

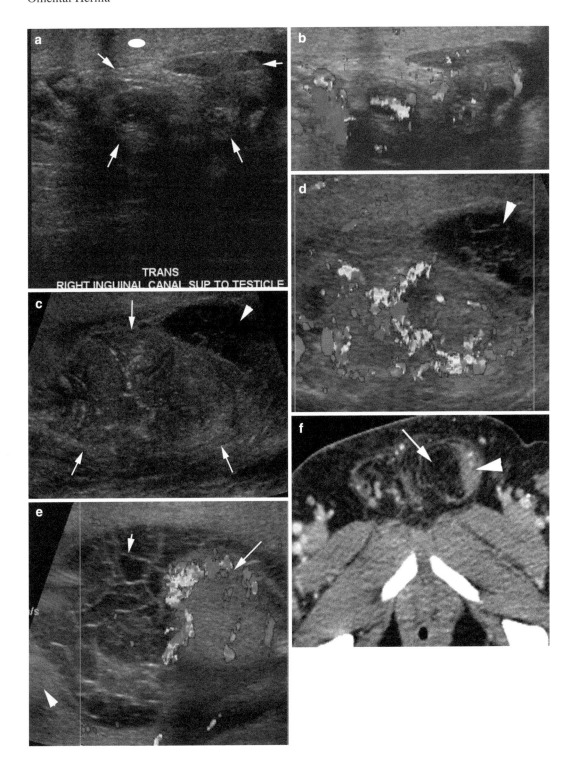

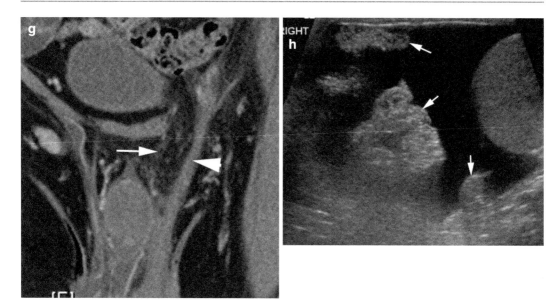

Fig. 19.37 (continued)

Diagnosis
Bowel Hernia

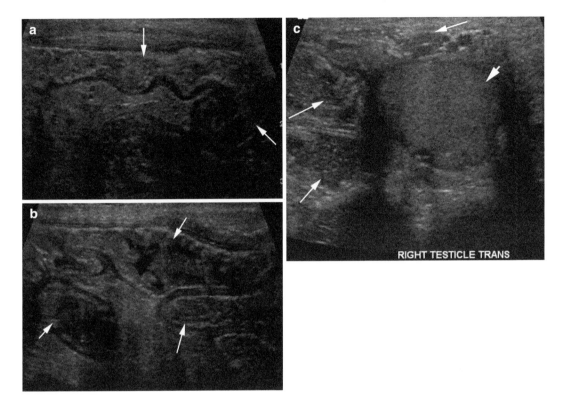

Fig. 19.38 Inguinoscrotal hernia of the bowel. (**a**, **b**) Grayscale US of the right inguinal region shows fluid-filled heteroechoic bowel loops extending through the inguinal canal (*arrows*). Wavy margins of the loops are from peristalsis. (**c**) Transverse grayscale US of the scrotum shows bowel loops (*thin long arrows*) surrounding the testes (*short thick arrow*)

Diagnosis
Sperm Granuloma

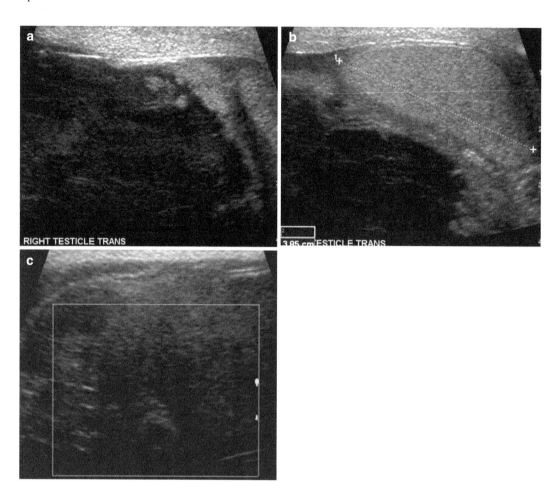

Fig. 19.39 Sperm granuloma in a patient with recent vasectomy and groin swelling. Sonogram of the right testis (**a**, **b**) shows a heteroechoic mass, mostly of low echogenicity, extending from the groin and is extrinsically compressing the testes (*caliper*). (**c**) Color Doppler study shows no flow within the mass

Testicular Malignancy

Diagnosis
Seminoma

Imaging Features
1. Homogeneous hypoechoic lesion but can be heterogeneous when large.
2. Cystic regions and calcification are less common.
3. Have internal vascularity.
4. Usually confined by tunica vaginalis.
5. Can have lymphatic and hematogenous spread.

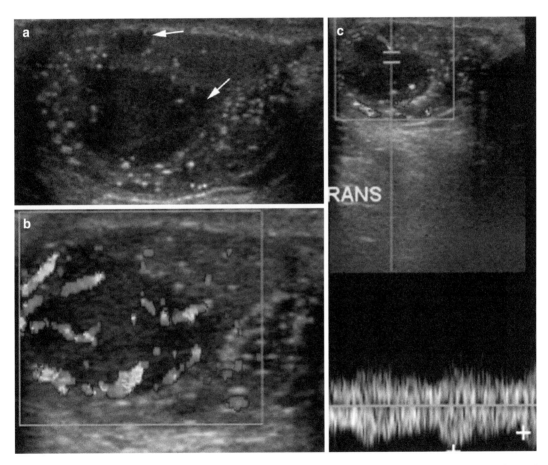

Fig. 19.40 Pure seminoma, surgery proven. (**a**) Grayscale US of the left testis shows diffuse microlithiasis with two low echogenic nodules (*arrows*). (**b**) Color Doppler shows increased vascularity within the larger mass. (**c**) Spectral study shows increase in flow in the mass

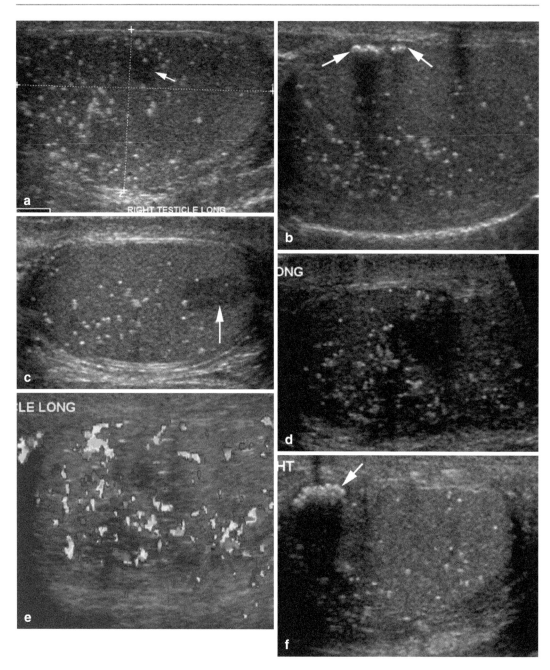

Fig. 19.41 Pure seminoma. Grayscale sonogram of the right testis (**a**) shows a focal area of low echogenicity (*arrow*) in the anterior testes (*calipers*) and diffuse microlithiasis throughout the testes. (**b**) Two months later macrocalcifications are seen in the same low echogenic area (*arrows*) indicating regressed seminoma. (**c**) One month later, a new low echogenic focus is seen in the lower pole (*arrow*). (**d**, **e**) Two months later, the seminoma have increased in size with multiple areas of low echogenicity in most of the testes and with increased vascularity. (**f**) The regressed area shows increased calcification (*arrow*)

Diagnosis
Immature Teratoma

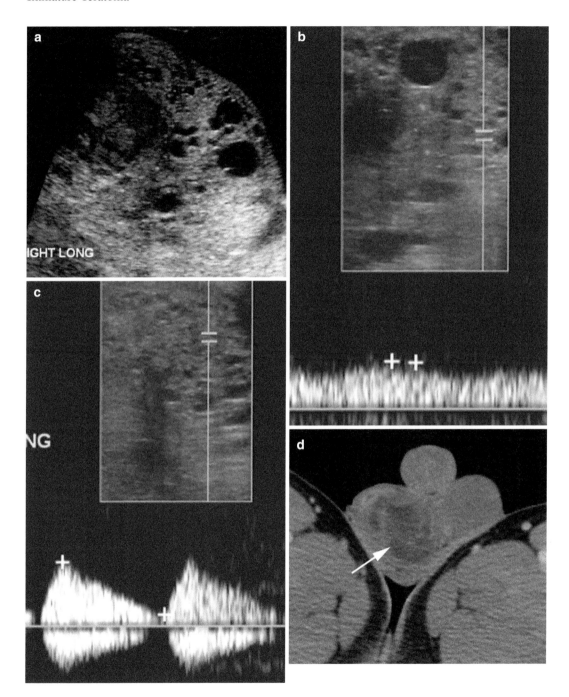

Fig. 19.42 Immature teratoma in two patients. Patient 1: (**a**) Grayscale sonogram shows heterogeneous mass with cystic spaces occupying the whole testis with hydrocele. Spectral flow study (**b**) shows prominent venous flow in some areas and (**c**) increased resistance to arterial flow with absent diastolic flow in some areas. Patient 2: (**d**) Axial CT at the scrotum shows a complex fatty mass on the right side (*arrow*). (**e**) Axial CT through the mid-abdomen shows metastasis to the retroperitoneal lymph node which has fat attenuation and septations similar to the testicular mass (*arrow*). (**f**, **g**) Grayscale and color Doppler sonogram show a large predominantly cystic mass (*arrow*) at the mediastinum of the testis with increased vascularity (*arrow*) in the inter-cystic spaces

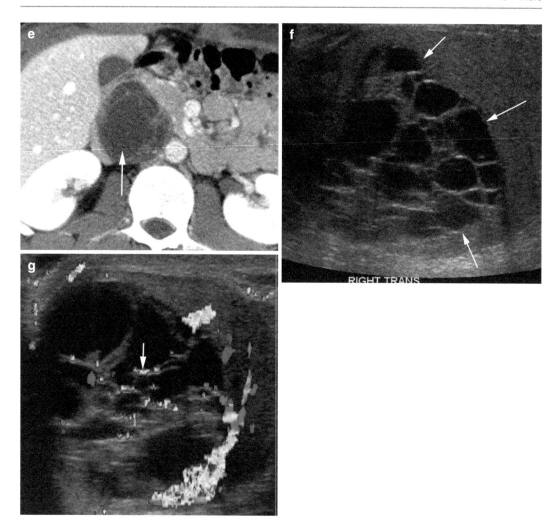

Fig. 19.42 (continued)

Diagnosis
Yolk Sac Tumor

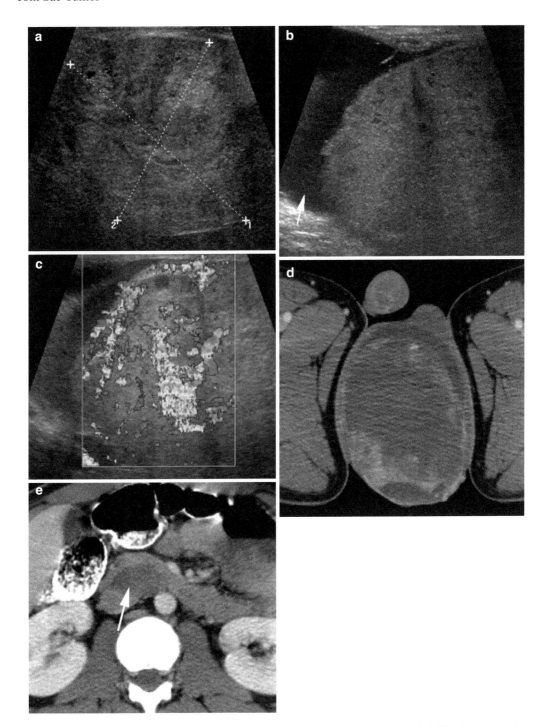

Fig. 19.43 Yolk sac tumor. History of weight loss and testicular mass. (**a**, **b**) Grayscale US shows a large heterogeneous mass (*calipers* in **a**) with small cystic spaces replacing the right testis with surrounding small hydrocele (*arrow*). (**c**) Color Doppler shows increased vascularity of tumor. (**d**) Axial CT of scrotum shows necrotic mass with peripheral enhancement replacing the right testis and with small hydrocele. (**e**) Axial CT of the mid-abdomen shows low-density lymph node metastasis in the right gonadal chain (*arrow*)

Diagnosis

Lymphoma

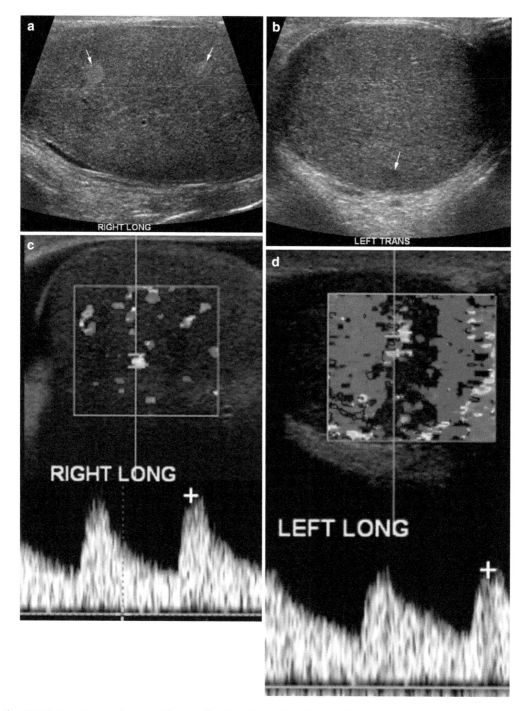

Fig. 19.44 Lymphoma of testes. History of enlarged testes. (**a**, **b**) Grayscale US shows mild diffuse hypoechoic testes with two focal areas of increased echogenicity in the right testis (*arrows* in **a**) and a small focus of decreased echogenicity (*arrow* in **b**) in the left testis. (**c**, **d**) Spectral study and (**e**, **f**) color Doppler study show diffuse increased flow and vascularity in both testis. (**g**) Axial CT shows uniform increased attenuation in both testis with increased vascularity of the right epididymis. (**h**) Coronal reformatted CT of the abdomen shows enlarged lymph nodes in the aortocaval region (*arrows*). (**i**, **j**) PET-CT fusion images show increased FDG uptake in the aortocaval lymph nodes. Right orchiectomy showed diffuse large B-cell lymphoma. (**k**) PET scan shows increased FDG uptake in the left testis

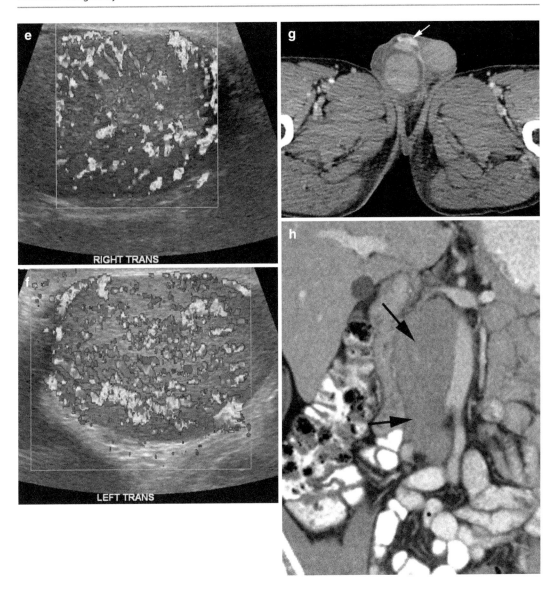

Fig. 19.44 (continued)

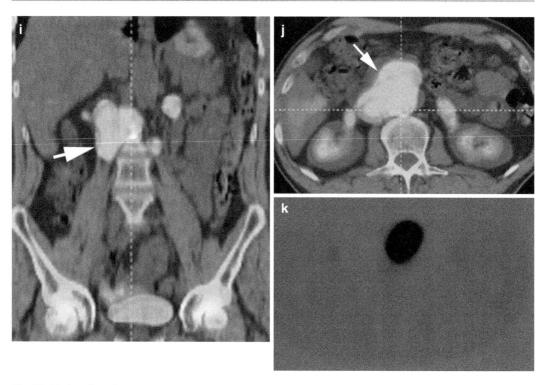

Fig. 19.44 (continued)

Diagnosis

Liposarcoma of Tunica Vaginalis

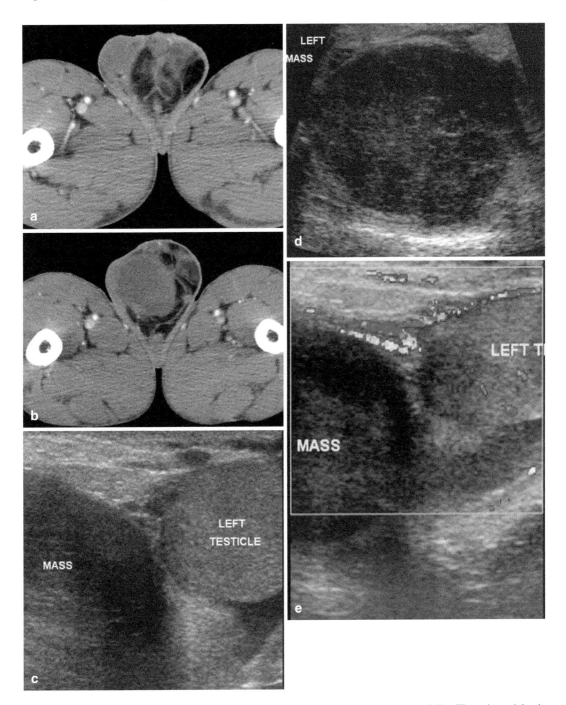

Fig. 19.45 Liposarcoma of tunica vaginalis. (**a**, **b**) Axial CT through the scrotum shows heterogeneous fatty mass surrounding the left testis. (**c**, **d**) Ultrasound shows heterogeneous extratesticular solid mass in the left scrotum displacing the testis medially. The echogenicity is lower than the testis. (**e**) Color Doppler shows no flow in the mass

Undescended, Retractile, and Ascending Testes

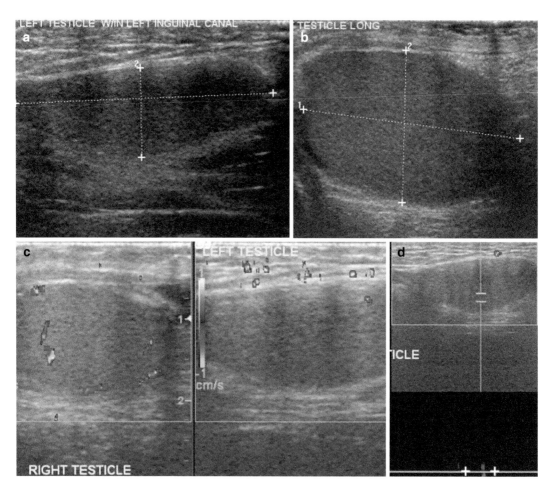

Fig. 19.46 Undescended testes in a 16-year-old with left inguinal pain. (**a**) US of the left inguinal canal shows the left testis (*calipers*) with uniform echogenicity. (**b**) US of the right scrotum shows the right testis (*calipers*) also with uniform echogenicity. Color Doppler (**c**) and spectral study (**d**) show absence of flow on the left side. At surgery, the left testis was viable and had intermittent torsion

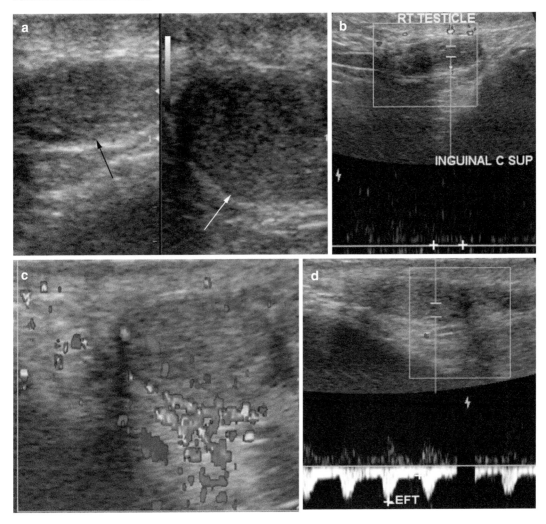

Fig. 19.47 Undescended testes with failed orchiopexy. Acute right inguinal pain in a 33-year-old man. History of orchidopexy at age 3 for bilateral undescended testes. (**a**) Grayscale US shows the small right testis in the right inguinal canal (*black arrow*) from failed orchidopexy. The left testis in the left scrotum (*white arrow*). Both testis have uniform echogenicity. (**b**) The right testis shows no spectral flow. (**c, d**) Color Doppler and spectral study show good flow in the left testis

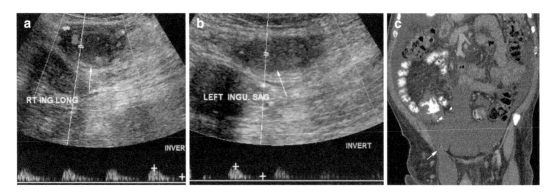

Fig. 19.48 Retractile or ascending testis: a 56-year-old patient has four children, comes with scrotal swelling, bilateral leg edema, and cirrhosis. (**a**, **b**) Color US shows both testis (*arrow*) in each inguinal canal, respectively, are small in size but with good flow and uniform normal echogenicity. Spectral waves show high resistance flow with poor diastolic flow bilaterally. (**c**) Coronal reformatted CT shows a large ascites extending to the right inguinal canal through patent processus vaginalis (*arrow*)

Bibliography

1. Alvarez DM, Bhatt S, Dogra VS. Sonographic spectrum of tunica albuginea cyst. J Clin Imgaging Sci. 2011;1:5. doi:10.4103/2156-7514.73503.

2. Avery LL, Scheinfeld MH. Imaging of penile and scrotal emergencies. Radiographics. 2013;33:721–40.

3. Baron KT, Babagbemi KT, Arleo EK, et al. Emergent complications of assisted reproduction: expecting the unexpected. Radiographics. 2013;33:229–44.

4. Brown DL, Dudiak KM, Laing FC. Adnexal masses: US characterization of reporting. Radiology. 2010;254: 2342–54.

5. Chang HC, Bhatt S, Dogra VS. Pearls and pitfalls in diagnosis of ovarian torsion. Radiographics. 2008;28: 1355–68.

6. Chen P, John S. Ultrasound of the acute scrotum. Appl Radiol. 2006;8–17.

7. Deurdulian C, Mittlestaedt CA, Chong WK, et al. US of acute scrotal trauma: optimal technique, imaging findings, and management. Radiographics. 2007;27: 357–69.

8. Dogra VS, Gottlieb RH, Oka M, et al. Sonography of the scrotum. Radiology. 2003;227:18–36.

9. Dogra VS, Rubens DJ, Gottlieb RH, et al. Torsion and beyond new twists in spectral Doppler evaluation of the scrotum. J Ultrasound Med. 2004;23: 1077–85.

10. Feldman MK, Katyal S, Blackwood MS. US artifacts. Radiographics. 2009;29:1179–89.

11. Forstner R, Hricak H, Occhipinti KA, et al. Ovarian cancer: staging with CT and MR imaging. Radiology. 1995;197:619–26.

12. Fried AM, Kenney CM, Stigers KB, et al. Benign pelvic masses: sonographic spectrum. Radiographics. 1996;16:321–34.

13. Garriga V, Serrano A, Marin A, et al. US of the tunica vaginalis testis: anatomic relationships and pathologic conditions. Radiographics. 2009;29:2017–32.

14. Green CL, Angtuaco TL, Shab HR, et al. Gestational trophoblastic disease: a spectrum of radiologic diagnosis. Radiographics. 1996;16:1371–84.

15. Jung SE, Lee JM, Rha SE, et al. CT and MR imaging of ovarian tumors with emphasis on differential diagnosis. Radiographics. 2002;22:1305–25.

16. Kawamoto S, Urban BA, Fishman EK. CT of epithelial ovarian tumors. Radiographics. 1999;19: S85–102.

17. Kim SH, Kim SH, Yang DM, et al. Unusual causes of tubo-ovarian abscess: CT and MR imaging findings. Radiographics. 2004;24:1575–89.

18. Kirsch JD, Scoutt LM. Imaging of ectopic pregnancy. Appl Radiol. 2010;3:10–25.

19. Kuligowska E, Deeds L, Lu K. Pelvic pain: overlooked and underdiagnosed gynecologic conditions. Radiographics. 2005;25:3–20.

20. Laing FC, Allison SJ. US of the ovary and adnexa: to worry or not to worry? Radiographics. 2012;32:1621–30.

21. Lalwani N, Prasad SR, Vikram R, et al. Histologic, molecular, and cytogenetic features of ovarian cancers: implications for diagnosis and treatment. Radiographics. 2011;31:625–46.

22. Lee JW, Kim S, Kwack SW, et al. Hepatic capsular and subcapsular pathologic conditions: demonstration with CT and MR imaging. Radiographics. 2008;28: I 307–23.

23. Levenson RB, Singh AK, Novelline RA. Fournier gangrene: role of imaging. Radiographics. 2008;27:519–28.

24. Levine D. Ectopic pregnancy. Radiology. 2007;245: 385–97.

25. Levine D, Brown DL, Andreotti RF, et al. Management of asymptomatic ovarian and other adnexal cysts imaged at US: Society of Radiologists in Ultrasound Consensus Conference Statement. Radiology. 2010; 256(3):943–54.

26. Outwater EK, Siegelman ES, Hunt JL. Ovarian teratomas: tumor types and imaging characteristics. Radiographics. 2001;21:475–90.

27. Park SB, Kim JK, Kim KR, et al. Imaging findings of complications and unusual manifestations of ovarian teratomas. Radiographics. 2008;28:969–83.

28. Rezvani M, Shaaban AM. Fallopian tube disease in the nonpregnant patient. Radiographics. 2011;31:527–48.

29. Rha SU, Byun JY, Jung SE, et al. CT and MR imaging features of adnexal torsion. Radiographics. 2002;22: 283–94.

30. Sam JW, Jacobs JE, Birnbaum BA. Spectrum of CT findings in acute pyogenic pelvic inflammatory disease. Radiogragphics. 2002;22:1327–34.

31. Sellmyer MA, Desser TS, Maturen KE, et al. Physiologic, histologic and imaging features of retained products of conception. Radiographics. 2013;33:781–96.

32. Shapiro E. Risk of retractile testes becoming ascending testes. Rev Urol. 2006;8(4):231–2.

33. Wagner BJ, Buck JI, Seidman JD, et al. Ovarian epithelial neoplasms: radiologic-pathologic correlation. Radiographics. 1994;14:1351–74.

34. Wagner BJ, Woodward PJ, Dickey GE, et al. Gestational trophoblastic disease: radiologic-pathologic correlation. Radiographics. 1996;16:131–48.

35. Westphalen ACA, Qayyum A. CT and MRI of adnexal masses. Appl Radiol. 2006;22–31.

36. Williams PL, Laifer-Narin SL, Ragavendra N. US of abnormal uterine bleeding. Radiographics. 2003;23: 703–18.

37. Winter T. Ultrasonography of the scrotum. Appl Radiol. 2006;9–18.

38. Woodward PJ, Hosseinzadeh K, Saenger JS. Radiologic staging of ovarian carcinoma with pathologic correlation. Radiographics. 2004;24:225–46.